Stress and Somatic Symptoms

Kyung Bong Koh

Stress and Somatic Symptoms

Biopsychosociospiritual Perspectives

Springer

Kyung Bong Koh
Department of Psychiatry
Yonsei University College of Medicine
Seoul, Korea

ISBN 978-3-030-02782-7 ISBN 978-3-030-02783-4 (eBook)
https://doi.org/10.1007/978-3-030-02783-4

Library of Congress Control Number: 2018959114

This Springer imprint is published by the registered company Springer Nature Switzerland AG
The registered company address is: Gewerbestrasse 11, 6330 Cham, Switzerland

Preface

This book primarily focuses on the assessment and treatment of patients with somatic symptoms, based on biopsychosociospiritual model. Basically, however, a broad spectrum of knowledge about stress is also needed for effective assessment and treatment of these patients because stress is closely related to the onset and course of disorders with somatic symptoms.

Although the role of religion in health and illness was overlooked for years, there is mounting evidence that religious cognitions and behaviors can offer effective resources for dealing with stress. In particular, much attention has focused on the role of spirituality as a coping mechanism to deal with life stress. Moreover, people may have greater spiritual needs during illnesses, especially terminal illnesses. Addressing the spiritual needs of patients may enhance recovery from illnesses and protect them against depression.

Treatment of disorders with somatic symptoms is challenging because they cannot be treated according to the existing biomedical model and patients with somatic symptoms are usually resistant to psychosocial approach. Therefore, specific assessment skills and treatment techniques are required to approach them effectively. In this regard, the importance of biopsychosociospiritual approach to patient-centered care is emphasized.

This book consists of four parts. Part 1 "Stress" explores stress, vulnerability, and resilience, intermediate mechanisms between stress and illness such as psychoneuroendocrinology and psychoimmunology, the measurement of stress, the relationship between stress and accidents, and cognitive behavioral approach to stress.

Part 2 "Somatization" deals with the concept, mechanisms, assessment, and treatment of somatization. Particularly interview techniques for physicians to learn for effective assessment and management of somatization are presented and discussed. In addition, somatic symptom and related disorders in DSM-5 are included. However, the approach to chronic pain is separately added to this part because pain is a major concern for patients with these disorders.

Part 3 "Specific Physical Disorders" mainly deals with common and distressing functional physical disorders such as functional dyspepsia and irritable bowel syndrome as well as major physical disorders such as stroke, Parkinson's disease, dementia, headache, cardiovascular diseases, diabetes, and cancer. Assessment and management of depression and anxiety in the medically ill and therapeutic approach for individuals at risk of coronary heart disease are also included. In addition, psychosocial issues of and therapeutic interventions for patients with specific cancers such as breast cancer, prostate cancer, and childhood cancer are addressed.

Part 4 "Religion, Spirituality, and Psychosomatic Medicine" emphasizes the importance of a biopsychosociospiritual perspective in an approach for patients with somatic symptoms, especially depressed patients with physical diseases and patients with terminal illnesses because of the growing need for spirituality in such patients. In addition, the role of spirituality as coping with stress and the relationship between religious involvement and mental/physical well-being are reviewed.

A considerable portion of all my chapters in the previously published book *Somatization and Psychosomatic Symptoms* edited by the author is included in some chapters of this book, because they are so essential in terms of the context of the book.

Overall, this book explores stress and a variety of issues relevant to the assessment and treatment of disorders with somatic symptoms in terms of biopsychosociospiritual perspectives. It will be of interest to researchers and healthcare practitioners such as psychiatrists, physicians, nurses, psychologists, and social workers dealing with stress, health, and mental health.

I am grateful to Ms. Katherine Chabalko, senior editor, Ms. Cynthya Pushparaj, production editor, and Ms. Kanimozhi Sekar, project manager, for their assistance throughout the process of editing and publication of this book. In addition, I thank my son, Jinwoo Koh, for his assistance in the preparation for the illustration, and my wife, Sungsook Cho, for her encouragement. I also thank God for enabling me to finish this work.

Seoul, Korea Kyung Bong Koh

Contents

Part I Stress

Part I
Stress

Chapter 1
Stress, Vulnerability, and Resilience

1.1 Introduction

In this chapter are reviewed definition of stress, causes of stress, vulnerability and resilience to stress, psychosocial factors associated with resilience, resilience and neuroendocrine stress responses, genetic influences on vulnerability and resilience, epigenetic mechanism of vulnerability and resilience, transcriptional mechanism of resilience, neural circuitry of resilience, and an integrated aspect of resilience.

1.1.1 Definition of Stress

The concept of stress was introduced by Cannon, who first identified stress reaction as the fight-or-flight response [1]. Later, the term was generally used by Selye who advocated the general adaptation syndrome [2]. In the past, stress was regarded as external stimuli or events threatening an organism or as an organism's responses to stressors [3, 4]. In addition, it referred to the interaction between an organism and the environment [5, 6].

These days stress is defined as external or internal stimuli that are meaningfully perceived by the person, activate emotions, and elicit physiological changes that threaten health and survival [4]. This stress concept emphasizes that an individual's stress responses depend on his/her subjective interpretation of an event rather than an event itself [7]. Therefore, the same event or situation may be differently perceived, resulting in quite different outcomes – health or illness. That is, what may be intolerable for one person may be acceptable to another.

K. B. Koh, *Stress and Somatic Symptoms*,
https://doi.org/10.1007/978-3-030-02783-4_1

1.1.2 Distress and Eustress

Hans Selye defined stress as "the nonspecific response of the body to any demand made upon it" [8]. He used the term "distress" for bad events (e.g., unemployment, the death of a loved one) to which we must adapt. Stress and distress are interchangeably used all too often because stress generally indicates the negative aspect. The term "eustress" was also introduced by Selye to describe good events (e.g., job promotion) to which we must adapt. Both events may trigger the same physiological arousal [1].

Too little stress (e.g., boredom) or too much stress is not good for health [9]. Optimal stress or moderate stress levels are defined as the maximal point where stress increases and health and performance also increase. Overload begins where stress continues to increase but health and performance begin to decrease [9, 10]. The aim of stress management is not to eliminate stress entirely but to control it so that an optimal level of arousal is maintained [9].

1.2 Causes of Stress

Major causes of stress are classified into psychosocial factors and environmental (bioecological) factors. This classification is based upon the direct causes of stress reaction [10].

1.2.1 Psychosocial Factors

There are four psychosocial factors such as adaptation (e.g., changes in job, school, and family), frustration (e.g., prejudice, discrimination relevant to religion, race, national origin, generation, and region, social status, sex, physical characteristics, socioeconomic hardship, bureaucracies), overload (e.g., occupational, academic and domestic), and deprivation (e.g., boredom, loneliness).

1.2.2 Environmental Factors

Environmental (bioecological) factors refer to stimuli, arising out of our relationship with our environment, that produce stress responses in most individuals through an innate biological mechanism. These stressors include biological rhythms (e.g., disturbed sleep-wakefulness cycle, menstruation), noise, pollution, and climate change.

1.3 Vulnerability and Resilience to Stress

Stress can seriously disturb the psychological and physiological balance of an individual, but traumatic stress does not affect everyone similarly. Vulnerable individuals poorly adapt to stressors and expose themselves to inappropriate responses that can become persistent states of stress, whereas resilient individuals can perceive adversity as minimally threatening and develop adaptive psychological and physiological responses [11]. In other words, resilience refers to a person's ability to adapt successfully to acute stress, trauma, or more chronic forms of adversity [12].

Several steps are intervened in the process between stressors and illnesses. Here we have options in cognitive appraisal and coping because they can be controlled. These two factors play important roles in determining vulnerability and resilience. Therefore, exposure to stressful events can be differently perceived by individuals and can cause persistent sequelae depending on the level of vulnerability or resilience of each person. Differences in individual vulnerability/resilience occur across sex, age, and culture. The underlying mechanisms of vulnerability and resilience are known to depend on a combination of genetic and nongenetic factors that interact in complex ways, but these mechanisms remain not fully understood [13].

The study of resilience originated with a group of researchers who directed their attention to the investigation of children capable of developing normally despite exposure to significant adversity [14]. For many years research focused on identifying the psychosocial determinants of stress resistance, such as positive emotions, the capacity for self-regulation, social competence with peers, and a close bond with a primary caregiver [15, 16].

1.3.1 Psychosocial Factors Associated with Vulnerability

1.3.1.1 Self-Perception or Self-Concept

Self-perception or self-concept refers to the image that a person holds of himself/herself. Such self-image plays an important role in personal stress. Poor self-image such as inferiority complex in relation to his/her own body, academic career, interpersonal relationship, and performance of task, may play a significant role in vulnerability or the onset of diseases [10].

1.3.1.2 Personality

1. Type A Personality

   Type A behavior is characterized by an intense sense of time urgency, confidence, aggressiveness, competitiveness, ambitiousness, and hyperactivity. Type A behavior is a style of behavior which constantly elicits stress responses, especially cardiovascular system arousal. Such behavior can be harmful because it leads to a psychophysiological condition which compromises the integrity of the cardiovascular system, resulting in coronary heart diseases [10].

2. Anxious Reactive Personality

   Anxiety is not only a symptom of stress but also a cause of further stress. Normal people experience stress at the anxious moment and are relieved when the stressor is removed. However, anxious reactive person continues to experience stress which lowers task performance even after the stressor is gone. In particular, perfectionists are vulnerable to anxiety even when facing minor events [10].

1.3.2 Psychosocial Factors Associated with Resilience

Early-life adversities, such as abuse or neglect, can increase the vulnerability to develop psychopathologies and cognitive decline later in life [17]. However, early-life adversity does not necessarily result in increased vulnerability to stress. Rather it can enhance stress resilience [18] and prepare the organism to perform optimally under stressful conditions in adulthood [19].

As mentioned earlier, resilience is linked to being able to perceive stressful events in less threatening ways, promoting adaptive coping strategies. Such cognitive reappraisal allows individuals to re-evaluate or reframe adverse experiences in a more positive light [20].

Active coping with stress such as participation in problem-solving and positive reassessment of aversive experiences can help produce long-term resilience [21]. In this respect, hardiness is proposed to be a resource that can neutralize the potentially harmful effects of stress [22]. Hardiness is a personality construct composed of three dimensions, such as commitment, control, and challenge. Commitment is a tendency to be involved. Control is a tendency to feel and act as if one is influential. Challenge is a tendency to believe that change is desirable. The combination of these dispositions seems to keep persons healthy despite encounters with stressful life events [23]. In contrast, passive coping such as denial, avoidance of conflicts, suppression of emotions, and behavioral disengagement is maladaptive and provides only short-term resilience to stress [21]. In addition, poor coping such as poor eating habit (hypoglycemia or excessive eating), excessive drinking and smoking, and reckless driving increases the risk of illnesses and accidents.

Resilient individuals are also characterized by dispositional optimism and high positive emotionality [24, 25]. Positive emotions promote adaptive coping and openness to social support [24], and are associated with greater flexibility of thinking and exploration, and decreased autonomic activity [26]. Social competence or the ability to mobilize social support is also linked to better health. Increased social support has buffering effects on mental and physical disorders and fosters adaptive coping strategies [20]. Other psychosocial characteristics associated with stress resilience include a sense of purpose in life, spirituality, and the ability to find meaning in the midst of trauma [20, 27–29].

1.3.3 Behavioral Factors Associated with Vulnerability

Preference for specific diet (e.g., food containing caffeine: coffee, tea, chocolate, and cocoa; sugar and sugar products: cake, pies, cookies, and candy; processed flour; salt) can increase vulnerability [10].

1.3.4 Behavioral Factors Associated with Resilience

Life habits (e.g., relaxation, meditation, exercise) and life satisfaction (e.g., humor, art, nature) can help enhance resilience.

1.4 Resilience and Neuroendocrine Stress Responses

Numerous hormones, neurotransmitters, and neuropeptides are involved in the acute psychobiological responses to stress. Differences in the function, balance, and interaction of these factors underlie interindividual variability in stress resilience [30].

1.4.1 Hypothalamic-Pituitary-Adrenal (HPA) Axis

Corticotropin-releasing hormone (CRH) is released by the hypothalamus in response to stress, leading to activation of the HPA axis and the release of cortisol [31]. The short-term actions of cortisol are protective and promote adaptation, whereas sustained exposure to abnormally high levels of cortisol can be harmful, causing immunosuppression and health problems [32]. In the brain, excessive cortisol is associated with atrophic effects in the hippocampus and amygdala [33, 34].

Resilience is associated with rapid activation of the stress response and its efficient termination [35]. Therefore, resilience can be related to the capacity to constrain stress-induced increases in CRH and cortisol through a negative feedback system, involving a balance of glucocorticoid and mineralocorticoid receptors [35–37].

1.4.2 Noradrenergic System

Stress releases noradrenaline from the brainstem nuclei, especially the locus ceruleus. Chronic hyper-responsiveness of the locus ceruleus is associated with anxiety disorders, whereas blockade of beta-adrenergic receptors in the amygdala can oppose the development of aversive memories in animals and humans [38, 39]. This suggests that reduced responsiveness of the locus ceruleus could promote resilience [30].

1.4.3 Serotonergic System

Serotonin modulates neural responses to stress, with both anxiogenic and anxiolytic effects depending on the brain region and receptor subtype involved [36]. Serotonin function is also closely linked to mood regulation [30]. Thus, it is suggested that serotonin could play a role in resilience.

1.4.4 Dopaminergic System

Dopamine neurons are activated in response to reward or the expectation of reward and generally inhibited by aversive stimuli. Dopamine signaling facilitates fear extinction, but its role in resilience per se is unclear [30].

1.4.5 Neuropeptide Y (NPY)

NPY acts against the anxiogenic effects of CRH in the amygdala, hippocampus, hypothalamus, and locus ceruleus, and resilience might be associated with maintaining a balance between NPY and CRH levels during stress [39]. In a study of resilient special forces soldiers, higher NPY levels during rigorous military training were associated with better performance [40].

1.5 Genetic Influences on Vulnerability and Resilience

Genetic factors affect vulnerability and resilience. For example, genetic makeup influences balance in the autonomic nervous system. General temperament is also genetically determined in part. Temperament refers to differences in activity levels (active vs. passive), emotionality (pleasant vs. unpleasant), and reactivity (hypersensitive vs. hyposensitive) [41].

Genes also control the codes for the structure and function of organs and body systems. Of most importance to stress are the cardiovascular system (risks for coronary heart disease, high blood pressure, arteriosclerosis), digestive system (risks for stomach and duodenal ulcer), kidneys, and nervous system (imbalance in autonomic system) [9].

Genetic predisposition for high stress reactivity amplifies effects of early-life adversity [42]. Therefore, complex interactions between an individual's genetic factor and his/her history of exposure to environmental stressors determine the degree of adaptability of neurochemical stress response systems to new adverse exposures, as well as the function of the neural circuitry involved in stress responses [30].

1.5.1 HPA Axis-Related Genes

Regulation of the HPA axis is affected by genetic factors. One study found that polymorphisms and haplotypes of the CRH type 1 receptor gene (CRHR1) moderate the influence of child abuse on depressive symptoms in adulthood, with certain alleles and haplotypes exerting protective effects [43].

1.5.2 Serotonin Transporter

The short allele of 5-HTTLPR is associated with decreased serotonin transporter availability and a resulting lower reuptake of serotonin from synaptic clefts. Carriers of the short allele showed elevated risk for depression on exposure to stressful life events, such as childhood maltreatment, compared with long-allele homozygotes in some but not all studies [44–46]. In contrast, the long allele of 5-HTTLPR was found to be associated with emotional resilience in college students [47].

1.5.3 Catechol-O-Methyltransferase (COMT)

A polymorphism relevant to resilience (Val158Met) has been found in the gene that codes for COMT, an enzyme that degrades dopamine and noradrenaline. Individuals with the low-functioning Met158 allele have higher circulating levels of these neurotransmitters. As a result, they tend to exhibit increased plasma adrenaline levels and higher anxiety levels in response to stress, leading to lower resilience to negative mood states [48].

1.5.4 Neuropeptide Y (NPY)

The level of NPY mRNA expression showed an inverse correlation with trait anxiety, as well as a direct correlation with the levels of stress-induced endogenous opioid release, which is implicated in the suppression of pain and stress responses [49].

1.6 Gene-Gene and Gene-Environment Interactions

A monoamine oxidase A (MAOA)-COMT interaction affects endocrine responses to a psychological challenge task [50], a 5-HTTLPR-COMT interaction affects limbic reactivity to unpleasant stimuli in healthy subjects [51], and a

5-HTTLPR-COMT-stressful life event interaction affects the risk for depression [52]. Social support seems to mitigate the effects of the short allele of 5-HTTLPR [53], and the 5-HTTLPR and BDNF Val66Met genotypes interact with stressful life events to predict risk for depression [54, 55].

1.6.1 Epigenetic Mechanisms of Vulnerability and Resilience

Epigenetic mechanisms are known to play important roles in gene-environment interactions that impact stress responses. Epigenetics is the ensemble of processes that induce heritable changes in gene expression without affecting the DNA sequence itself. Epigenetic mechanisms occur primarily at the chromatin and involve multiple mechanisms including DNA methylation [13]. Epigenetic mechanisms can be influenced by environmental factors such as diet, culture, and stress. Their dysregulation has been implicated in stress-related neurodevelopmental and psychiatric disorders [56–58].

Memes (replicable memory, i.e., information) associated with early stress and nurturance also cause epigenetic changes and determine genetic vulnerability or resilience for later stress. With imitation, information (memory) could be transferred from one brain to other brains in the form of memes. With the acquisition of language in humans, memory became spreadable memes. There are endemic memes we call culture that are introduced into the brains of children from early life. Such endemic memes may be protective or pathogenic [59].

The findings that epigenetic changes underlie lifelong differences in behavior suggest that drugs influencing DNA methylation and related epigenetic mechanisms might promote resilience in humans [60].

1.6.2 Transcriptional Mechanisms of Resilience

The findings of animal research underscore the view that resilience is not simply the absence of maladaptive changes that occur in vulnerable individuals; rather, it is mediated by adaptive changes [30]. As one example, the ventrolateral region of the periaqueductal gray (vlPAG) in the midbrain area has long been known to be associated with passive responses to stress [61], which can predict vulnerability over resilience. On the other hand, it was reported that the induction of a transcriptional factor, FOSB, in vlPAG neurons in resilient animals suppressed the expression of the neuropeptide substance P in these cells, which in turn reduced substance P transmission to target regions such as the nucleus accumbens and promoted resilience. These findings suggest the use of substance P antagonists such as neurokinin 1 receptor antagonists as a way to promote resilience in humans [62].

1.7 Neural Circuitry of Resilience

The neural regulation of emotion can be studied in humans by monitoring stress responses during functional imaging studies [63]. Neural circuitry of fear, reward, emotional regulation, and social behavior was reviewed in order to explore neural circuitry of resilience.

1.7.1 Neural Circuitry of Fear

Brain imaging studies in healthy participants have shown that acquisition of fear conditioning is associated with activation in the amygdala [64], whereas extinction of fear memory involves both the ventromedial prefrontal cortex (vmPFC) and amygdala [64, 65]. In particular, the vmPFC seems to mediate the shifting of fear to a different stimulus under stressful conditions [66]. Thus, it is suggested that the neural circuitry of fear plays an important role in resilience.

1.7.2 Neural Circuitry of Reward

In fMRI studies, patients with major depressive disorder and posttraumatic stress disorder (PTSD) have shown reduced striatal activation during the performance of reward-related tasks. These findings suggest reward system dysfunction in these patients [67–69]. Trait optimism is linked to reward circuit function. The level of activation in the rostral anterior cingulate cortex (ACC) was positively correlated with dispositional optimism [70].

1.7.3 Neural Circuitry of Emotional Regulation

A greater capacity for emotional regulation has been related to stress resilience [71]. fMRI studies have shown increased activation in the lateral and medial PFC regions and decreased amygdala activation during cognitive reappraisal, with increased activation in the lateral PFC associated with reappraisal success [72, 73]. It has thus been suggested that the PFC regulates the intensity of emotion responses by modulating the activation of the amygdala.

An fMRI study found that resilient women with a history of sexual trauma were more successful at cognitively enhancing emotional responses to aversive pictures than women with PTSD after sexual trauma and healthy, non-traumatized controls. This increased capacity to enhance emotional responses was associated with increased PFC activation [74].

1.7.4 Neural Circuits of Social Behavior

Social competence and openness to social support are core characteristics of resilient individuals [30]. The capacity for empathy enables individuals to generate appropriate emotional responses in social contexts and might be related to social competence [75, 76]. Some studies have shown a surge of interest in the so-called mirror neuron system; cortical neurons are similarly activated in the same areas of the brain when an animal performs a task or observes another animal of the same species performing the task [77]. It is possible that this system, acting in conjunction with limbic brain regions, has a central role in empathy, that is, understanding others' emotion and intentions [76].

In humans, the vmPFC is activated both when people think about their own mental states and when they think about those of other people, and patients with lesions of this region have deficits in social emotions such as shame, guilt, and empathy [78].

The neuropeptide oxytocin seems to facilitate social attachment by improving a person's ability to infer the mental states of others [79], enhancing the reward value of social stimuli, and reducing potential fear responses [80]. Imaging studies have demonstrated that mutual cooperation induces activation in reward circuitry regions, which are modulated by oxytocin [81]. An fMRI study of married women demonstrated that holding hands with their husband attenuated neural responses to the threat of receiving a shock [82].

1.8 An Integrated Aspect of Resilience

Beginning in development, an individual's genes and gene-environment interactions shape the neural circuitry and neurochemical function that are expressed in psychological strengths and behaviors characteristic of resilient individuals. Various genetic polymorphisms affect a person's limbic reactivity and prefrontal-limbic connectivity, influencing their initial responses to negative or traumatic events, as well as their capacity for cognitive reappraisal of those events. Thus, the functional capacity of the brain structures involved in the integrated circuits that mediate mood and emotion determines stress resilience [30].

1.9 Conclusions

Causes of stress are classified into psychosocial factors and environmental (bioecological) factors. Vulnerability refers to poorly adapting to stressors and showing inappropriate responses that can become persistent states of stress. In contrast, resilience is linked to being able to perceive stressful events in less threatening ways, promoting adaptive coping strategies. Differences in individual vulnerability and resilience occur across sex, age, and culture. The underlying mechanisms of vulnerability and resilience are known to depend on a combination of genetic and nongenetic factors. Psychosocial factors, behavioral factors, neuroendocrine stress responses, genetic and epigenetic mechanisms, and neural circuitry are likely to be involved in vulnerability and resilience to stress. In particular, the functional capacity of the brain structures involved in the integrated circuits that mediate mood and emotion determines stress resilience.

References

1. Greenberg JS. Coping with stress: a practical guide. Dubuque: Wm C Publishers; 1990.
2. Selye H. The stress of life. New York: McGraw-Hill; 1956.
3. Derogatis LR, Coons HL. Self-report measures of stress. In: Goldberg L, Breznitz S, editors. Handbook of stress – theoretical and clinical aspects. 2nd ed. New York: The Free Press; 1993.
4. Lipowski ZJ. Psychosomatic medicine and liaison psychiatry. New York: Plenum Medical Book Co; 1985.
5. Lazarus RS. Patterns of adjustment. New York: McGraw-Hill; 1976.
6. Lazarus RS. The stress and coping paradigm. Edisdorfer C, Cohen D, Kleinman A, et al.. Models for clinical psychopathology. New York; Spectrum; 1981
7. Reiser MF. Psychophysiology of stress and its sequelae. In: Reiser MF, editor. Mind, brain, body: toward a convergence of psychoanalysis and neurobiology. New York: Basic Books; 1984.
8. Selye H. Stress without distress. New York: J.B. Lippincott; 1974.
9. Rice PL. Stress and health: principles and practice for coping and wellness. Pacific Grove: Brooks/Cole Publishing Co; 1987.
10. Girdano DA, Everly G. Controlling stress and tension: a holistic approach. New Jersey: Prentice-Hall; 1979.
11. Del Giudice M, Ellis BJ, Shirtcliff EA. The adaptive calibration model of stress responsivity. Neurosci Biobehav Rev. 2011;35:1562–92.
12. Rutter M. Implications of resilience concepts for scientific understanding. Ann N Y Acad Sci. 2006;1094:1–12.
13. Franklin TB, Saab BJ, Mansuy IM. Neural mechanisms of stress resilience and vulnerability. Neuron. 2012;75:747–61.
14. Masten AS. Ordinary magic. Resilience processes in development. Am Psychol. 2001;56:227–38.
15. Masten AS, Coatsworth JD. The development of competence in favorable and unfavorable environments. Lessons from research on successful children. Am Psychol. 1998;53:205–20.
16. Rutter M. Resilience in the face of adversity. Protective factors and resistance to psychiatric disorder. Br J Psychiatry. 1985;147:598–611.
17. Yam KY, Naninck EF, Schmidt MV, et al. Early-life adversity programs emotional functions and the neuroendocrine stress system: the contribution of nutrition, metabolic hormones and epigenetic mechanisms. Stress. 2015;18:328–42.
18. Santarelli S, Zimmermann C, Kalideris G, et al. An adverse early life environment can enhance stress resilience in adulthood. Psychoneuroendocrinology. 2017;78:213–21.
19. Oomen CA, Soeters H, Audureau N, et al. Severe early life stress hampers spatial learning and neurogenesis, but improves hippocampal synaptic plasticity and emotional learning under high-stress conditions in adulthood. J Neurosci. 2010;30:6635–45.

20. Southwick SM, Vythilingam M, Charney DS. The psychobiology of depression and resilience to stress: implications for prevention and treatment. Annu Rev Clin Psychol. 2005;1:255–91.
21. Sherrer MV. The role of cognitive appraisal in adaptation to traumatic stress in adults with serious mental illness: a critical review. Trauma Violence Abuse. 2011;12:151–67.
22. Antonovsky A. Health, stress and coping. San Francisco: Jossey-Bass; 1982.
23. Cotton DHG. Stress management: an integrated approach to therapy. New York: Brunner/Mazel; 1990. p. 80–110.
24. Ong AD, Bergeman CS, Bisconti TL, et al. Psychological resilience, positive emotions, and successful adaptation to stress in later life. J Pers Soc Psychol. 2006;91:730–49.
25. Tugade MM, Fredrickson BL. Resilient individuals use positive emotions to bounce back from negative emotional experiences. J Pers Soc Psychol. 2004;86:320–33.
26. Fredrickson BL. The role of positive emotions in positive psychology. The broaden-and-build theory of positive emotions. Am Psychol. 2001;56:218–26.
27. Alim TN, Feder A, Graves RE, et al. Trauma, resilience, and recovery in a high-risk African-American population. Am J Psychiatry. 2008;165:1566–75.
28. Ryff CD, Keyes CL. The structure of psychological well-being revisited. J Pers Soc Psychol. 1995;69:719–27.
29. Pargement KI, Koenig BW, Perez L. Patterns of positive and negative religious coping with major life stressors. J Sci Study Relig. 1998;37:710–24.
30. Feder A, Nestler EJ, Charney DS. Psychobiology and molecular genetics of resilience. Nat Rev/Neurosci. 2009;10:446–57.
31. Heim C, Nemeroff CB. The role of childhood trauma in the neurobiology of mood and anxiety disorders: preclinical and clinical studies. Biol Psychiatry. 2001;49:1023–39.
32. Karlamangla AS, Singer BH, McEwen BS, et al. Allostatic load as a predictor of functional decline. MacArthur studies of successful aging. J Clin Epidemiol. 2002;55:696–710.
33. McEwen BS, Milner TA. Hippocampal formation: shedding light on the influence of sex and stress on the brain. Brain Res Rev. 2007;55:343–55.
34. Brown ES, Woolston DJ, Frol AB. Amygdala volume in patients receiving chronic corticosteroid therapy. Biol Psychiatry. 2008;63:705–9.
35. de Kloet ER, Joels M, Holsboer F. Stress and the brain: from adaptation to disease. Nat Rev Neurosci. 2005;6:463–75.
36. Charney DS. Psychobiological mechanisms of resilience and vulnerability: implications for successful adaptation to extreme stress. Am J Psychiatry. 2004;161:195–216.
37. de Kloet ER, Deriik RH, Meijer OC. Therapy insight: is there an imbalanced response of mineralocorticoid and glucocorticoid receptors in depression? Nat Clin Pract Endocrinol Metab. 2007;3:168–79.
38. Charney DS. Neuroanatomical circuits modulating fear and anxiety behaviors. Acta Psychiatr Scand Suppl. 2003;417:38–50.
39. Sajdyk TJ, Shekhar A, Gehlert DR. Interactions between NPY and CRF in the amygdala to regulate emotionality. Neuropeptides. 2004;38:225–34.
40. Morgan CA, Wang S, Southwick SM, et al. Plasma neuropeptide Y concentrations in humans exposed to military survival training. Biol Psychiatry. 2000;47:902–9.
41. Fuller JL, Thompson WR. Foundations of behavior genetics. St. Louis: Mosby; 1978.
42. McIlwrick S, Rechenberg A, Matthes M, et al. Genetic predisposition for high stress reactivity amplifies effects of early-life adversity. Psychoneuroendocrinology. 2016;70:85–97.
43. Bradley RG, Binder EB, Epstein MP, et al. Influence of child abuse on adult depression: moderation by the corticotropin-releasing hormone receptor gene. Arch Gen Psychiatry. 2008;65:190–200.
44. Caspi A, Sugden K, Moffitt TE, et al. Influence of life stress on depression: moderation by a polymorphism in the 5-HTT gene. Science. 2003;301:386–9.
45. Kendler KS, Kuhn JW, Vittum J, et al. The interaction of stressful life events and a serotonin transporter polymorphism in the prediction of episodes of major depression: a replication. Arch Gen Psychiatry. 2005;62:529–35.

46. Gillespie NA, Whitfield JB, Williams B, et al. The relationship between stressful life events, the serotonin transporter (5-HTTLPR) genotype and major depression. Psychol Med. 2005;35:101–11.
47. Stein MB, Campbell-Sills L, Gelernter J. Genetic variation in 5-HTTLPR is associated with emotional resilience. Am J Med Genet B Neuropsychiatr Genet. 2009;150B:900–6.
48. Heinz A, Smolka MN. The effects of catechol O-methyltransferase genotype on brain activation elicited by affective stimuli and cognitive tasks. Rev Neurosci. 2006;17:359–67.
49. Zhou Z, Zhu G, Hariri AR, et al. Genetic variation in human NPY expression affects stress response and emotion. Nature. 2008;452:997–1001.
50. Jabbi M, Korf J, Kema IP, et al. Convergent genetic modulation of the endocrine stress response involves polymorphic variations of 5-HTT, COMT and MAOA. Mol Psychiatry. 2007;12:483–90.
51. Smolka MN, Buhler M, Schumann G, et al. Gene-gene effects on central processing of aversive stimuli. Mol Psychiatry. 2007;12:307–17.
52. Mandelli L, Serretti A, Marino E, et al. Interaction between serotonin transporter gene, catechol-O-methyltransferase gene and stressful life events in mood disorders. Int J Neuropsychopharmacol. 2007;10:437–47.
53. Kaufman J, Yang B-Z, Douglas-Palumberi H, et al. Social supports and serotonin transporter gene moderate depression in maltreated children. Proc Natl Acad Sci U S A. 2004;101:17316–21.
54. Kim JM, Stewart R, Kim SW, et al. Interactions between life stressors and susceptibility genes (5-HTTLPR and BDNF) on depression in Korean elders. Biol Psychiatry. 2007;62:423–8.
55. Kaufman J, Yang B-Z, Douglas-Palumberi H, et al. Brain-derived neurotrophic factor-5-HTTLPR gene interactions and environmental modifiers of depression in children. Biol Psychiatry. 2006;59:673–80.
56. Franklin TB, Mansuy IM. The involvement of epigenetic defects in mental retardation. Neurobiol Learn Mem. 2011;96:61–7.
57. Kubota T, Miyake K, Hirasawa T. Epigenetic understanding of gene-environment interactions in psychiatric disorders: a new concept of clinical genetics. Clin Epigenetics. 2012;4:1.
58. McEwen BS, Eiland L, Hunter RG, et al. Stress and anxiety: structural plasticity and epigenetic regulation as a consequence of stress. Neuropharmacology. 2012;62:3–12.
59. Leigh H. Genes, memes, culture, and psychosomatic medicine: an integrative model. In: Koh KB, editor. Somatization and psychosomatic symptoms. New York: Springer; 2013.
60. Krishnan V, Han M-H, Graham DL, et al. Molecular adaptations underlying susceptibility and resistance to social defeat in brain reward regions. Cell. 2007;131:391–404.
61. Bandler R, Shipley MT. Columnar organization in the midbrain periaqueductal gray: modules for emotional expression? Trends Neurosci. 1994;17:379–89.
62. Berton O, Covington IIIHE, Ebner K, et al. Induction of FosB in the periaqueductal gray by stress promotes active coping responses. Neuron. 2007;55:289–300.
63. Dedovic K, Renwick R, Najmeh KM, et al. The Montreal imaging stress task: using functional imaging to investigate the effects of perceiving and processing psychosocial stress in the human brain. J Psychiatry Neurosci. 2005;30:319–25.
64. Delgado MR, Olsson A, Phelps EA. Extending animal models of fear conditioning to humans. Biol Psychol. 2006;73:39–48.
65. Milad MR, Quinn BT, Pitman RK, et al. Thickness of ventromedial prefrontal cortex in humans is correlated with extinction memory. Proc Natl Acad Sci U S A. 2005;102:10706–11.
66. Schiller D, Levy I, Niv Y, et al. From fear to safety and back: reversal of fear in the human brain. J Neurosci. 2008;28:11517–25.
67. Pizzagalli DA, Holmes AJ, Dillon DJ, et al. Reduced caudate and nucleus accumbens response to rewards in unmedicated subjects with major depressive disorder. Am J Psychiatry. 2008;166:702–10.
68. Sailer U, Robinson S, Fischmeister F, et al. Altered reward processing in the nucleus accumbens and mesial prefrontal cortex of patients with posttraumatic stress disorder. Neuropsychologia. 2008;46:2836–44.

69. Drevets WC, Price JL, Furey ML. Brain structural and functional abnormalities in mood disorders: implication for neurocircuitry models of depression. Brain Struct Funct. 2008;213:93–118.
70. Sharot T, Riccardi AM, Raio CM, et al. Neural mechanisms mediating optimism bias. Nature. 2007;450:102–5.
71. Ressler KJ, Mayberg HS. Targeting abnormal neural circuits in mood and anxiety disorders: from the laboratory to the clinic. Nat Neurosci. 2007;10:1116–24.
72. Goldin PR, McRae K, Ramel W, et al. The neural bases of emotion regulation: reappraisal and suppression of negative emotion. Biol Psychiatry. 2008;63:577–86.
73. Ochsner KN, Ray RD, Cooper JC, et al. For better or for worse: neural systems supporting the cognitive down- and up-regulation of negative emotion. NeuroImage. 2004;23:483–99.
74. New AS, Fan J, Murrough JW, et al. A functional magnetic resonance imaging study of deliberate emotion regulation in PTSD and resilience. Biol Psychiatry. 2009;66:656–64.
75. Iarocci G, Yager J, Elfers T. What gene-environment interactions can tell us about social competence in typical and atypical populations. Brain Cogn. 2007;65:112–7.
76. Storm EE, Tecott LH. Social circuits: peptidergic regulation of mammalian social behavior. Neuron. 2005;47:483–6.
77. Rizzolatti G, Craighero L. The mirror-neuron system. Annu Rev Neurosci. 2004;27:169–92.
78. Pfeifer JH, Iacoboni M, Mazziotta JC, et al. Mirroring others' emotions relates to empathy and interpersonal competence in children. NeuroImage. 2008;39:2067–85.
79. Domes G, Heinrichs M, Michel A, et al. Oxytocin improves mind-reading in humans. Biol Psychiatry. 2007;61:731–3.
80. Skuse DH, Gallagher L. Dopaminergic neuropeptide interactions in the social brain. Trends Cogn Sci. 2009;13:27–35.
81. Rilling JK, Gutman DA, Zeh TR, et al. A neural basis for social cooperation. Neuron. 2002;35:395–405.
82. Coan JA, Schaefer HS, Davidson RJ. Lending a hand: social regulation of the neural response to threat. Psychol Sci. 2006;17:1032–9.

Chapter 2
Measurement of Stress

2.1 Introduction

Measurement of stress is crucial for assessment and management of patients with somatic symptoms as well as those with psychological symptoms, because stress is closely associated with the onset and progress of each of somatic and psychological symptoms. In addition, stress measurement is required for examining the relationship between stress and biological variables [1].

Stress measures have been developed in a variety of forms and contents. However, a considerable number of measures focus on cognitive processes (e.g., appraisal and coping) and emotional state (e.g., anxiety, depression), because these elements are emphasized as being central to the definition of stress. Therefore, these two are primary targets for stress measurement [1].

Biological markers (e.g., neurotransmitters, cortisol, neuropeptides) have been explored as more objective measures of stress, but their specificity has not been found. Otherwise, phenomenological approaches, such as clinicians' ratings and consensual judgments of stimulus values, have been tried. However, it is not only difficult for them to evaluate the personal valences that stressors may have for each individual, but bias may occur in the observers' evaluative processes. As a result, self-report stress measures are adopted as a major assessment tool due to their advantages despite their subjective quality being criticized [1].

Most of studies have been done on the frequency and the amount of life changes (e.g., *Social Readjustment Rating Scale*) [2]. This chapter reviews stress measures available for assessing the relationship between stress and diseases.

K. B. Koh, *Stress and Somatic Symptoms*,
https://doi.org/10.1007/978-3-030-02783-4_2

2.2 Theories of Stress

Theories of stress consist of three types: stimulus-oriented theories, response-oriented theories, and interactional theories [3]. Stimulus-oriented theories view stress as the stimulus provided by the organism's environment [1]. If the event leads to psychological distress, behavioral disruption, or deterioration in performance, then it is characterized as a stressor. These stressors include daily hassles and chronic daily events [4–6].

Response-oriented theories define the presence of stress as the response of the individual or organism to the environment or the events. Stress responses may be neurobiological (e.g., hormones, neurotransmitters, neuropeptides), physiological (e.g., blood pressure, muscle tension), and psychological (e.g., anxiety, depression) [1]. Response-oriented theories of stress find their modern beginnings in the work of Cannon [7, 8], but response-oriented definition was elucidated in Selye's theory of *general adaptation syndrome* [9, 10].

Interactional theories emphasize the characteristics of the organism as major mediating mechanisms between the environmental stimuli and the responses they invoke. The perceptual, cognitive, and physiological characteristics of the individual affect the responses to his/her environmental stimuli [11, 12]. In other words, these theories emphasize reciprocal interactions between the individual's characteristics (perceptual, cognitive, and emotional) and the external environment [1].

2.3 Self-Report Measures of Stress

2.3.1 Stimulus-Oriented Measures

Stimulus-oriented measures address the characteristics of the environmental stimuli or life events that impinge upon the individual. The *Social Readjustment Rating Scale* [2] was developed to rate the extent of adaptation to recent life changes. On the other hand, the *Global Assessment of Recent Stress (GARS)* is a self-report instrument developed to examine the relationship between recent life events and physiological responses [13].

2.3.2 Response-Oriented Measures

As already mentioned by Cannon [8] and Seyle [9], stress theory is a theoretical underpinning of response-oriented measurement. However, the majority of measures arise from clinical research on psychopathology. Therefore, the self-report instruments that have been utilized most prominently as presumptive measures of stress are psychopathological scales including mood and affect. Among them, there are *Minnesota Multiphasic Personality Inventory (MMPI)* [14], *Symptom Checklist-90-Revised*

(SCL-90-R) [15], and *Stress Response Inventory (SRI)* [16]. In addition, *Beck Depression Inventory* [17] and *State-Trait Anxiety Inventory* [18] are known as unidimensional symptom inventories designed to assess either depression or anxiety.

2.3.3 Interaction-Oriented Measures

As mentioned previously, interaction-oriented measures are based on the hypotheses that in addition to environmental stimuli, perceptual, cognitive, personality, and other characteristics of the individual interact to mediate responses to stress. As such scales, there are *Jenkins Activity Survey* [19] and *Ways of Coping Checklist* [20]. The Jenkins Activity Survey is a self-report screening instrument developed to measure a specific pattern of behavior such as type A behavior thought to have a high association with proneness to coronary heart disease.

By now, three categories of variables which need to be assessed are (1) stressors, (2) stress responses, and (3) personal characteristics, behavior patterns, and coping styles. The purpose of these measures is to clearly define problem areas so that therapy can be planned appropriately, then identify the individual's initial status, and assess its progress over the course of therapy [21].

2.4 Approaches to Stress Measurement

There are three approaches to stress measurement, such as interview, self-rating measures, and direct observation. Each of these approaches has its own strengths and weaknesses. Direct observation or self-monitoring may be unrealistically time-consuming if used to record major life events, which occur infrequently and which can be listed in an interview. Interviews are of limited utility for eliciting information about physiological symptoms, descriptions of which may be difficult to verbalize; checklists work well in that case. Questionnaires identifying specific thought patterns may not contain items relevant to a specific individual; self-monitoring and recording are more useful in this instance [21].

2.5 Measurement of Stressors

2.5.1 Major Life Events

2.5.1.1 Social Readjustment Rating Scale

This most well-known of the life events scales over 40 major life events, such as death of a spouse, change of job, divorce, etc., each of which has been assigned a mean value of between 11 and 100 life change units. Clients are asked to rate the extent of adaptation to recent life changes compared with marriage (50 units). The total score has some predictive value in terms of anticipating diseases or illnesses [2].

2.5.2 Minor Life Events

2.5.2.1 Hassles Scale

The Hassles Scale consists of 117 irritants ranging from minor annoyance to fairly major problems. Subjects are asked to identify the hassles which have occurred in the past month and rate each one as being somewhat severe, moderately severe, or extremely severe. Clinically, the Hassles Scale provides a complement to the major life event approach [22].

2.5.3 Mixed Life Events

2.5.3.1 Global Assessment of Recent Stress (GARS) Scale

This scale is an instrument developed for assessing the severity of recent stressors in seven areas and one overall area during the last week, which includes major and minor life events. This constitutes eight subscales, such as work/job/school, interpersonal area, changes in relationships, sickness/injury, financial area, unusual happenings, change/no change in routine, and overall global. Each item is rated on a 10-point scale, ranging from 0 (not at all) to 9 (extremely severe). It helps examine the relationship between stressors and physiological variables [13].

2.5.4 Appraisal of Stressful Situations

Appraisal of specific stressful situations might best be determined by asking the question: "What makes the situation so stressful for you?" In addition, discussion of specific situations in an interview, as well as recording of stressful situations as they may occur, can generate individual examples of cognitive appraisal [21].

2.5.4.1 Dysfunctional Attitude Scale

This is a 40-item scale designed to identify cognitive distortions which may be related to depression. Each item is rated on a seven-point scale according to the extent to which the client agrees with the item. The items were selected to measure seven value systems, such as approval, love, achievement, perfectionism, entitlement, omnipotence, and autonomy. This scale can be clinically used to examine areas in which the client is emotionally vulnerable and to identify tendencies toward nonadaptive thinking. Since automatic thoughts are sometimes difficult for clients to verbalize spontaneously, this scale may be useful in identifying cognitive distortions [23].

2.5.4.2 Rational Behavior Inventory

This is a 37-item scale designed to measure irrational and absolutistic beliefs. Eleven factors including guilt, perfectionism, and need for approval were identified from this scale. This instrument was developed in order to assess if clients are good candidates for cognitive therapy and to assess the progress of such therapy [24].

2.6 Measures of Stress Responses

2.6.1 Physiological Responses

2.6.1.1 Direct Observation

This system is most useful for symptoms which occur fairly often and at discrete intervals [21].

2.6.1.2 Self-Rating Measures

1. Self-Rating Anxiety Scale
   This is a 20-item measure that includes 15 somatic and 5 affective symptoms of stress. The frequency of each symptom is rated by the client on a 4-point scale. However, the total score represents the sum of 5 affective as well as the 15 physiological symptoms. This total score is useful if one is attempting to formulate a DSM diagnosis or to compare a client's overall level of anxiety with a reference group. It may be useful to assess global change over time [25].
2. Somatic Stress Response Scale
   This is a 32-item scale designed to examine the relationship between stress and somatic responses. This scale consists of five subscales, such as cardiorespiratory, somatic sensitivity, gastrointestinal response, general somatic response, and genitourinary response. Each item is rated on a five-point scale, ranging from 0 (not at all) to 4 (absolutely) [26].

2.6.2 *Cognitive Responses*

By asking repeatedly such questions as "What did you think about that?," "How did that make you feel?," "What were you thinking while that was going on?," and "Why is that so important to you?," the therapist can get an idea of the sequence of thoughts and behaviors that the client is experiencing [21].

2.6.2.1 Direct Observation

Usually this is done in conjunction with the recording of specific stressful events identified earlier. For example, the client may be asked to note each time he or she felt stressed, what was happening, and what he or she was saying to himself or herself at this time [21]. Meichenbaum [27] recommended the therapist to keep recording requirements to a minimum and to avoid the exercise itself becoming a stressor.

2.6.2.2 Self-Rating Measures

1. Automatic Thoughts Questionnaire (ATQ)

   This is a 30-item instrument that measures the frequency of automatic negative statements about the self. The scale deals with four aspects of automatic thoughts: (1) personal maladjustment and desire for changes ("I wish I were a better person"), (2) negative self-concepts and negative expectations ("I am no good"), (3) low self-esteem ("I hate myself"), and (4) helplessness ("I can't finish anything"). The primary object of this scale is to differentiate depressed from nondepressed subjects and to measure changes in cognitions attributable to clinical interventions [28].
2. Cognitive-Somatic Anxiety Questionnaire (CSAQ)

   This is a 14-item scale which assesses both cognitive and somatic aspects of anxiety. Since it focuses only on symptoms, it is appropriate for the measurement of the stress responses. Cognitive items emphasize persistent thoughts, imagining terrifying scenes, worry, and concentration. Somatic items include references to gastrointestinal complaints, increased heart rate, and so on. This scale may help differentiate clients with predominantly cognitive symptoms from those with predominantly somatic symptoms, although the items are not comprehensive due to a brief scale [29].
3. Social Anxiety Thoughts Questionnaire (SAT)

   This is a 21-item scale designed to measure the cognitive aspects of social anxiety. The items include self-defeating and negative thoughts related to general discomfort, concern about others' awareness of distress, fear of negative evaluations, and perceptions of performance anxiety. This is a questionnaire which may serve as a starting point for the discussion of cognitive distortions or self-defeating statements for clients whose stress is associated with social situations. This scale may also be useful to assess changes over time since it is an instrument which refers to thoughts that have occurred for the past 1 week [30].

4. Stress-Induced Cognition Scale

   This is a 21-item scale designed to measure cognitive stress responses, such as extreme-negative thought, aggressive-hostile thought, and self-depreciative thought experienced for the last week. Each item is rated on a five-point scale, ranging from 0 (not at all) to 4 (absolutely) [31].

2.6.3 Behavioral Responses

2.6.3.1 Direct Observation

One method consists of keeping a structured diary (e.g., recording a specified behavior, along with the antecedents and consequences of the behavior). Another method is the frequency count (e.g., the number of cigarettes smoked per day) [21].

2.6.3.2 Self-Rating Measures

There are many scales which assess behaviors, such as smoking, eating habits, social skills, and assertiveness [21].

1. Assertion Inventory

   This 40-item scale was designed to measure three aspects of assertion: discomfort with assertion, probability of engaging in assertive behavior, and identification of problem situations. This scale can be used to classify individuals as "assertive," "unassertive," "anxious performer," or "does not care." It has also been used to measure changes during therapy [32].

2. Assertive Behavior Survey Schedule (ABSS)

   In contrast to the above scale, this is not primarily a measurement scale but rather a descriptive scale. It might be considered a structured interview technique. The client is asked to anticipate his or her reaction in six situations requiring assertion. Then, he or she should answer the questions about the anticipated consequences of acting assertively with a variety of people (e.g., parents, friends). Finally, the client is asked to identify his or her general behavioral tendency in a situation of inequality with other important persons in his or her life. This scale would not be helpful to assess changes over time, because it provides descriptive information [33].

2.6.4 *Multidimensional Responses*

2.6.4.1 Self-Rating Measures

There are some scales which are widely used for multiple purposes, although they do not measure any specific elements of stress responses.

1. Symptom Checklist-90-Revised (SCL-90-R)
   This is a 90-item scale for assessing psychopathology during the last week and constitutes somatization, interpersonal sensitivity, obsessive-compulsive, anxiety, depression, hostility, phobia, paranoid ideation, and psychoticism. Each item is rated on a 5-point scale, ranging from 0 (never at all) to 4 (very severe).
2. Perceived Stress Questionnaire (PSQ)
   This is a 30-item scale designed to assess perceived stress during the last month and constitutes 7 subscales, such as harassment, overload, irritability, lack of joy, fatigue, worries, and tension. This scale is an instrument which deals with stressors and stress responses at the same time [34].
3. Stress Response Inventory (SRI)
   This is a 39-item scale developed by Koh et al. [16], which deals with four stress responses, such as emotional, somatic, cognitive, and behavioral responses. It has seven subscales, such as tension, aggression, somatization, anger, depression, fatigue, and frustration. Each item is rated on a five-point scale, ranging from 0 (not at all) to 4 (absolutely).

2.6.5 *Personality and Personal Styles*

In those cases in which stressors are more related to a function of the individual than to the situations, personality assessment may help examine the individual's personality structure [21].

2.6.5.1 State-Trait Anger Expression Inventory-2 (STAXI-2)

The STAXI-2 [35] is a 57-item inventory which measures the intensity of anger as an emotional state at a particular moment (State Anger) and the disposition to experience angry feelings as a personality trait (Trait Anger). The instrument includes six subscales: state anger, trait anger, anger expression-in, anger expression-out, anger control-in, and anger control-out. Each item is rated on a four-point scale, ranging from 0 (not at all) to 3 (almost always). This instrument was developed to assess how different anger components contribute to the development of medical conditions such as hypertension and coronary heart disease.

2.6.6 *Personal Resources*

2.6.6.1 Coping Style

1. Revised Version of Ways of Coping Scale
   Folkman et al. [36] have developed the revised version of the Ways of Coping [20] which has 50 items and consists of 8 subscales, such as confrontation, distancing, self-controlling, seeking social support, accepting responsibility, escape-avoidance, planned problem-solving, and positive reappraisal.
2. Anger Coping Scale
   This is a 19-item scale designed to assess coping strategies for anger. This scale consists of five subscales, such as behavioral aggression, problem-solving coping, verbal aggression, tension-releasing coping, and anger suppression. Each item is rated on a 5-point scale, ranging from 0 (not at all) to 4 (absolutely) [37].

2.6.6.2 Intellectual Levels and Social Factors

Clients who have less skill in the verbal area may well benefit more from behavioral approaches, whereas intelligent individuals may be offended by behavioral approaches so that cognitive approaches may be more effective for them. Social support is known to be a moderator of stress, but the nature of social support is complex [21].

2.7 Conclusions

The assessment of stress is essential in clinical approaches as well as in psychosomatic research, particularly for exploring the relationship between stress and diseases. Such assessment has been done in terms of stimulus-oriented, response-oriented, and interaction-oriented measurement. Three categories of variables which need to be assessed are stressors, stress responses (cognitive, physiological, and behavioral), and personal characteristics (personal resources, behavioral patterns, and coping styles). The purpose of stress assessment in these three aspects is to make clear the client's problem areas and help the therapist plan therapeutic approaches appropriately. In addition, such assessment can be used to evaluate changes between pre-treatment and posttreatment states. There are three approaches to stress measurement, such as interview, paper-and-pencil measures (use of rating scales or checklists), and direct observation. Each of these approaches has its own strength and weakness. Therefore, the therapist needs to be aware of both the strengths and weaknesses of the assessment tools to select the tool specifically fit for the individual.

Stress Response Inventory

DIRECTIONS: A number of statements which people have used to describe themselves under stress are given below. Read each statement carefully, and then circle under the statement that best indicates how you have been feeling or what you have been *experiencing during the past seven (7) days including today*. There are no right or wrong answers. Do not spend too much time on any one statement, but make sure to answer all the given statements. One example is given below.

(Example)

	Not at all	Somewhat	Moderately	Very much	Absolutely
I have no appetite			O		

****

	Not at all	Somewhat	Moderately	Very much	Absolutely
1. I make many mistakes at work					
2. I don't feel like talking					
3. My chest feels tight					
4. I feel angry					
5. I feel agitated and restless					
6. I suffer from indigestion					
7. My stomach hurts					
8. I feel like screaming					
9. I often sigh					
10. I feel dizzy					
11. Everything bothers me					
12. I have distracting thoughts					
13. I am easily fatigued					
14. I feel totally exhausted					
15. I have lost my self-confidence					
16. I feel tense					
17. My body trembles					
18. I feel like hitting someone					
19. I have lost incentive to do anything					
20. I feel like crying					
21. I feel on edge					
22. I have no future in my current work					
23. I often stare blankly					
24. I hate someone					
25. I can't get that thought out of my head					
26. My voice is louder than it usually is					

	Not at all	Somewhat	Moderately	Very much	Absolutely
27. I easily get impatient					
28. I act violently (such as reckless driving, cursing, fighting)					
29. I feel like breaking something					
30. I talk less than I used to					
31. My head hurts or it feels heavy					
32. My heart throbs					
33. I feel like killing someone					
34. My face gets flushed or it feels hot					
35. I feel bored					
36. I have lost my patience					
37. My face looks rigid					
38. I am useless (or unworthy)					
39. I don't like moving any part of my body					

References

1. Derogatis LR, Coons HL. Self-report measures of stress. In: Goldberg L, Breznitz S, editors. Handbook of stress – theoretical and clinical aspects. 2nd ed. New York: The Free Press; 1993. p. 200–33.
2. Holmes TH, Rahe RH. The social readjustment rating scale. J Psychosom Res. 1967;1:213–8.
3. Lazarus RS. Psychological stress and the coping process. New York: McGraw-Hill; 1966.
4. Vingerhoets AJ, Marcelissen FH. Stress research: its present status and issues for future developments. Soc Sci Med. 1988;26:279–91.
5. Delongis A, Coyne JC, Dakof G, et al. Relationship of daily hassles uplifts and major life events to health status. Health Psychol. 1982;1:119–36.
6. Lazarus RA, Delongis A. Psychological stress and coping in aging. Am Psychol. 1983;38:245–54.
7. Cannon WB. Bodily changes in fear, hunger, pain, and rage: an account of recent researches into the function of emotional excitement. 2nd ed. New York: Appleton; 1929.
8. Cannon WB. The wisdom of the body. 2nd ed. New York: Norton; 1932.
9. Selye H. The physiology and pathology of exposure to stress. Montreal: Acta; 1950.
10. Selye H. The evolution of the stress concept. Am J Cardiol. 1970;26:289–99.
11. Lazarus RS. Patterns of adjustment. New York: McGraw-Hill; 1976.
12. Lazarus RS. The stress and coping paradigm. In: Edisdorfer C, Cohen D, Kleinman A, et al., editors. Models for clinical psychopathology. New York: Spectrum; 1981.
13. Linn MW. A global assessment of recent stress (GARS) scale. Int J Psychiatry Med. 1985;15:47–59.
14. Derogatis LR, Rickels K, Rock AF. The SCL-90 and MMPI: a step in the validation of a new report scale. Br J Psychiatry. 1976;128:280–9.
15. Derogatis LR, Lipman RS, Covi L. SCL-90: an outpatient psychiatric rating scale: preliminary report. Psychopharmacol Bull. 1973;9:13–27.
16. Koh KB, Park JK, Kim CH, et al. Development of the stress response inventory and its application in clinical practice. Psychosom Med. 2001;63:668–78.

17. Beck AT, Ward C, Mendelson M, et al. An inventory for measuring depression. Arch Gen Psychiatry. 1961;4:53–63.
18. Spielberger CD, Gorsuch RC, Lushene RE. Manual for the state-trait anxiety inventory. Palo Alto: Consulting Psychologists Press; 1970.
19. Jenkins CD, Rosenman RH, Friedman M. Development of an objective psychological test for the determination of the coronary-prone behavior pattern in employed men. J Chronic Dis. 1967;20:371–9.
20. Folkman S, Lazarus RS. An analysis of coping in a middle-aged community sample. J Health Soc Behav. 1980;21:219–39.
21. Cotton DHG. Stress management: an integrated approach to therapy. New York: Brunner/Mazel; 1990. p. 80–110.
22. Kanner AD, Coyne JC, Schaefer C, et al. Comparison of two modes of stress measurement: daily hassles and uplifts versus major life events. J Behav Med. 1981;4:1–39.
23. Weissman AN. Assessing depressogenic attitudes: a validation study. Paper presented at the 51st Annual Meeting of the Eastern Psychological Association, Hartford; 1980
24. Shorkey CT, Whiteman VL. Development of the rational behavior inventory: initial validity and reliability. Educ Psychol Meas. 1977;37:527–34.
25. Zung WK. A rating instrument for anxiety disorders. Psychosomatics. 1971;12:371–9.
26. Koh KB, Park JK, Cho SH. Development of the somatic stress response scale and its application in clinical practice. Yonsei Med J. 2005;46:614–24.
27. Meichenbaum D. A cognitive-behavior modification approach to assessment. In: Hersen M, Bellack AS, editors. Behavioral assessment: a practical handbook. New York: Pergamon Press; 1976. p. p143–71.
28. Hollon SD, Kendall PC. Cognitive self-statements in depression: development of an automatic thoughts questionnaire. Cogn Ther Res. 1980;4:383–95.
29. Schwartz GE, Davidson RJ, Goleman DT. Patterning of cognitive and somatic processes in self-regulation of anxiety: effects of meditation versus exercise. Psychosom Med. 1978;40:321–8.
30. Hartman LM. Cognitive components of anxiety. J Clin Psychol. 1984;40:137–9.
31. Koh KB, Park JK, Cho SH. Development of the stress-induced cognition scale. Yonsei Med J. 2006;47:384–92.
32. Gambrill ED, Richey CA. An assertion inventory for use in assessment and research. Behav Ther. 1975;6:550–61.
33. Hersen M, Bellack AS. Behavioral assessment: a practical handbook. New York: Peragamon Press; 1976.
34. Levenstein S, Prantera C, Varvo M, et al. Development of the perceived stress questionnaire: a new tool for psychosomatic research. J Psychosom Res. 1993;37:19–32.
35. Spielberger CD. Manual for the state-trait anger expression inventory–2. Odessa: Psychological Assessment Resources; 1999.
36. Folkman S, Lazarus RS, Dunkel-Schetter C, et al. Dynamics of a stressful encounter: cognitive appraisal, coping, and encounter outcomes. J Pers Soc Psychol. 1986;50:992–1003.
37. Koh KB, Park JK. Development of the anger coping scale. J Korean Neuropsychiatr Assoc. 2005;44:477–88.

Chapter 3
Stress and Neuroendocrine Function

3.1 Introduction

In this chapter are reviewed history of psychoneuroendocrinology, the rationale for using endocrine markers in stress research, and measures of hormones such as catecholamines and cortisol. In addition, general adaptation syndrome, the relationship between stressors and hormones, emotion and hormones, duration of exposure to stress and changes of hormones, effects of gene-environment interaction on neuroendocrine functions, and coping and hormones were also addressed.

3.2 History of Psychoneuroendocrinology

Cannon [1] laid groundwork for the hypothesis that secretion of stress-induced epinephrine, called sympathin, works on physiological functions such as heart rate, respiration rate, blood pressure, and metabolism of fat and carbohydrate in order to prepare the body for fight-flight responses. Later, Selye [2] had interest in adrenal cortical responses to stress. His general adaptation syndrome mainly referred to responses to physical stress, but he found that psychological stress also can stimulate secretion of adrenocorticotropic hormone (ACTH) and corticosteroid. His findings later became a catalyst for a number of studies in this field [3]. Thus, he is considered the father of psychoneuroendocrinology [4].

K. B. Koh, *Stress and Somatic Symptoms*,
https://doi.org/10.1007/978-3-030-02783-4_3

3.3 Studies on the Effects of Psychological Stress on Hormones

Researchers tried to exclude any physical trauma in their experiments to determine if hormone responses were the result of psychological stress. An example is monkeys' emotional and endocrine response to a red light when the red light has been previously associated with an electric shock. The monkeys secreted significant amounts of cortisol, even though they learned to avoid the electric shock by pressing a pedal upon seeing the red light. These animal experiments demonstrated that psychological stress alone can be a strong enough stimulus for corticosteroid secretion. Thus, the researchers turned their attention to humans. Corticosteroid secretion was measured in healthy persons exposed to psychologically stressful situations (e.g., parents of children dying with leukemia, patients waiting for surgery) as well as experimentally stressful situations [3].

3.4 Why Are Endocrine Markers Used in Stress Research?

The rationale for using endocrine markers in stress research is based on the observation that most systems in the body show changes during stress and that changes of endocrine markers are associated with stress. Conceptually, the central role of sympathetic nervous system (SNS) and hypothalamic-pituitary-adrenal (HPA) activation in stress responses provides justification for measuring hormonal changes [5].

3.5 Measures of Hormones

3.5.1 Catecholamines

Circulating levels of catecholamines can be measured by assaying blood samples, but the half-life of epinephrine and norepinephrine is very short (1–3 min) [6]. In particular, epinephrine is very fast acting and gets out of the bloodstream quickly. However, norepinephrine appears to clear out of the bloodstream more slowly [7]. Baselines for catecholamines cannot be taken right after venipuncture because the SNS-stimulating effects of the venipuncture will affect epinephrine and norepinephrine right away [5].

For studies of the effects of chronic stress, these blood measures are not useful because of considerable fluctuation and interindividual variability in epinephrine and norepinephrine levels. However, measurement of urinary epinephrine and norepinephrine or assay of metabolites provide longer, more stable indices of SNS activity than do blood measures. Radioenzymatic assay (REA) and high-performance liquid chromatography (HPLC) are used to measure levels of catecholamines [5].

3.5.2 *Cortisol*

The HPA axis is not as rapidly responsive as is the SNS. The half-life of cortisol (about 70 min) is longer than that of catecholamines. The effects of venipuncture on cortisol might not be evident for at least 10–15 min after the venipuncture, so an immediate postdraw sample would provide a useful baseline for cortisol [5]. In addition, measures of salivary cortisol offer a less reactive, less expensive, and more accessible method of measuring stress-related HPA response in humans than do traditional blood and urine measures [5, 8, 9].

3.5.2.1 Advantages of Cortisol Measurement in Stress Research

Corticosteroids are usually assayed by radioimmunoassay (RIA) techniques. These assays yield reliable determinations of cortisol in plasma, urine, and saliva [10]. Cortisol is neither very sensitive to movement and effort nor immediately responsive and unstable. Consequently, blood-sampled measures of cortisol reflect more stable arousal and can be used to represent an hour or more of mood and experience [5].

3.5.3 *Other Hormones*

Prolactin, thyroid hormones, growth hormone, insulin, gonadal hormones, and other peptides show changes associated with stress. In some cases, however, research is not clear on the direction of change [11].

As a whole, systematic incorporation of neuroendocrine measures in research can provide a valuable tool for probing a basic level of stress response [5].

3.6 General Adaptation Syndrome

According to Selye's view, any organism shows the same physiological responses after exposure to physical stressors such as hot, cold, or trauma. He called these stress responses the "general adaptation syndrome." This syndrome consists of three stages, which can be summarized as follows [2, 7, 12, 13].

Stage 1. Alarm reaction. It refers to changes of the body occurring after the first exposure to a stressor. At the same time, its resistance is diminished. But the body quickly mobilizes defensive resources and makes self-protective adjustments. If the defensive reactions are successful, the body returns to normal activity. Most short-term stress is resolved in this stage. This may be seen as an acute stress reaction. At this time, secretion of adrenocorticotropic hormone (ACTH) from the anterior pituitary is increased and epinephrine is secreted from the adrenal medulla.

Stage 2. Stage of resistance. Resistance ensues until one can adapt to continued exposure to the stressor. The bodily signs characteristic of the alarm reaction virtually disappear and resistance rises above normal. It is also called counter-shock phase. This stage is characterized by hypertrophy and hyperactivity of the adrenal cortex and degradation of the thymus and other lymphoid tissues. At this time, the adrenal cortex is stimulated by ACTH and cortisol secretion is increased.

Stage 3. Stage of exhaustion. Following long-term exposure to the same stressor, to which the body had become adjusted, eventually adaptation energy is exhausted. The signs of the alarm reaction reappear, but now they are irreversible, and the individual may die. At this stage, cortisol or energy resource is depleted, and then the body's resistance breaks down.

Adaptation may be a lifesaving process, but it must also be recognized as a type of disease process. At first, hormones secreted from anterior lobe of the pituitary and the adrenal cortex after exposure to a stressor help increase the body's resistance but later hypersecretion of the hormones can result in diseases including hypertension, myocardiopathy, and arthritis. Selye referred to these stress-related diseases as "diseases of adaptation." He viewed diseases of adaptation as a product of hyperactive response of the adrenal cortex to a stressor, which means the body's overdefense can do harm to the body itself [12].

Despite powerful influence of this syndrome, one major weakness is that it does not encompass the psychosocial factors of critical importance to understanding human stress [7].

3.7 Stressors and Hormones

Acute stressors stimulate adrenal medulla through the SNS and release epinephrine or norepinephrine, increasing cardiac output, pulse rate and respiration rate, and causing metabolic changes such as alteration in blood glucose. Therefore, blood flow to the large active muscles increases, but blood flow to internal (e.g., digestive) organs not needed for rapid activity decreases [7]. Because of these physiological changes of the SNS activated by the hypothalamus, people have been able to perform incredible feats in emergencies [14].

Chronic stressors stimulate the hypothalamic-pituitary-adrenal (HPA) axis [15]. Corticotropin-releasing hormone (CRH) secreted from the hypothalamus acts at the anterior pituitary to trigger release of adrenocorticotropic hormone (ACTH). Once ACTH is released, it acts at the adrenal cortex to stimulate the synthesis and release of glucocorticoids. In the short term, glucocorticoids can act to promote energy use, increase cardiovascular activity (in the service of the fight-flight response), and inhibit functions such as growth, reproduction, and immunity. This HPA axis is subject to negative feedback control by its own end products (i.e., ACTH and cortisol) at multiple levels, including the anterior pituitary, hypothalamus, and hippocampus [16].

3.7.1 Catecholamines

Catecholamines such as epinephrine and norepinephrine were increased in people exposed to stressors, such as public speech, examination, mental arithmetic, and exercises (e.g., cycling, treadmill, race) [17–28]. They were also increased in patients with phobic symptoms exposed to phobic stimuli [25].

3.7.2 Cortisol and ACTH

Loss of control and anticipatory behavior in humans and animals showed correlations with increased levels of cortisol [26]. For example, cognitive conflict and frustration in a brief period of experiment increased urine cortisol levels, and loss of control in relation to environmental stimuli increased cortisol secretion [27]. In addition, cortisol production was increased in air traffic controllers [28], and urine cortisol levels were increased in residents living near a nuclear power plant with nuclear leakage [29].

Psychological stressors, such as patients waiting for surgery, exercises (e.g., cycling, treadmill, race), parachute training, and competitive oral test, were reported to increase plasma cortisol levels [21, 22, 30–34]. Medical students' examination stress increased blood and urine cortisol levels, and public speech and excessive mental work increased salivary cortisol levels [18, 35–38]. Anticipation for difficult surgery was also associated with increased levels of salivary cortisol. However, no increase in salivary cortisol levels in pop musicians during performance was reported. Therefore, it was proposed that cortisol does not secrete automatically in response to any stressors but rather secrete in differentiated state [39].

In contrast, studies that examine the effects of stressors on ACTH are sparse. Some studies found that noise stress, competitive oral test, and preexamination stress increased blood ACTH levels [34, 40, 41].

3.7.3 Growth Hormone

Some studies found that serum growth hormone was increased in response to acute stressors [42]. For example, patients experiencing anxiety while undergoing cardiac catheterization or gastroscopy showed an increase in serum levels of growth hormone [43, 44]. Growth hormone is known to react strongly to anxiety. Growth hormone can be released in even overanxious patients who anticipate injection of insulin or arginine necessary for growth hormone test. Practically patients need to take rest for at least 1 h before the test in order to reach baseline level [3]. Another study reported that blood levels of growth hormone were increased in overdefensive people, although they had low levels of anxiety [42].

3.7.4 Prolactin

Prolactin is normally increased during sleep and is gradually decreased during wakefulness. It is also increased in women while breast feeding or stimulating nipples. Plasma levels of prolactin were reported to be increased in responses to stress, such as undergoing gastroscopy or rectoscopy, waiting for surgery, exercises (e.g., cycling, treadmill, race), parachute training, and competitive oral test [3, 21, 22, 34, 45]. However, medical students' examinations increase serum cortisol levels, but do not increase serum prolactin levels. This suggests that an increase in prolactin levels may require a stronger stimulus than an increase in cortisol levels [36].

3.7.5 Testosterone

Testosterone is counterresponsive to stress. For example, a monkey who was the alpha male in one group showed decreased levels of serum testosterone when moved to another alien group. However, serum testosterone level returned to normal soon when the monkey was moved to the previous group. Urine levels of testosterone were decreased in new recruits poorly adapted to military basic training than those well adapted to the training [3].

3.7.6 Estrogen

It is uncertain whether estrogen is responsive to stress or not. Long-term avoidance stress experiments in monkeys showed suppression of estrogen secretion which later returned to normal secretion after removal of the stressors. However, there were limitations in the reliability of the biochemical technique at the time of such experiments. Nonetheless, it is well-known for ovulation to be suppressed at situations in which psychological stress is severe. In particular, amenorrhea without ovulation was frequently noted in women at concentration camps during World War II. In addition, girls entering dormitories or attending camps for the first time after admission to school showed amenorrhea [3].

3.7.7 Luteinizing Hormone

Luteinizing hormone regulates testosterone secreted by the testes and estrogen secreted by the ovaries. Testosterone reacts to stress, and its effect can be mediated by changes in secretion of luteinizing hormone. Therefore, it can be presumed that luteinizing hormone is vulnerable to stress. However, the effect of psychological stress on luteinizing hormone remains uncertain. To date, it has been reported that long-distance running, postoperative state, and medical students' pretest in men decrease luteinizing hormone levels [46–48]. Stressful situations, such as social obedience in monkeys, also suppressed secretion of luteinizing hormone [49]. However, there was another report that no changes in luteinizing hormone levels occurred during physical or psychological stress [50].

3.7.8 Thyroid Hormone

Thyroid hormone is known to be associated with exposure to stressors [11]. However, the meaning of changes in the hormone levels is not always clear [5].

3.8 Emotion and Hormones

3.8.1 Catecholamines

In general, epinephrine is found in connection with fear, while norepinephrine is found when anger occurs [7].

3.8.2 Cortisol

Secretion of cortisol is known to be associated with emotional variables. Depression elevated plasma corticosteroid levels [51, 52], but remission of depression returned the hormone to normal levels [53, 54]. Anxiety also seemed to stimulate secretion of cortisol intensely [55, 56]. Phobic stimuli in patients with phobic disorder increased plasma cortisol and urine cortisol levels [25, 54]. High levels of subjective anxiety in medical students were associated with increased levels of plasma cortisol [57].

Levels of 24 h urine cortisol were significantly lower in patients with posttraumatic stress disorder (PTSD) compared with normal controls, contrasting with hypercortisolemia seen as a typical response to stressors [58, 59]. However, another study found that patients with PTSD had higher levels of 24 h urine cortisol than controls [60]. Such differences might be due to differences in methodology of data collection, data analyses, and patterns of subject groups, which should be considered in future studies [61]. In addition, no significant correlations were found between the levels of anxiety caused by an anxiety-provoking film and release of salivary cortisol [62]. Medical students' interpersonal sensitivity during an examination period had a significant and negative correlation with serum cortisol levels [36].

3.9 Duration of Exposure to Stress and Changes of Hormones

Stress is generally related to hyperactivity of the HPA axis followed by increased glucocorticoid levels [63]. However, chronic and repetitive stress conditions can lower HPA axis activity [61]. For example, chronic stressors, such as injection of formaldehyde in rats, exposure to ether, forced swimming, exposure to noise, immobilization, and exposure to cold, gradually weaken adrenocortical responses [64–72]. It takes 2–6 weeks for such adaptation to stressors to occur [61].

Low cortisol levels after exposure to chronic stressors are presumed to be due to high negative feedback sensitivity as a compensatory mechanism for preventing harmful sequela of chronically increased glucocorticoid at the levels of the hypothalamus, pituitary, and hippocampus. This phenomenon might be chronic adaptation to HPA activation induced by stress [73], which is consistent with the relationship between hormone responses to stress and coping mechanisms in human studies [74–76]. Prolactin levels are also known to be rapidly increased two or three times after exposure to psychological stressors and then decreased after repetitive exposure to the stressors [77].

It has been assumed that repeated exposure to a wide range of stressors differing in nature and intensity results in a reduced response of prototypical stress markers (i.e., plasma levels of ACTH and adrenaline) after an acute challenge with the same stressor. This reduction has been considered to be a habituation-like phenomenon. In adult male rats, however, adaptation of the HPA axis to repeated stress does not follow some of the critical rules of habituation [78].

3.10 Effects of Gene-Environment Interaction on Neuroendocrine Functions

During early life, brain development is affected by endogenous modulators including stress hormones as well as by exogenous factors such as nutrition and maternal care. There has been evidence that exposure to both early-life stress and early-life under-/malnutrition similarly leads to life-long alterations in the neuroendocrine stress system and modify emotional functions [79].

It has long been understood that stress during early life can have a significant and lasting influence on the development of the neuroendocrine system and its neural regulators, partially by modifying epigenetic regulation of gene expression, with implications for health in later life [80, 81]. However, evidence is accumulating that epigenetic plasticity also extends to adulthood. This has been proposed as a mechanism by which psychological trauma later in life can exert long-lasting effects on HPA axis function, brain plasticity, neuronal function, and behavioral adaptation to neuropsychological stress [81].

3.11 Coping and Hormones

Stress responses depend on individuals' ability to deal with stressors rather than harmful nature of stressors. That is, coping strategies are more important determinants in experiencing stress than the nature of stressors [82, 83]. If individuals cope with environmental stressors successfully, they will not be able to experience stress. For example, people who do not defend themselves effectively are known to secrete more cortisol during psychological stress than those who do [84]. A significant and negative correlation was also reported between an individual's coping style of "comforting cognition" and cortisol response during mental stress [38]. Therefore, individuals whose blood corticosteroid levels do not increase can be considered to cope with stressors effectively [45].

Generally adrenal responses to stressors in humans do not occur so dramatically as in animals, because humans minimize responses to threatening stimuli through psychological defenses or coping mechanisms, even though they have stress responses [3]. When parents whose children are dying with leukemia psychologically cope well and show emotional stability, 17-hydroxycorticosteroid levels do not increase. In contrast, in parents who do not cope effectively and show severe emotional distress, this hormone levels markedly increase [4].

Most women with potential of breast cancer waiting for surgery coped well with stress through denial, prayer, and intellectualization. Even in severe stressful situations, they did not show psychological distress and increased secretion of cortisol. In only a small number of subjects who did not defend themselves effectively and showed anxiety, it was predicted to increase cortisol secretion [3].

3.12 Conclusions

Measurement of stress hormones, general adaptation syndrome, the relationship between stressors/emotion and hormones, coping and hormones, and effects of gene-environment interaction on neuroendocrine functions were reviewed in order to examine the relationship between stress and endocrine functions. Among hormones, catecholamines such as epinephrine and norepinephrine and cortisol were used in most stress-related studies. Salivary cortisol has more advantage than blood or urine samples of cortisol in such studies. Pituitary hormones such as ACTH, prolactin and growth hormone, and target hormones such as testosterone and cortisol are known to be sensitive to stress. These hormones affect a number of biochemical and physiological processes widely, so the close relationship between stress and hormones could provide important clues on the psychobiological mechanisms of diseases. Systematic incorporation of neuroendocrine measures in research can provide a valuable tool for probing a basic level of stress response.

References

1. Cannon WB. The emergent function of the adrenal medulla in pain and the major emotion. Am J Phys. 1914;33:356–72.
2. Selye H. The stress of life. New York: McGraw-Hill; 1976.
3. Sachar EJ. Hormonal changes in stress and mental illness. In: Krieger DT, Hughes JC, editors. Neuroendocrinology. New York: HP Publishing Co; 1980. p. 177–83.
4. Stoudemire A, McDaniel JS. Psychological factors affecting medical condition (psychosomatic disorders). In: Kaplan HI, Sadock BJ, editors. Comprehensive textbook of psychiatry. 6th ed. Baltimore: Williams & Wilkins; 1995. p. 1463–545.
5. Baum A, Grunberg N. Measurement of stress hormones. In: Cohen S, Kessler RC, Gordon LU, editors. Measuring stress. New York: Oxford Univ. Press; 1995. p. 175–92.
6. Berne RM, Levy MN. Physiology. St. Louis: Mosby; 1983. p. 1033–68.
7. Rice PL. Stress and health: principles and practice for coping and wellness. Pacific Grove: Brooks/Cole Publishing Co; 1987. p. 17–33. p37-60.
8. Kirschbaum C, Hellhammer DH. Salivary cortisol in psychobiological research: an overview. Neuropsychobiology. 1989;22:150–69.
9. Vining RF, McGinley RA. Transport of steroid from blood to saliva. In: Read GF, Riad-fahmy D, Walker RF, editors. Radioimmunoassays of steroids in saliva. Cardiff: Alpha Omega; 1984. p. 56–63.
10. Walker RF, Riad-fahmy D, Read GF. Adrenal status assessed by direct radioimmunoassay of cortisol in whole saliva or parotid saliva. Clin Chem. 1978;24:1460–3.
11. Mason JW, Kosten TR, Southwick SM, et al. The use of psychoendocrine strategies in post-traumatic stress disorder. J Appl Soc Psychol. 1990;20:1822–46.
12. Girdano DA, Everly G. Controlling stress and tension: a holistic approach. New Jersey: Prentice-Hall; 1979.
13. Koh KB. Stress and psychosomatic disorders. Seoul: Ilchokak; 2011.
14. Greenberg JS. Coping with stress: a practical guide. Dubuque: Wm C Publishers; 1990.
15. Fawzy FI. Behavior and immunity. In: Kaplan HI, Sadock BJ, editors. Comprehensive textbook of psychiatry. Baltimore: Williams & Wilkins; 1995.
16. Kaplan HI, Sadock BJ. Synopsis of psychiatry: behavioral sciences & clinical psychiatry. 9th ed. Philadelphia: Lippincott Williams & Wilkins; 2003. p. 823.
17. Dimsdale JE, Moss J. Short-term catecholamine response to psychological stress. Psychosom Med. 1980;42:493–7.
18. Frankenhauser M, Von Wright MR, Collins A, et al. Sex differences in psychoneuroendocrine reactions to examination stress. Psychosom Med. 1978;40:334–43.
19. Lane JD, White AD, Williams RB Jr. Cardiovascular effects of mental arithmetic in type A and type B females. Psychophysiology. 1984;21:39–46.
20. Moss AJ, Wanar B. Tachycardia in house officers presenting cases at grand rounds. Ann Int. 1970;72:255–6.
21. Oleshansky M, Zotlick J, Herman R, et al. Neuroendocrine responses to maximal treadmill exercise. Psychiatry Res. 1986;16(Special Suppl):72.
22. Hartley LH, Mason JW, Hogan RP, et al. Multiple hormonal responses to graded exercise in relation to physical training. J Appl Physiol. 1972;33:602–6.
23. Grossman A, Bouloux P, Price P, et al. The role of opioid peptides in the hormonal responses to acute exercise in man. Clin Sci. 1984;67:483–91.
24. Fraioli F, Moretti C, Paolucci D, et al. Physical exercise stimulates marked concomitant release of β-endorphin and adrenocorticotropic hormone (ACTH) in peripheral blood in man. Experientia. 1980;36:987–9.
25. Nesse RM, Curtis GC, Thyer BA, et al. Endocrine and cardiovascular responses during phobic anxiety. Psychosom Med. 1985;47:320–32.
26. Mason JW. A review of psychoendocrine research on the pituitary-adrenal cortical system. Psychosom Med. 1968;30:576–607.

27. Lundberg U, Frankenhaeuser M. Psychophysiological reactions to noise as modified by personal control over stimulus intensity. Biol Psychol. 1978;6:51–9.
28. Rose RM, Jenkins CD, Hurst MW. Air traffic controller health change study. Boston: Boston University School of Medicine; 1978.
29. Schaeffer MC, Baum A. Adrenal cortical response to stress at three mile island. Psychosom Med. 1984;46:227–37.
30. Corenblum B, Taylor PJ. Mechanism of control of prolactin release in response to apprehension stress and anesthesia-surgery stress. Fertil Steril. 1981;36:712–5.
31. Smallridge RC, Whorton NE, Burman KD, et al. Effects of exercise and physical fitness on the pituitary-thyroid axis and on prolactin secretion in male runners. Metabolism. 1985;34:949–54.
32. De Meirleir KL, Baeyens L, L'Hermite-Baleriaux M, et al. Exercise-induced prolactin release is related to anaerobiosis. J Clin Endocrinol Metab. 1985;60:1250–2.
33. Noel GL, Diamond RC, Earll JM, et al. Prolactin, thyrotropin, and growth hormone released during stress associated with parachute jumping. Aviat Space Environ Med. 1976;47:543–7.
34. Meyerhoff JL, Oleshansky MA, Mougey EH. Psychological stress increases plasma levels of prolactin, cortisol, and POMC-derived peptides in man. Psychosom Med. 1988;50:295–303.
35. Lovallo WR, Pincomb GA, Edwards GA, et al. Work pressure and the type A behavior pattern exam stress in male medical students. Psychosom Med. 1986;48:125–33.
36. Koh KB. The relationship of examination stress with serum cortisol and prolactin levels. Korean J Psychosom Med. 1995;3:159–65.
37. Lehnert H, Beyer J, Walger P, et al. Salivary cortisol in normal men: the effects of corticotropin-releasing factor and different psychological stimuli. In: Weiner H, Florin I, Murison R, et al., editors. Frontiers of stress research. Toronto: Hans Huber; 1989. p. 392–4.
38. Bohnen N, Nicolson N, Sulon J, et al. Coping style, trait anxiety and cortisol reactivity during mental stress. J Psychosom Res. 1991;35:141–7.
39. Jezova D, Slezark V, Alexandrova M, et al. Professional stress in surgeons and artists as assessed by salivary cortisol. In: Kvetnansky R, McCarty R, Julius A, editors. Stress-neuroendocrine and molecular approaches. Philadelphia: Gordon and Breach Science Publishers; 1992. p. 953–62.
40. Breier A, Albus M, Pickar D, et al. Controllable and uncontrollable stress in humans: alterations in mood and neuroendocrine and psychophysiological function. Am J Psychiatry. 1987;144:1419–25.
41. Koh KB, Choi EH, Song JE, et al. Effect of coping on endocrinoimmune functions in different stress situations. Psychiatry Res. 2006;143:223–34.
42. Kosten TR, Jacobs S, Mason J, et al. Psychological correlates of growth hormone response to stress. Psychosom Med. 1984;46:49–57.
43. Creene WA, Conrow C, Schalch DS, et al. Psychological correlates of growth hormone and adrenal secretory response to patients undergoing cardiac catheterization. Psychosom Med. 1970;32:599–614.
44. Kurokawa N, Suematsu H, Tamai H. Effect of emotional stress on human growth hormone secretion. J Psychosom Res. 1977;21:231–5.
45. Levine S. Cortisol changes following repeated experiences with parachute training. In: Ursin H, Baade E, Levine S, editors. Psychobiology of stress. New York: Academic Press; 1978.
46. Kuoppasalmi K, Naveri H, Horkonen M, et al. Plasma cortisol, androstenedione, and testosterone and luteinizing hormone in running exercise of different intensities. Scand J Clin Lab Invest. 1980;40:403–9.
47. Carstensen H, Amer I, Wide L, et al. Plasma testosterone, LH, FSH during the first 24 hours after surgical operations. J Steroid Biochem. 1973;4:605–11.
48. Johansson GG, Laakso ML, Peder M, et al. Examination stress decreases plasma level of luteinizing hormone in male students. Psychosom Med. 1988;50:286–94.
49. Rose RM. Overview of endocrinology of stress. In: Brown GM, Koslow SH, Reichlin S, editors. Neuroendocrinology and psychiatric disorder. New York: Raven Press; 1984. p. 95–122.
50. Rose RM. Psychoendocrinology. In: Wilson JD, Foster DW, editors. Textbook of endocrinology. Philadelphia: WB Saunders Co; 1985. p. 653–81.

51. Board F, Wadeson R, Persky H, et al. Psychological stress and endocrine functions. Psychosom Med. 1956;18:324–33.
52. Kugler J, Kalveram KT. Is salivary cortisol related to mood states and psychosomatic symptoms? In: Weiner H, Florin I, Murison R, et al., editors. Frontiers of stress research. Toronto: Hans Huber Publishers; 1989. p. 388–91.
53. Board F, Wadeson R, Persky H. Depressive affect and endocrine functions. Arch Neurol Psychiatr. 1957;78:612–20.
54. Gibbons JL, McHugh PR. Plasma cortisol in depressive illness. J Psychiatr Res. 1962;1:162–71.
55. Frankenhauser M. A psychobiological framework for research on human stress and coping. In: Appley MH, Trumbull R, editors. Dynamics of stress – physiological, psychological and social perspectives. New York: Plenum Press; 1986. p. 101–16.
56. Kirschbaum C, Hellhammer DH, Strasburger CJ, et al. Relationship between salivary cortisol, electrodermal activity, and anxiety under mild experimental stress in children. In: Weiner H, Florin I, Murison R, et al., editors. Frontiers of stress research. Toronto: Hans Huber Publishers; 1989. p. 383–7.
57. Baker GHB, Irani MS, Byrom NA, et al. Stress, cortisol concentrations, and lymphocyte subpopulations. In: Freedman DX, Lourie RS, Meltzer HY, et al., editors. The 1987 year book of psychiatry and applied mental health. Chicago: Year Book Medical Publishers; 1985. p. 217–8.
58. Mason JW, Giller EL, Kosten TR, et al. Urinary free-cortisol levels in post-traumatic stress disorder patients. J Nerv Ment Dis. 1986;174:1145–59.
59. Yehuda R, Southwick SM, Nussbaum G. Low urinary cortisol excretion in PTSD. J Nerv Ment Dis. 1990;178:366–9.
60. Pitman R, Orr S. Twenty-four urinary cortisol and catecholamine excretion in combat-related post-traumatic stress disorder. Biol Psychiatry. 1990;27:245–7.
61. Yehuda R, Resnick H, Kahana B, et al. Long-lasting hormonal alterations to extreme stress in humans: normative or maladaptive? Psychosom Med. 1993;55:287–97.
62. Hubert W, de Jong-Meyer R. Emotional stress and saliva cortisol response. J Clin Chem Clin Biochem. 1989;27:235–7.
63. Yehuda R, Giller EL, Southwick SM, et al. Hypothalamic- pituitary-adrenal dysfunction in posttraumatic stress disorder. Biol Psychiatry. 1991;30:1031–48.
64. Stark E, Fachet J, Makara GB, et al. An attempt to explain differences in the hypophyseal-adrenocortical response to repeated stressful stimuli by their dependence of differences in pathways. Acta Med Acad Sci Hung. 1968;25:251–60.
65. Miculaj L, Mitrius A, Murgas K, et al. Adrenocortical activity during and after stress with respect to adaptation. In: Nemeth S, Bratislava, editors. Hormones, metabolism and stress—recent progress and perspectives. Bratislava: Publishing House of the Slovak Academy of Science; 1973. p. 115–28.
66. Riegle CD. Chronic stress effects on adrenocortical responsiveness in young and aged rats. Neuroendocrinology. 1973;11:1–5.
67. Katz RJ, Roth A, Carrol BJ. Acute and chronic stress effects on open field activity in the rat: implications for a model of depression. Neurosci Biobehav Rev. 1981;5:247–51.
68. Armario A, Restrepo C, Cstellanos JM, et al. Dissociation between adrenocorticotropin and corticosterone responses to restrain after previous chronic exposure to stress. Life Sci. 1985;36:2085–92.
69. Kawakami M, Seto K, Kimura F. Influence of repeated immobilization stress upon the circadian rhythmicity of adrenocorticoid biosynthesis. Neuroendocrinology. 1972;9:207–14.
70. Natelson BH, Ottenweller JE, Cook J. Effect of stressor intensity on habituation of the adrenocortical stress response. Physiol Behav. 1988;43:41–8.
71. Pitman DL, Ottenweller JE, Natelson BH. Plasma corticosterone levels during repeated presentation of two intensities of restraint stress: chronic stress and habituation. Physiol Behav. 1988;43:47–56.

72. Daniels-Severs A, Goodwin A, Keil LC, et al. Effect of chronic crowding and cold on the pituitary-adrenal system: responsiveness to an acute stimulus during chronic stress. Pharmacology. 1973;9:348–53.
73. Meaney MJ, Aitken DH, van Verkel C. Effect of neonatal handling on age-related impairments associated with the hippocampus. Science. 1988;239:766–8.
74. Mason JW. A review of psychoendocrine research on the sympathetic-adrenal medullary system. Psychosom Med. 1968;30:631–53.
75. Wolff CT, Friedman SB, Hofer MA, et al. Relationship between psychological defenses and mean urinary 17-OHCS excretion rates: a predictive study of parents of fatally ill children. Psychosom Med. 1964;26:576–91.
76. Knight RB, Atkins A, Eagle J. Psychological stress, ego defenses, and cortisol production in children hospitalized for elective surgery. Psychosom Med. 1979;41:40–9.
77. Reus VI. Psychoneuroendocrinology. In: Kaplan HI, Sadock BJ, editors. Comprehensive textbook of psychiatry. 5th ed. Baltimore: Williams & Wilkins; 1989. p. 105–11.
78. Rabasa C, Gagliano H, Pastor-Ciurana J, et al. Adaptation of the hypothalamus-pituitary-adrenal axis to daily repeated stress does not follow the rules of habituation: A new perspective. Neurosci Biobehav Rev. 2015;56:35–49.
79. Yam KY, Naninck EF, Schmidt MV, et al. Early-life adversity programs emotional functions and the neuroendocrine stress system: the contribution of nutrition, metabolic hormones and epigenetic mechanisms. Stress. 2015;18:328–42.
80. Dirven BCJ, Homberg JR, Kozicz T, et al. Epigenetic programming of the neuroendocrine stress response by adult life stress. J Mol Endocrinol. 2017;59:R11–31.
81. McIlwrick S, Rechenberg A, Matthes M, et al. Genetic predisposition for high stress reactivity amplifies effects of early-life adversity. Psychoneuroendocrinology. 2016;70:85–97.
82. Holroyd KA, Lazarus RS. Stress, coping and somatic adaptation. In: Goldberger L, Breznitz S, editors. Handbook of stress: theoretical and clinical aspects. New York: Free Press; 1982.
83. Vogel WH. Coping, stressors and health consequences. Neuropsychobiology. 1985;13:129–35.
84. Vickers RR. Effectiveness of defenses; a significant predictor of cortisol excretion under stress. J Psychosom Res. 1988;32:21–9.

References

Chapter 4
Stress, Emotion, and Immunity

4.1 Introduction

Psychological stress can alter one's immune function and increase susceptibility to physical diseases [1–3]. It can be assumed that negative events (stressors) lead to negative affective states (distress), producing alterations in human immunity [4].

Immunosuppression has been reported in human subjects who experience symptoms of anxiety and depression in response to situations such as examinations, bereavement, separation, and divorce [5–11]. In animals, immunosuppression has also been demonstrated in response to a variety of stressors [5, 12, 13]. In contrast, stress-reducing interventions such as relaxation may enhance immune function [14].

In this chapter are reviewed the effects of coping strategies and stress management techniques on immune function, as well as the relationship of stress and emotion with immunity.

4.2 Stress and Immune Regulation

A number of studies have indicated that academic stress, such as an examination period for medical students, downregulates immune functions such as lymphocyte proliferation, natural killer (NK)-cell activity, salivary immunoglobulin A (IgA), latency of herpes virus and Epstein-Barr virus, production of interferon-γ (IFN-γ), interleukin-2 (IL-2) receptor gene expression, and mucosal wound healing [15–24].

However, immune activation has been reported in response to examination stress in other studies. For example, salivary IgA levels were reported to be enhanced in students during an acute stress of an imminent examination [25]. The levels of phytohemagglutinin (PHA)-stimulated IL-2 production and lymphocyte proliferative

K. B. Koh, *Stress and Somatic Symptoms*,
https://doi.org/10.1007/978-3-030-02783-4_4

responses to PHA were also shown to be significantly higher during an examination period than during a non-examination period [26–28]. Similarly, in another study, students with reactions to examination stress had significantly higher numbers of leukocytes, neutrophils, and monocytes during the examination period than those without stress reactions [29].

Such activated immune response may be associated with the intensity and/or duration of stress. Immune response may be enhanced when the stressful condition is mild to moderate in intensity. Mild, brief, and controllable states of challenged homeostasis may actually be perceived as pleasant or exciting, which could be positive stimuli for emotional and intellectual growth and development [12]. Biologically immune activation may be associated with increased epinephrine release from the adrenal medulla by sympathetic nervous system activation or direct links of norepinephrine neurons that synapse upon immune target cells [30].

In contrast, stressful situations in which psychological and physical distress is more severe, protracted, and uncontrollable are likely to lead to overt disease states [31], apparently resulting from immunosuppression.

Therefore, immune activation can be considered to be a transient phenomenon that occurs prior to the downregulation of the immune function, which reflects the body's defensive response to stress [32]. It is also possible that arousal/hypervigilance associated with examinations play a role in activating immunity. From these perspectives, immune activation may be a biological signal warning an impending danger to health, as well as the body's physiological defense against stress [33].

4.3 Stress and Inflammatory Responses

Stress modulates inflammatory responses [34, 35]. Previous research has suggested that psychological stressors or perceived stress levels are associated with increased production of proinflammatory cytokines, such as IL-1, IL-6, tumor necrosis factor α (TNF-α), and IFN-γ [36–39]. In addition, a meta-analytic study found that brief stressors such as academic examinations changed the profile of cytokine production via a decrease in levels of IFN-γ and increases in levels of IL-6 and IL-10 [40]. However, one previous study reported reduced lipopolysaccharide (LPS)-stimulated expression of proinflammatory cytokines, such as IL-6 and TNF-α [41]. This is in line with the finding of Koh et al.'s study [42] in which only PHA was used to stimulate lymphocytes and reduced IL-6 production levels were found during an academic stress period. These contrasting differences might depend on cognitive stress appraisals such as the perceived levels of challenge or threat, control expectancy [41], and the intensity and duration of stressors or coping ability [28, 43]. Koh et al. [42] also reported that vacation associated with low stress is more likely to have a counter-stress effect on proinflammatory cytokines (e.g., increased IL-6 and TNF-α production) than on an anti-inflammatory cytokine (e.g., IL-10 production).

4.4 Emotion and Immunity

4.4.1 *Anxiety and Immunity*

A 72-h stimulation with anti-CD3+ induced significantly lower expression of CD25+ in generalized anxiety disorder patients compared to controls [44]. Patients with panic disorder had significantly lower levels of CD4+ than healthy controls and depressive disorder patients [45]. In addition, a reduced cell-mediated immune function (e.g., lymphocyte proliferative response to PHA and IL-2 production) was found in patients with anxiety disorders compared to normal controls [46]. However, lymphocyte proliferative response to mitogens varies within a wide range; decreased, normal, and increased responses have been observed in panic disorder patients compared with normal controls [47–51]. Moreover, IgA levels are increased in panic disorder patients compared to normal controls [52].

Patients with obsessive compulsive disorder do not differ from normal controls in plasma concentration of IL-1β, IL-6, soluble IL-6 receptor, sIL-2R, or transferrin receptor [53]. Subjects suffering from posttraumatic stress disorder (PTSD) after a hurricane had lower NK-cell activity when compared to normal controls [54]. In another study, however, combat veterans with PTSD had enhanced cell-mediated immunity compared with healthy civilians and servicemen in a test of cell-mediated immunity [55]. Such unexpected findings suggest that the arousal/hypervigilance associated with PTSD may be more influential on immune functioning than the anxiety symptoms which often accompany PTSD.

As opposed to a clinical level of anxiety, subclinical anxiety seen in people suffering from familial traumatic injury [56] or medical students during examination stress [57] may be associated with increased immune function (e.g., mitogen-induced lymphocyte proliferation, NK-cell activity). Such immune enhancement in subclinical anxiety may be considered a transient phenomenon occurring prior to the downregulation of immune function, reflecting the body's defense against a stressor. Thus, immune alteration may occur differently depending on clinical or subclinical levels of anxiety and the levels of hypervigilance [32].

4.4.2 *Depression and Immunity*

Many studies have suggested that depressed patients exhibit decreased immune functions in a variety of immune measures when compared to non-depressed controls [58–61]. Examinations of the impact of depression on T-cell responses in humans found that, in the context of bereavement or severe major depressive disorder, proliferation of peripheral blood mononuclear cells in response to the T-cell mitogens, PHA and concanavalin A (Con A), was significantly reduced [5, 58, 62–64].

The degree of immunosuppression may be related to the severity of depression in depressive disorders [61]. For example, lymphocyte responses to PHA and pokeweed mitogen (PWM) in patients with melancholic and psychotic depression were significantly lower than those with minor depression [65]. Compared to patients with non-melancholic depression, patients with melancholia demonstrated reduced in vivo cell-mediated immunity as assessed by delayed-type hypersensitivity skin responses [66]. However, the mechanisms of T-cell alterations in depression in humans have yet to be established.

Depression enhances the production of proinflammatory cytokines, including IL-6 [67–70]. There is growing evidence that the production of proinflammatory cytokines stimulated by depression can influence a spectrum of conditions associated with aging, including cardiovascular disease, osteoporosis, arthritis, type 2 diabetes, certain cancers, periodontal disease, frailty, and functional decline. Therefore, processes such as prolonged infection and delayed wound healing that fuel sustained proinflammatory cytokine production may be promoted by depression [71].

4.5 Coping Strategies and Immunity

Coping strategies represent specific actions that people take in order to deal with a given problem or stressor [72]. An individual's coping strategies are known to affect the stress responses [73] such as endocrine and immune functions. Coping by accepting the reality of stressful situations proved protective for patients with hepatitis B, whereas coping by substance use increased the risk of having an inadequate count of hepatitis B antibody [74]. In the context of personal relationships and immune function, lonelier medical students had lower NK-cell activity than students who were not as lonely [75]. Medical students who reported greater social support showed stronger immune response to hepatitis B vaccine than those with less support [76]. In an experimental study, expressing emotionally traumatic events that had not previously been disclosed to others was associated with increased proliferative response to PHA [21].

A few studies reported relationships between coping and immunity in different stress situations and at different perceived stress levels. Law students who were optimistic showed higher numbers of CD4+ cells in less conflictual situations and lower numbers of CD4+ cells in more conflictual situations [77]. In another study, however, in a stress condition optimism was inversely related to IL-6 responses in healthy men, suggesting that optimism may promote health by counteracting stress-induced increases in inflammation [78].

In addition, higher levels of active coping were significantly related to greater increases in proliferative response to PHA and Con A at high stress levels. In contrast, at low stress levels, active coping was not significantly related to proliferative responses, whereas avoidance was associated with greater proliferative response to Con A [79]. In another study [28], positive reappraisal and seeking social support were associated with alteration of immune function (reduced IL-2 production and lymphocyte proliferative response to PHA) in medical students during a chronic stress period, suggesting their counter-stress effects on immune function; in particular, positive reappraisal was found to reverse stress-induced immune responses.

4.6 Stress Reduction and Immunity in Healthy Individuals

Stress management techniques such as relaxation and meditation may affect immune function. In one study, a single 20-min session of relaxation training resulted in significant increases in salivary IgA concentrations from the prerelaxation period to the postrelaxation period, in contrast to a non-relaxation control group [80]. Stress reduction has also been shown to diminish inflammatory responses [81, 82]. Koh et al. [83] reported significant reductions in the change (stress period value minus baseline period value) in the levels of IL-6 and TNF-α production and significant enhancement in the change in the levels of the IL-10 production in a relaxation group of medical students compared with a non-relaxation group (Fig. 4.1). These results suggest that relaxation is associated with reduction in stress-induced proinflammatory cytokine alterations but with enhancement in stress-induced anti-inflammatory cytokine alteration. Therefore, relaxation is more likely to have counter-stress effect on proinflammatory cytokines than on anti-inflammatory cytokine.

Healthy individuals experiencing job-related stress who participated in mindfulness meditation showed greater antibody responses to the influenza vaccine when compared to a control group [84]. Within the meditation group, increased meditation practice was correlated with decreased stress-induced IL-6 levels. These data suggest that engagement in meditation may reduce stress-induced immune responses [85]. However, one study found that stress reduction techniques such as relaxation did not affect IL-6 levels in healthy individuals [86].

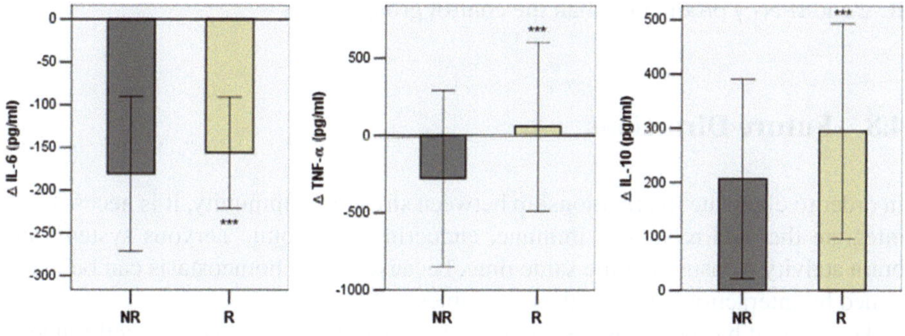

Fig. 4.1 Effects of relaxation on the changes in proinflammatory and anti-inflammatory cytokines production. *R* relaxation group, *NR* non-relaxation group. ***Indicates significant reductions in the change (stress period value minus baseline period value) in the levels of IL-6 and TNF-α production and significant enhancement in the change in the levels of the IL-10 production in a relaxation group compared with a non-relaxation group. (From Koh et al. [83])

4.7 Stress Reduction and Immunity in Patients with Physical Diseases

Stress management techniques may affect immune function in patients with physical diseases. A study of the effects of relaxation on immunity in human immunodeficiency virus (HIV)-positive men showed that lower stress levels achieved after relaxation practice were associated with greater decreases in herpes simplex virus type 2 IgG [87]. A randomized study of relaxation, meditation, and hypnosis training in asymptomatic HIV-positive men found improved T-cell counts in the treatment group which were maintained at a 1-month follow-up [88]. Geriatric patients who received relaxation training reported decreases in distress symptoms coupled with increased NK-cell cytotoxicity and decreased antibody titers to latent herpes simplex virus [89]. In addition, psychological intervention, including relaxation, improved T-cell blastogenesis in breast cancer patients [90]. However, it was reported that relaxation and visualization therapy did not affect lymphocyte proliferation in breast cancer patients undergoing radiotherapy [91].

A mindfulness-based stress reduction (MBSR) program that incorporated relaxation, meditation, gentle yoga, and daily home practice also increased NK-cell activity in HIV-positive men [92] and buffered CD4+ T lymphocyte declines in HIV-1 infected adults [93]. Over time, women with breast cancer showed enhanced NK-cell activity and reduced levels of IL-4 and IL-10 production in the MBSR group compared with the non-MBSR group [94].

A combined program of light-to-moderate-intensity aerobic and resistance exercise offsets the apparent decrement in NK-cell activity associated with weight loss in obese women [95]. T-cell proliferation in response to PHA and Con A remained stable or increased after psychological intervention (strategies to reduce stress, improve mood, alter health behaviors, and maintain adherence to cancer treatment and care) in patients with breast cancer [96]. In addition, breast cancer patients receiving cognitive behavioral stress management showed greater Th1 cytokine IL-2 and IFN- γ production than the control group [97].

4.8 Future Directions

In order to elucidate the relationship between stress and immunity, it is necessary to integrate the data related to immune, endocrine, autonomic nervous system, and brain activity measured at the same time, because bodily homeostasis can be maintained by interaction between these variables [98].

However, it has been suggested that genetic factors are related to T-cell function in depression. For example, several genes that play roles in T-cell function are associated with major depressive disorder and responses to antidepressants. Single nucleotide polymorphisms (SNPs) in the genes PSMB4 (proteasome beta4 subunit, which is important for antigen processing) and TBX21 (T bet, which is important in T-cell differentiation) are associated in a dose-dependent fashion with the likelihood of being diagnosed with depression [99]. Therefore, the addition of genetic factors to the other variables such as immune, endocrine, autonomic nervous system, and brain activity will be required to examine the relationship between depression and immunity.

On the other hand, activated T cells may play an important neuroprotective role in the context of stress and inflammation [100–102]. For example, generation of autoreactive T cells through immunization with central nervous system (CNS)-specific antigens reverses stress-induced decreases in hippocampal neurogenesis as well as depressive-like behavior in rodents. T regulatory cells may also play a role in depression through the downregulation of chronic inflammatory responses. Based on the hypothesis that T cells may subserve neuroprotective and anti-inflammatory functions during stress and inflammation, impaired T-cell function may directly contribute to the development of depression. Further elucidation of T-cell pathology may lead to new insights into immune system contributions to depression. Moreover, enhancement of T-cell function may represent an alternative strategy to treat depression [103].

4.9 Conclusions

Immune responses may depend on the intensity and/or duration of stress and coping ability. Immune activation may be a biological signal warning an impending danger to health, as well as the body's physiological defense against stress. Immune alteration may occur differently depending on clinical or subclinical levels of anxiety and the levels of hypervigilance. The degree of immunosuppression seems to be related to the severity of depression in depressive disorders. This literature review reveals evidence that relaxation and mindfulness-based stress reduction are effective interventions to counter the effects of stress on immunity. The ability of such interventions to improve immunity has been demonstrated for HIV-infected men, for breast cancer patients as well as for healthy individuals experiencing stress. In order to elucidate the relationship between stress and immunity, it is necessary to integrate the data related to immune, endocrine, autonomic nervous system, and brain activity. However, genetic factors need to be added to the above variables to examine the relationship between depression and immunity.

References

1. Elliot GR, Eisengdorfer C. Stress and human health: analysis and implications of research. In: A study by the institute of medicine and the national academy of sciences. New York: Springer Verag; 1982.
2. Herberman RB. NK cells and other natural effector cells. New York: Academic; 1982.
3. Levy L. Psychosocial stress and disease: a conceptual model. In: Gunderson EK, Rahe RH, editors. Life stress and illness. Springfield: Thomas; 1974.

4. Herbert TB, Cohen S. Depression and immunity: a meta-analytic review. Psychol Bull. 1993;113:472–86.
5. Bartrop RW, Luckhurst E, Lazarus L. Depressed lymphocyte function after bereavement. Lancet. 1977;1:834–6.
6. Tecoma ES, Huey LY. Psychic distress and the immune response. Life Sci. 1985;36:1799–812.
7. Calabrese JR, Skwerer RG, Barna B, et al. Depression, immunocompetence, and prostaglandins of the E series. Psychiatry Res. 1986;17:41–7.
8. Perez M, Farrant J. Immune reactions and mental disorders (editorial). Psychosom Med. 1988;18:11–3.
9. Hickie I, Silove D, Hickie C. Is there immune dysfunction in depressive disorders? Psychol Med. 1990;20:755–61.
10. Khansari DN, Murugo AH, Faith RE. Effects of stress on the immune system. Immunol Today. 1990;11:170–5.
11. Kiecolt-Glaser JK, Glaser R. Stress and the immune system: human studies. In: Tasman A, Riba MB, editors. American psychiatric press review of psychiatry, vol. 11. Washington, DC: American Psychiatric Press; 1992.
12. Weiss JM, Sundar S. Effects of stress on cellular immune responses in animals. In: Tasman A, Riba MB, editors. Am psychiatric press review of psychiatry, vol. 11. Washington, DC: Am Psychiatr Press; 1992.
13. Kelley KW. Immunological consequences of changing environmental stimuli. In: Moberg G, editor. Animal stress. Bethesda: Am Psychological Soc; 1985.
14. Kiecolt-Glaser JK, Glaser R. Psychological influences on immunity. Psychosomatics. 1986;27:621–4.
15. Glaser R, Rice J, Speicher CE, et al. Stress depresses interferon production and natural killer (NK) cell activity in humans. Behav Neurosci. 1986;100:675–8.
16. Glaser R, Rice J, Sheridan J, et al. Stress-related immune suppression: health implications. Brain Behav Immun. 1987;1:7–20.
17. Marchesi GF, Cotani P, Santone G, et al. Psychological and immunological relationships during acute academic stress. New Trends Exp Clin Psychiatry. 1989;5:5–22.
18. Glaser R, Kennedy S, Lafuse WP, et al. Psychological stress-induced modulation of interleukin-2 receptor gene expression and interleukin-2 production in peripheral blood leukocytes. Arch Gen Psychiatry. 1990;47:702–12.
19. Dobbin JP, Harth M, Mccain GA, et al. Cytokine production and lymphocyte transformation during stress. Brain Behav Immun. 1991;5:339–48.
20. Glaser R, Pearson GR, Jones JF, et al. Stress-related activation of Epstein-Barr virus. Brain Behav Immun. 1991;5:219–32.
21. Fawzy FI. Behavior and immunity. In: Kaplan HI, Sodock BJ, editors. Comprehensive textbook of psychiatry. Baltimore: Willams & Wilkins; 1995.
22. Deinzer R, Schuller N. Dynamics of stress-related decrease of salivary immunoglobulin A (sIgA): relationship to symptoms of the common cold and studying behavior. Behav Med. 1998;23:161–9.
23. Marucha DT, Kiecolt-Glaser JK, Favagehi M. Mucosal wound healing is impaired by examination stress. Psychosom Med. 1998;60:362–5.
24. Rojas IG, Padgett DA, Sheridan JF, et al. Stress-induced susceptibility to bacterial infection during cutaneous wound healing. Brain Behav Immun. 2002;16:74–84.
25. Bosch JA, Brand HS, Ligtenberg AJM, et al. The response of salivary protein levels and S-IgA to an academic examination are associated with daily stress. J Psychophysiol. 1998;4:170–8.
26. Kang D, Coe CL, McCarthy DO. Academic examinations significantly impact immune responses, but not lung function, in healthy and well-managed asthmatic adolescents. Brain Behav Immun. 1996;10:164–81.
27. Koh KB. The relationship of stress-induced hypothalamic-pituitary-adrenal axis function with cell-mediated immunity. J Kor Neuorpsychiatr Assoc. 2001;40:857–66.

28. Koh KB, Choe E, Song JE, et al. Effect of coping on endocrinoimmune functions in different stress situations. Psychiatry Res. 2006;143:223–34.
29. Maes M, van Bockstaele DR, Gastel AV, et al. The effects of psychological stress on leukocyte subset distribution in humans: evidence of immune activation. Neuropsychobiology. 1999;39:1–9.
30. Sadock BJ, Sadock VA. Synopsis of psychiatry – behavioral sciences/clinical psychiatry. 9th ed. Philadelphia: Lippincott Williams & Wilkins; 2003.
31. Chrousos GP. The concept of stress and stress system disorders. JAMA. 1992;267:1244–52.
32. Koh KB. Emotion and immunity. J Psychosom Res. 1998;45:107–15.
33. Koh KB. Emotion, interventions, and immunity. In: Koh KB, editor. Somatization and psychosomatic symptoms. New York: Springer; 2013. p. 299–315.
34. Chrousos GP. The hypothalamic-pituitary-adrenal axis and immune-mediated inflammation. New Engl J Med. 1995;332:1351–62.
35. Sternberg EM, Chrousos GP, Wilder RL, et al. The stress response and the regulation of inflammatory disease. Ann Intern Med. 1992;117:854–66.
36. Maes M, Song C, Lin A, et al. The effects of psychological stress on humans: increased production of pro-inflammatory cytokines and a Th1-like response in stress-induced anxiety. Cytokine. 1998;10:313–8.
37. Maes M, Song C, Lin A, et al. Immune and clinical correlates of psychological stress-induced production of interferon—γ and IL-10 in humans. In: Plotnikoff NP, Faith RE, Murgo AJ, et al., editors. Cytokines, stress and immunity. Boca Raton: Raven Press; 1998.
38. Goebel MU, Mills PJ, Irwin MR, et al. Interleukin-6 and tumor necrosis factor- α production after acute psychological stress, exercise, and infused isoproterenol: differential effects and pathways. Psychosom Med. 2000;62:591–8.
39. Steptoe A, Willemsen G, Owen N, et al. Acute mental stress elicits delayed increases in circulating inflammatory cytokine levels. Clin Sci. 2001;101:185–92.
40. Segerstrom SC, Miller GE. Psychological stress and the human immune system: a meta-analytic study of 30 years of inquiry. Psychol Bull. 2004;130:601–30.
41. Wirtz PH, von Kanel R, Emini L, et al. Variations in anticipatory cognitive stress appraisal and differential proinflammatory cytokine expression in response to acute stress. Brain Behav Immun. 2007;21:851–9.
42. Koh KB, Lee Y, Beyn KM, et al. Effects of high and low stress on proinflammatory and anti-inflammatory cytokines. Psychophysiology. 2012;49:1290–7.
43. Koh KB. Stress and psychosomatic medicine. Seoul: Ilchokak; 2011.
44. La Via MF, Munno I, Lydiard RB, et al. The influence of stress intrusion on immunodepression in generalized anxiety disorder patients and controls. Psychosom Med. 1996;58:138–42.
45. Marazziti D, Ambrogi F, Vanacore R, et al. Immune cell imbalance in major depressive and panic disorders. Neuropsychobiology. 1992;26:23–6.
46. Koh KB, Lee BK. Reduced lymphocyte proliferation and interleukin-2 production in anxiety disorders. Psychosom Med. 1998;60:479–83.
47. Schleifer SJ, Keller SE, Scotte BJ, et al. Lymphocyte function in panic disorder. Biol Psychiatry. 1990;27(Suppl):66A.
48. Surman OS, Williams J, Sheehan DV, et al. Immunological response to stress in agoraphobia and panic attacks. Biol Psychiatry. 1986;21:768–74.
49. Brambilla F, Bellodi L, Perna G, et al. Psychoimmunoendocrine aspects of panic disorder. Neuropsychobiology. 1992;26:12–22.
50. Andreoil A, Keller SE, Taban C, et al. Immune function in major depressive disorder: relation to panic disorder comorbidity. Biol Psychiatry. 1990;27(Suppl):9A–95A.
51. Koh KB, Lee Y. Reduced anxiety level by therapeutic interventions and cell-mediated immunity in panic disorder patients. Psychother Psychosom. 2004;73:286–92.
52. Ramesh C, Yeragani VK, Balon R. A comparative study of immune status in panic disorder patients and controls. Acta Psychiatr Scand. 1991;84:396–7.

53. Maes M, Meltzer HY, Bosmans E. Psychoimmune investigation in obsessive-compulsive disorder: assays of plasma transferrin, IL-2 and IL-6 receptor, and IL-1β and IL-6 concentrations. Neuropsychobiology. 1994;30:57–60.
54. Ironson G, Wynings C, Schneiderman N, et al. Posttraumatic stress symptoms, intrusive thoughts, loss, and immune function after Hurricane Andrew. Psychosom Med. 1997;59:128–41.
55. Watson PB, Muller HK, Jones IH, et al. Cell-mediated immunity in combat veterans with post-traumatic stress disorder. Med J Aust. 1993;159:513–6.
56. Schleifer SJ, Keller SE, Scott BJ, et al. Familial traumatic injury and immunity. In: Am Psychiatric Assoc, New Research, May (Abstract). San Francisco: Am Psychiatric Assoc; 1989.
57. Koh KB. The relationship between stress and natural killer-cell activity in medical college students. Kor J Psychosom Med. 1995;3:3–10.
58. Kronfol A, Silva J, Gredin J, et al. Impaired lymphocyte function in depressive illness. Life Sci. 1983;33:241–7.
59. Kronfol Z, House JD. Depression, cortisol, and immune function. Lancet. 1984;1:1026–7.
60. Krueger RB, Levy EM, Cathcart ES. Lymphocyte subsets in patients with major depression: preliminary findings. Advances. 1984;1:5–9.
61. Stein M, Keller SE, Schleifer SJ. Stress and immunomodulation: the role of depression and neuroendocrine function. J Immunol. 1985;135:827–33.
62. Schleifer SJ, Keller SE, Camereno M, et al. Suppression of lymphocyte stimulation following bereavement. JAMA. 1983;250:374–7.
63. Schleifer SJ, Keller SE, Meyerson AT, et al. Lymphocyte function in major depressive disorder. Arch Gen Psychiatry. 1984;41:484–6.
64. Stein M, Miller AH, Trestman RL. Depression, the immune system, and health and illness. Arch Gen Psychiatry. 1991;48:171–7.
65. Maes M, Bosmans E, Suy E, et al. Impaired lymphocyte stimulation by mitogens in severely depressed patients. Br J Psychiatry. 1989;155:793–8.
66. Hickie I, Hickie C, Lloyd A, et al. Impaired in vivo immune responses in patients with melancholia. Br J Psychiatry. 1993;162:651–7.
67. Dentino AN, Pieper CF, Rao KMK, et al. Association of interleukin-6 and other biologic variables with depression in older people living in the community. J Am Geriatr Soc. 1999;47:6–11.
68. Maes M, Bosmans E, De Jongh, et al. Increased serum IL-6 and IL-1 receptor antagonist concentrations in major depression and treatment resistant depression. Cytokine. 1995;9:853–8.
69. Maes M, Lin A, Delmeire L, et al. Elevated serum interleukin-6 (IL-6) and IL-6 receptor concentrations in posttraumatic stress disorder following accidental man-made traumatic events. Biol Psychiatry. 1999;45:833–9.
70. Wright CE, Strike PC, Brydon L, et al. Acute inflammation and negative mood: mediation by cytokine activation. Brain Behav Immun. 2005;19:345–50.
71. Kiecolt-Glaser JK, Glaser R. Depression and immune function: central pathways to morbidity and mortality. J Psychosm Res. 2002;53:873–6.
72. Menaghan EG. Measuring coping effectiveness: a panel analysis of marital problems and coping efforts. J Health Soc Behav. 1982;23:220–34.
73. Holroyd KA, Lazarus RS. Stress, coping and somatic adaptation. In: Goldberger L, Breznitz S, editors. Handbook of stress: theoretical and clinical aspects. New York: Free Press; 1982.
74. Burns VE, Carroll D, Ring C, et al. Stress, coping, and hepatitis B antibody status. Psychosom Med. 2002;64:287–93.
75. Kiecolt-Glaser JK, Garner W, Speicher C, et al. Psychosocial modifiers of immunocompetence in medical students. Psychosom Med. 1984;46:7–14.
76. Glaser R, Kiecolt-Glaser JK, Bonneau R, et al. Stress-induced modulation of the immune response to recombinant hepatitis B vaccine. Psychosom Med. 1992;54:22–9.

77. Segerstrom SC. Optimism, goal conflict, and stressor-related immune change. J Behav Med. 2001;24:441–67.
78. Brydon L, Walker C, Wawrzyniak AJ, et al. Dispositional optimism and stress-induced changes in immunity and negative mood. Brain Behav Immun. 2009;23:810–6.
79. Stowell JR, Kiecolt-Glaser JK, Glaser R. Perceived stress and cellular immunity: when coping counts. J Behav Med. 2001;24:323–39.
80. Green RG, Green ML. Relaxation increases salivary immunoglobulin A. Psychol Rep. 1987;61:623–9.
81. Laidlaw TM, Booth RJ, Large RG. Reduction in skin reactions to histamine after a hypnotic procedure. Psychosom Med. 1996;58:242–8.
82. Kabat-Zinn J, Wheeler E, Light T, et al. Influence of a mindfulness meditation-based stress reduction in patients with moderate to severe psoriasis undergoing phototherapy (UVB) and photochemotherapy (PUVA). Psychosom Med. 1998;60:625–32.
83. Koh KB, Lee Y, Beyn KM, et al. Counter-stress effects of relaxation on proinflammatory and anti-inflammatory cytokines. Brain Behav Immun. 2008;22:1130–7.
84. Davidson RJ, Kabat-zinn J, Schumacher J, et al. Alterations in brain and immune function produced by mindfulness meditation. Psychosom Med. 2003;65:564–70.
85. Pace TW, Negi LT, Adame DD, et al. Effect of compassion meditation on neuroendocrine, innate immune and behavioral responses to psychosocial stress. Psychoneuroendocrinology. 2009;34:87–98.
86. Lutgendorf SK, Logan H, Costanzo E, et al. Effects of acute stress, relaxation, and a neurogenic inflammatory stimulus on interleukin-6 in humans. Brain Behav Immun. 2004;18:55–64.
87. Cruess S, Antoni M, Cruess D, et al. Reductions in herpes simplex virus type 2 antibody titers after cognitive behavioral stress management and relationships with neuroendocrine function, relaxation skills, and social support in HIV-positive men. Psychosom Med. 2000;62:828–37.
88. Taylor DN. Effects of a behavioral stress-management program on anxiety, mood, self-esteem, and T-cell count in HIV positive men. Psychol Rep. 1995;76:451–7.
89. Kiecolt-Glaser JK, Glaser R, Williger D. Psychosocial enhancement of immunocompetence in a geriatric population. Health Psychol. 1985;4:25–41.
90. Andersen BL, Golden-Kreutz D, Emery CF, et al. Distress reduction from a psychological intervention contributes to improved health for cancer patients. Brain Behav Immun. 2007;21:953–61.
91. Nunes DF, Rodriguez AL, da Silva Hoffmann F, et al. Relaxation and guided imagery program in patients with breast cancer undergoing radiotherapy is not associated with neuroimmunomodulatory effects. J Psychosom Res. 2007;63:647–55.
92. Robinson FP, Mathews HL, Witek-Janusek L, et al. Psycho-endocrine-immune response to mindfulness-based stress reduction in individuals infected with the human immunodeficiency virus: a quasiexperimental study. J Altern Complement Med New York. 2003;9:683–94.
93. Creswell JD, Myers HF, Cole SW, et al. Mindfulness meditation training effects on CD4+ T lymphocytes in HIV-1 infected adults: a small randomized controlled trial. Brain Behav Immun. 2009;23:184–8.
94. Witek-Janusek L, Albuquerque K, Chroniak KR, et al. Effect of mindfulness based stress reduction on immune function, quality of life and coping in women newly diagnosed with early stage breast cancer. Brain Behav Immun. 2008;22:969–81.
95. Scanga CB, Verde TJ, Paolone AM, et al. Effects of weight loss and exercise training on natural killer cell activity in obese women. Med Sci Sports Exerc. 1998;30:1666–71.
96. Andersen BL, Farrar WB, Golden-Kreutz DM, et al. Psychological, behavioral, and immune changes after a psychological intervention: a clinical trial. J Clin Oncol. 2004;22:3570–80.
97. Antoni MH, Lechner S, Diaz A, et al. Cognitive behavioral stress management effects on psychosocial and physiological adaptation in women undergoing treatment for breast cancer. Brain Behav Immun. 2009;23:580–91.
98. Daruna JH, Morgan JE. Psychosocial effects on immune function: neuroendocrine pathways. Psychosomatics. 1990;31:4–12.

99. Wong ML, Dong C, Maestre-Mesa J, et al. Polymorphisms in inflammation-related genes are associated with susceptibility to major depression and antidepressant response. Mol Psychiatry. 2008;13:800–12.
100. Lewitus GM, Schwartz M. Behavioral immunization: immunity to self-antigens contributes to psychological stress resilience. Mol Psychiatry. 2009;14:532–6.
101. Lewitus GM, Wilf-Yarkoni A, Ziv Y, et al. Vaccination as a novel approach for treating depressive behavior. Biol Psychiatry. 2009;65:283–8.
102. Rook GA, Lowry CA. The hygiene hypothesis and psychiatric disorders. Trends Immunol. 2008;29:150–8.
103. Miller AH. Depression and immunity: a role for T cells? Brain Behav Immun. 2010;24:1–8.

Chapter 5
Stress and Illness

5.1 Introduction

About 71% of medical inpatients were found to have psychological factors affecting other medical conditions (PFAOMC, previously called psychosomatic disorders) in Korea. These results suggest that a considerable number of patients with physical diseases are affected by stressors [1]. A majority of PFAOMC seem to be related to cumulative effects of chronic ordinary stressors rather than an acute severe stressor, leading to destructive changes in tissues or physiology of organs.

PFAOMC patients have lower levels of perceived stress than patients with depressive or anxiety disorders [2], which suggests that PFAOMC patients are likely to be unaware of when to get stressed so that unwittingly cumulated stress can cause or exacerbate physical diseases.

PFAOMC includes a variety of physical diseases and symptoms, such as tension headache, migraine, hypertension, coronary heart disease, hyperventilation syndrome, diabetes mellitus, gastric or duodenal ulcer, ulcerative colitis, irritable bowel syndrome, rheumatoid arthritis, neurodermatitis, cancer, pain during menstruation, and so on [3].

Somatoform disorders (somatic symptom and related disorders in DSM-5) [4] are also stress-related disorders. Patients with these disorders continue to complain of somatic symptoms despite no abnormal findings on physical examination or laboratory tests and tend to exaggerate their somatic symptoms. In addition, stress can cause mental disorders such as anxiety disorders, depressive disorders, adjustment disorders, acute psychosis, suicidal attempt, and so on. However, the magnitude of correlation between stress and these disorders is known to be smaller than that between stress and physical symptoms or physical diseases [3].

Holmes and Rahe [5] constructed the Social Readjustment Rating Scale which ranks the relative degree of adjustment required by life-changing events. Individuals with 200 or more life-change units accumulated in a single year are considered to be at high risk of developing a physical disease in that year. The death of a spouse

K. B. Koh, *Stress and Somatic Symptoms*,
https://doi.org/10.1007/978-3-030-02783-4_5

ranked the highest, followed by the death of a close family member, being fired from work, and divorce in the United States in 1978 [6], whereas the death of a spouse followed by the death of a close family member, divorce, and marital reconciliation in Korea in 1982 [7]. However, the death of a spouse was found to rank the highest, followed by divorce, the death of a close family member, and marital separation in the United States in 1994 [6]. These results suggest that the magnitude of intensity of life events is different from country to country and changes over time [3].

5.2 Mechanisms Linking Stress to Illness

There is no question about the coexistence of psychological factors and physical diseases, because many data support this. Our concern is by what mechanisms psychosocial factors affect physical diseases. Among a number of explanations for this, it is noteworthy that the perception of life events elicits emotional state, especially when inner conflicts or external conditions interfere with resolving the events, which causes physiological changes, leading to physical diseases [3].

Psychological factors also can alter behavior, which induces physical changes. That is, exercises, ingestion of fat and salt, drinking alcohol, smoking cigarettes, and use of drugs can play important roles in the onset of physical pathology. In addition, general stress responses associated with past traumatic experiences can affect the existing vulnerable organs associated with genetic defects, previous tissue injury, external physical factors, and so on, leading to physical diseases [3].

5.2.1 Relationship Between Stress and Physical Diseases

Reiser [8] posited that hormones, and other chemical materials related to stress, simultaneously caused both physical (e.g., internal organs) and psychological changes, leading to the weakening of self-defense and ego functions. As a result, such individuals are forced to rely on ineffective coping strategies which intensify their stress responses. This process initiates a brain feedback loop (e.g., giving feedback to the brain) that ultimately threatens the body's homeostasis and causes injury to tissues, including internal organs [9].

Based on these assumptions and findings, the relationship between stress and physical diseases can be summarized as follows [10].

Stressor → cognitive appraisal → coping → psychological responses (emotional responses) → physiological responses (neuroendocrine system: hypothalamic-pituitary-adrenal axis, sympathetic-adrenal-medullary axis, endogenous opium, immune system) → physical diseases.

Cerebral cortex perceives stressors and evaluates if they are threats to the body or not (appraisal and reappraisal of the stressor). Among the variables affecting the appraisal, there are physical ones (e.g., gender and age), psychological ones (e.g., personality and the existing psychopathology), and environmental ones (e.g., social support and economic status). Then individuals choose coping methods. Emotional responses, such as anxiety, depression, and anger, follow their chosen coping. Acute stressors stimulate the adrenal medulla through the sympathetic nervous system and release epinephrine or norepinephrine, increasing cardiac output, pulse rate and respiration rate, and causing metabolic changes such as alteration in blood glucose. However, chronic stressors stimulate hypothalamic-pituitary-adrenal (HPA) axis and release cortisol, lowering immune functions and increasing the risk of physical diseases. In addition, the pituitary releases pro-opiomelanocortin (POMC)-induced peptides such as enkephalin and endorphin, probably affecting immune functions [10].

5.2.2 Stress and Coping Model

Rahe [6] proposed stress and coping model. This model consists of six steps that take place between a person's initial experience of a significant recent life event and the diagnosis of an illness.

1. Life event perception step: The intensity of stress depends on individuals' perception of life events and can be affected by their past experiences of events, current social support, and individuals' assets such as income and education.
2. Psychological defense step: Psychological defenses such as repression and denial can help prevent psychophysiological responses. Otherwise, a variety of psychophysiological responses occur.
3. Psychophysiological response step: Psychophysiological responses can be divided into recognizable symptoms such as changes in mood, headache, and muscular tension, and unrecognizable symptoms such as increases in blood pressure and serum lipid.
4. Response management (coping skill utilization) step: Coping skills include life habits (e.g., medication, food, relaxation, meditation, exercise), social support, responses to stressors (positive response vs. negative response such as avoidance and self-reproach), and life satisfaction (e.g., optimism, humor, art, family, nature, and spiritual life).
5. Illness behavior step: Preoccupation with somatic symptoms leads to sick role, not going to work but instead doctor shopping to seek medical help.
6. Illness evaluation step: Diagnoses are made by physicians.

Most persons successfully manage the 1st, 2nd, and 4th step and do not develop an illness. However, when psychological defenses (the 2nd step) or coping skills (the 4th step) are ineffective, a person is at high risk for near-future illness (the 5th and 6th step).

5.3 Stress and the Brain

It is an important foundation for understanding the mechanisms linking stress and diseases to identify anatomical sites related to stress and physiological functions of each site. The role of the brain related to stress known to date is as follows:

The diencephalon that regulates emotions is made up of the thalamus and hypothalamus. The thalamus relays sensory impulses from other parts of the nervous system to the cerebral cortex. The hypothalamus, a key structure in stress reactivity, is the primary activator of the autonomic nervous system (ANS), which controls basic body processes such as hormone balance, temperature, and the constriction and dilation of blood vessels [11]. The structures of the brain and their locations are shown in Fig. 5.1.

5.3.1 Reticular Activating System (RAS)

The RAS may be viewed as the gate sentry of the brain. In general, the RAS is involved in communication between the brain and body, gating (selection of sensory information for processing by the cortex), and vigilance [12].

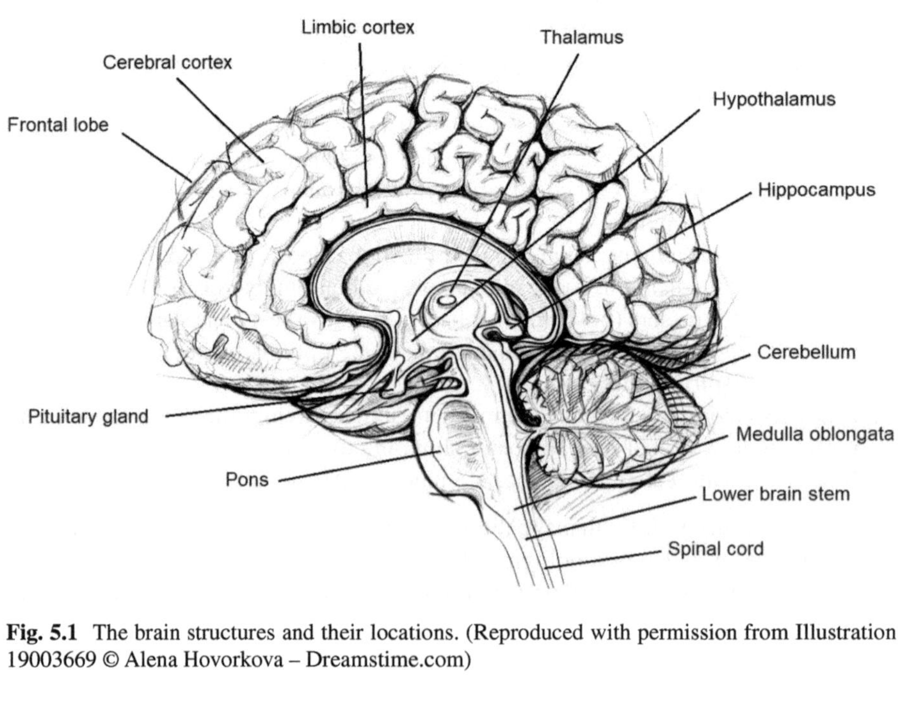

Fig. 5.1 The brain structures and their locations. (Reproduced with permission from Illustration 19003669 © Alena Hovorkova – Dreamstime.com)

5.3.2 *Visceral Brain*

The visceral brain comprises the thalamus, hypothalamus, and limbic system [12].

5.3.2.1 Thalamus

The thalamus is the major relay center for every sensory system except the sense of smell. Its function is to evaluate the emotional content of information provided by the senses [13]. Physical damage to the thalamus can cause overreaction to emotional stimuli (e.g., uncontrollable weeping or laughing). Another important function of the thalamus is related to the perception of pain. Each of the pain pathways terminates in the thalamus [14].

5.3.2.2 Limbic System

The limbic system includes the thalamus, hypothalamus, amygdala, hippocampus, and septum. This system seems to be associated with emotions in response to physical and psychological signals [11, 12].

The amygdala and septum serve to balance aggressive tendencies: the former starting and the latter moderating aggression. The amygdala and septum have also been implicated as major reward centers in the brain. The hippocampus is involved in long-term memory and learning [12].

5.3.2.3 Hypothalamus

The hypothalamus has powerful effects on nearly every visceral system in the body through its connection to the pituitary [12]. The role of the hypothalamus in stress is most clearly revealed in four specific functions: (1) initiating activity in the ANS, (2) stimulating the secretion of adrenocorticotropic hormone (ACTH) from the anterior pituitary, (3) stimulating the thyroid gland to produce thyroxin, and (4) producing oxytocin and vasopressin or antidiuretic hormone (ADH) [12]. Oxytocin and vasopressin activated by the anterior hypothalamus are secreted from the posterior pituitary which is under control of the ANS [15, 16] (Fig. 5.2).

5.3.3 *Autonomic Nervous System (ANS)*

The ANS controls heart activity, blood pressure, digestion, urinary and bowel elimination, and many other body functions. The ANS is controlled by the brain stem, hypothalamus, and spinal cord. The ANS has sympathetic and parasympathetic nerves. These two systems work in a dynamic but antagonistic way. However,

ANS→ Adrenal Medulla→ E, NE

↗

Posterior

Stressor→ Cerebral Cortex→ Thalamus→ Hypothalamus

Anterior→ ANS→ Pituitary→ Oxytocin/Vasopressin

↘

CRH / TRH→ Pituitary→ ACTH/TTH→

Adrenal Cortex / Thyroid→ Cortisol/Thyroxin

Fig. 5.2 Stress and the brain. *ANS* autonomic nervous system, *E* epinephrine, *NE* norepinephrine, *CRH* corticotropin-releasing hormone, *ACTH* adrenocorticotropic hormone, *TRH* thyrotropin-releasing hormone, *TTH* thyrotropic hormone (thyrotropin)

undesirable effects of prolonged sympathetic arousal can lead to diseases such as hypertension and peptic ulcers. When the emergency is over, the hypothalamus activates the parasympathetic system which starts repairing destructive effects from the emergency state [12].

5.3.4 Pituitary Gland

The pituitary secretes six important hormones from its anterior region and two from its posterior region. All of its secretions are under the direct control of the hypothalamus [12]. In general, cortisol provides the fuel for battle (fight or flight). Its primary function is to increase the blood glucose so we have the energy for action [11].

Aldosterone increases blood pressure so we can transport food and oxygen to the active parts of our body, such as limbs and organs [11]. Epinephrine increases both the rate and the strength of heart contractions, resulting in increased blood pressure. By a feedback loop to the hypothalamus, it tends to increase the secretion of ACTH and other hormones, followed by enhanced HPA activity [12].

The thyroid gland is also involved in the stress reaction. Activated by thyrotropic hormone (TTH) from the pituitary, it secretes thyroxin, which increases the basal metabolic rate, free fatty acids, rate of gluconeogenesis, gastrointestinal motility (e.g., diarrhea), respiration rate and depth, heart rate, blood pressure, and anxiety [11].

The relationship between stress and the brain as mentioned above can be summarized as follows. When we encounter a stressor, the body part (e.g., eyes, nose, muscles) first notes that the stressor passes a message along the nerves to the brain. During the process, the diencephalon recognizes fear, and then the cerebral cortex perceives and evaluates the stressor as threatening or nonthreatening. These messages associated with the stressor pass through the RAS either from or to the limbic system and the thalamus. The limbic system is where emotion evolves, and the thalamus serves as the switchboard, determining what to do with the incoming messages. The hypothalamus then comes into play, which activates the endocrine system and ANS [11].

In case of the activated endocrine system, the anterior part of the hypothalamus releases corticotropin-releasing hormone (CRH), which stimulates the anterior pituitary to secrete adrenocorticotropic hormone (ACTH). ACTH then activates the adrenal cortex, followed by increased secretion of cortisol (glucocorticoids). In case of the ANS activation, however, the posterior part of the hypothalamus stimulates the adrenal medulla via the ANS pathway, followed by increased release of catecholamines, such as epinephrine (adrenaline) and norepinephrine (noradrenaline) [11, 12] (Fig. 5.2).

5.4 Stress and the Immune System

The body's initial responses to stress that are often seen in the endocrine and immune systems help protect the body from infection and diseases. However, increased cortisol secretion induced by chronic stress suppresses the immune system and increase the risk of infections and diseases [11].

A body of research on the relationship between psychosocial stress and immunity has suggested that stress alters the way in which the immune system works [17]. Severe and protracted stressful situations cause immunosuppression and are likely to lead to overt disease [18]. In contrast, immune response may be enhanced when the stressful condition is brief in duration and mild to moderate in intensity [19].

The recent evidence indicates that activation of the immune response system and release of common proinflammatory mediators link chronic stress and systemic illness [20].

5.5 Stress and Memes

As already mentioned in Chap. 1, memes (replicable memory, i.e., information) associated with early stress cause epigenetic changes and determine genetic vulnerability or resilience for later stress. In the course of development, memes that are stored in the brain undergo Darwinian natural selection, and some memes become dominant, while others become attenuated or dormant. Later stress may result in hormonal changes leading to an attenuation of hippocampal function followed by an attenuation of protective dominant memes, allowing a massive infusion of stress memes that in turn awaken dormant pathologic memes. This cascade may result in mental and stress-related psychosomatic illness [21].

5.6 Conclusions

The mechanisms linking stress to illness were reviewed. Cognitive appraisal of stressors, coping with stress, emotional responses, physiological changes related to the hypothalamic-pituitary-adrenal (HPA) axis, sympathetic-adrenal-medullary (SAM) axis, endogenous opium, and immune system can be involved in the development of illnesses. Stress and coping model with emphases on individuals' cognition toward stressors and coping consists of six steps: life event perception, psychological defense, psychophysiological response, response management (coping skill utilization), illness behavior, and illness evaluation steps. To explore the role of the brain in the relationship between stress and illnesses, the functions of each of the reticular activating system (RAS), limbic system, hypothalamus, autonomic nervous system (ANS), and pituitary, and their interactions were reviewed. In addition, the relationship between stress and memes was discussed. More details on the relationship between stress and immune system were already described in the chapter "Stress, Emotion, and Immunity."

References

1. Koh KB. The prevalence of psychosomatic disorders and stress perception in medical inpatients. J Korean Neuropsychiatr Assoc. 1988;27:525–34.
2. Koh KB. Stress perception of patients with psychosomatic disorders. J Korean Neuropsychiatr Assoc. 1988;27:514–23.
3. Koh KB. Stress and psychosomatic medicine. Ilchokak: Seoul; 2011.
4. American Psychiatric Association (APA). Statistical and diagnostic manual of mental disorders. 5th ed. Washington, DC: Am Psychiatric Publishing; 2013.
5. Holmes TH, Rahe RH. The social readjustment rating scale. J Psychosom Res. 1967;11:213.
6. Rahe RH. Stress and psychiatry. In: Kaplan HI, Sadock BJ, editors. Comprehensive textbook of psychiatry. 6th ed. Baltimore: Williams & Wilkins; 1995.
7. Hong K, Chung D. Social readjustment rating scale: methodological study. J Korean Neuropsychiatr Assoc. 1982;21:123–36.
8. Reiser MF. Psychophysiology of stress and its sequelae. In: Reiser MF, editor. Mind, brain, body: toward a convergence of psychoanalysis and neurobiology. New York: Basic Books; 1984.
9. Oken D. Current theoretical concepts in psychosomatic medicine. In: Kaplan HI, Sadock BJ, editors. Comprehensive textbook of psychiatry, vol. 2. 5th ed. Baltimore: Williams & Wilkins; 1989.
10. Fawzy FI. Behavior and immunity. In: Kaplan HI, Sadock BJ, editors. Comprehensive textbook of psychiatry. Baltimore: Williams & Wilkins; 1995.
11. Greenberg JS. Coping with stress: a practical guide. Dubuque: Wm C Publishers; 1990.
12. Rice PL. Stress and health: principles and practice for coping and wellness. Pacific Grove: Brooks/Cole Publishing Co; 1987. p. 17–33. p37–60.
13. Grossman S. Essentials of physiological psychology. New York: Wiley; 1973.
14. Melzack R, Wall P. Pain mechanisms: a new theory. Science. 1965;50:971–9.
15. Standring S. Gray's anatomy. The anatomical basis of clinical practice. 41st ed. Amsterdam: Elsevier Health Sciences; 2015. p. 358.
16. Marieb E. Anatomy & physiology. Glenview: Pearson Education; 2014.

17. Locke SE. Stress, adaptation, and immunity: studies in humans. Gen Hosp Psychiatry. 1982;4:49–58.
18. Chrousos GP. The concept of stress and stress system disorders. JAMA. 1992;267:1244–52.
19. Weiss JM, Sundar S. Effects of stress on cellular immune responses in animals. In: Tasman A, Riba MB, editors. Am psychiatr press review of psychiatry, vol. 11. Washington, DC: Am Psychiatr Press; 1992.
20. Duric V, Clayton S, Leong ML, et al. Comorbidity factors and brain mechanisms linking chronic stress and systemic illness. Neural Plast. https://doi.org/10.1155/2016/5460732.
21. Leigh H. Genes, memes, culture, and psychosomatic medicine: an integrative model. In: Koh KB, editor. Somatization and psychosomatic symptoms. New York: Springer; 2013.

Chapter 6
Stress and Accidents: Interventions for Accidental Injuries

6.1 Introduction

Accidents are often likely to be associated with the victim's emotional state and life events, although they look like occurring by chance. In a single moment, unanticipated and unprepared for, accident victims begin a complicated process of injury, coping, and rehabilitation. Accidents are a major public health issue [1].

Among the most difficult patients to manage, and very expensive to the government and insurance companies, are those who as a result of an injury fail to regain function as productive members of society. Their disability continues even when there is no evidence, or minimal evidence, of the persistence of any objective physical findings. These patients continue to complain of a variety of physical symptoms, and no medical intervention proves helpful. The problem of disability is not merely a medical issue, because it is determined by a wide variety of factors, including intrapsychic and interpersonal issues and social and economic factors [2].

In this chapter are reviewed psychosocial assessment and management of accidental injuries as well as psychological factors of accidents including stress.

6.2 Causes and Risk Factors of Accidents

Causes of accidents can largely be divided into dynamic, environmental, life experiences, personality, and time factors. In addition, etiological factors of frequently recurrent accidents are associated with universal risk, unusual physical environment, personal maladaptation and irresponsibility, trigger episode, and behavior in a trigger state [3].

Universal risk is defined as a risk factor for accidents people can ubiquitously face. Unusual physical environment can be seen as a human-made risk factor. For example, workers who have dangerous jobs or work at dangerous workplaces are

K. B. Koh, *Stress and Somatic Symptoms*,
https://doi.org/10.1007/978-3-030-02783-4_6

more likely to cause accidents than those who do not. Psychological and physiological maladaptation of an individual to an environment and irresponsibility are main causes of accidents. Accidents tend to occur when workers ignore safety rules at workplaces requiring them. Trigger episodes are causes of all accidents, indicating temporary imbalance, imprudent decision, or miscalculated action. For example, a driver rushed a car to a slippery side of the road in rain or snow, or a staff overloaded a ship with too many people and huge luggage [3].

The majority of accidents are known to be associated with human factors, particularly individuals' maladaptation to the environment. Traffic accidents seem to occur by chance, but when seen in depth, there are many defects in human factors, such as people's involvement in making a car or driving a car [3].

6.3 Psychological Factors

6.3.1 Unconscious Motivation of Accidents

Regarding unconscious motivation of accidents, Freud explained that accidents can occur as a self-punishment to alleviate guilt, as an excuse to avoid an unpleasant situation, and as a symbolic castration. He considered serious or fatal accidents in terms of a death instinct [4]. People who attempted suicide [5] and showed self-destructive tendencies [6] had higher frequency of accidents than the control population.

6.3.2 Personality

A high frequency of accidents in some workers, known as accident-prone persons, was seen as related to an individual's personality traits [7, 8]. The term "accident proneness" was first used by Farmer and Chambers [9, 10] who defined it as "a personal idiosyncrasy predisposing the individual who possess it in a marked degree to a relatively high accident rate." These accident-prone persons have personality traits, such as impulsiveness and resentment against authority, that make them vulnerable to accidents under stress that threatens their sense of independence [7, 8].

The personality traits prevalent in accident-prone persons are known to be masochism, depression and grief, and counterdependent impulsiveness. In masochism, severe guilt feelings associated with angry feelings toward important others are relieved by self-punishment, or by being hurt. However, even without masochistic personality features, rage toward spouse, lover, or parent is often followed by self-injury. Unresolved grief and associated guilt feelings play a role in determining an individual's seemingly chance injuries. Individuals who have greater difficulty with dependent feelings have trouble during periods of stress, such as times of separation [1].

6.3.3 Stress

Accidental injuries seem to occur by chance but are related to psychological stressors prior to them when seen in depth [1, 11, 12]. This has been confirmed by several studies. It has been reported that injuries by traffic accidents are mainly associated with life changes, stress related to job and interpersonal relationship, and recent emotional problems [13, 14]. In one study, two thirds of the drivers who died in traffic accidents were known either to have been recently given positions of increased responsibility or to have been considering such changes [15]. Another study reported that injuries during the movement of machinery and working at heights were positively correlated with physical and mental stress [16]. In addition, 20% of 96 drivers involved in fatal injuries were noted to have been acutely upset as the result of violent quarrels with wives or girlfriends in the 6-h period prior to their accidents [11]. Lack of sleep related to stress may also play an important role in accidental injuries [16]. Moreover, psychological stressors induce alcohol abuse and precipitate accidental injuries [17, 18]. Vulnerabilities to accidental injuries differ from individual to individual but are dependent on the degree of stress [19–21].

There were differences in the kinds of pre-death stressors between people who died by accidental injuries and those who died by suicide [15]. In the former, individuals assumed new responsibilities, which made them tense and anxious, whereas in the latter, they experienced the loss of a significant person, a sense of failure, and feelings of not being cared for before committing suicide. In general, emotional instability was associated with being neglected or criticized by others in the former group but with experiences of loss in the latter.

6.3.4 Psychopathology

Studies found that the psychopathology of individuals having a high incidence of accidents included impulsivity, aggressiveness, paranoid traits, unmet dependency needs, and depressive tendencies [15, 17, 22, 23]. In addition, they are known to have exhibitionistic tendency and conflict with authority and overuse projection. Persons involved in traffic accidents manifest excessive hostility and dyscontrol of it, less anxiety tolerance, less conformity, more difficulty with authority, more hyperactivity, and a tendency toward risk taking, indicating all age-related traits associated with psychological immaturity [24]. Drivers involved in fatal injuries tended to be more depressed and have more suicidal tendency, individual conflicts, and job and financial stress than those not involved in injuries [11]. Airmen involved in accidents displayed poorer control of hostility, lower tension tolerance, higher separation anxiety, and higher dependency needs when compared with those not involved in accidents [23].

Regarding general life patterns before accidental injuries, people who died by accidents tended to be active, exhibitionistic, and nonintegrative with others, whereas people who died after committing suicide tended to be depressed, self-punitive, and integrative with other important persons [15].

Psychological factors of accidental injuries can be explored by thorough psychiatric interviews. Victims of accidents and people involved in accidents are known to experience anger, guilt, grief, or loneliness prior to the time of the accidents [25].

6.4 Accident Process

A series of psychological events causing an accident are called an accident process. That is, accidents do not occur by chance, but in association with a psychological process [12, 26, 27]. Generally people face a variety of stressors (e.g., financial problems) which lead to accidents during their lives [1, 12]. At the time of their accidents, many skilled workers seem suddenly to do things which even novices would not make the mistake of doing. Something threatening happens inside of workers, and they seek pain or injury as a solution. Since such personal need is unacceptable to them, they blame the impending danger on their machines or on other parts of their environment. They experience conflicts because they chase help away while they seek aid [12].

Accidents and accidental injuries can become a means to resolve their difficult life problems. They do not give up their symptoms, showing resistance to and uncooperative attitude toward therapeutic management including pain remission and rehabilitation [12].

Not infrequently, victims of accidents had physical diseases such as peptic ulcer, hypertension, and rheumatoid arthritis, as well as depression prior to accidents. These diseases can help rationalize chronicity of accident-related disorders because accidents along with physical defects were accepted socially as well as personally. Such a vicious cycle needs to be broken for successful treatment. To do so, it is necessary to check physical changes as well as depression before accidents [27]. Likewise, the general public should always try to evaluate physical changes as well as psychological status indicating stress in order to prevent accidents.

In conclusion, a variety of emotional factors and life stressors can be implicated as important causes of many fortuitous accidents. Accidents usually result from the momentary convergence of psychological vulnerability, transient life stressors, and the physical opportunity for the accident at one point in time [1].

Case

A 26-year-old male patient had been working as a welder for 2 years before his accident and was aware of the danger of his workplace where he was looking at a big L-type pipe loosely tied up with wire. However, one day, despite the risk, he took his helmet off while working. He unwittingly pulled the wire, resulting in the pipe falling down and hitting his head. Then he lost consciousness and was transferred to a hospital where he was diagnosed with a skull fracture, epidural hematoma, and cerebral contusion. He underwent brain surgery at the department of neurosurgery and then received treatment for several months. Even after being discharged from the hospital, he continued to complain of headaches, nausea, vomiting, decreased reactionary ability, and diminished memory and calculation abilities. He was therefore transferred to the department of psychiatry.

He recalled that he had been working overly hard for nearly 1 month at the time of the accident, finishing his welding job early and continuing working at other places to make more money, because he was under economic pressure. On the day of the accident, he started work as soon as he finished his lunch and was tired due to his constant work overload.

This case shows a clear accident process, indicating that the accident occurred while the patient was working without taking any risk measures due to stressors such as his financial burden and fatigue, although he was aware of the dangerous conditions at his workplace.

6.5 Therapeutic Processes for Accident Victims

A detailed and investigative psychological interview will often elicit evidence indicating the psychological determinants and permit the consideration of various therapeutic options. The time and effort involved in eliciting detailed history from accident victims are more than justified by the pain and cost of their injuries to themselves, to their families, and to society [1].

Early discovery of the anxieties, stressors, and conflicts involved in the accident process will increase the likelihood that psychiatric treatment can be directed to these underlying factors, possibly avoiding enduring disability. Psychological consultation with those involved in the physical rehabilitation and treatment of these patients can increase the effectiveness of their work and minimize the possibility of increasing disability for the patients [28].

The patients may be aware of the role of recent upsets or angry feelings in accident causation and be troubled by this. A chance to talk openly with a psychiatrist is likely to relieve some emotional distress and to facilitate coping with hospitalization [1].

Preexisting psychopathology such as unresolved grief, depression, or acute situational disturbances are likely to predispose the patients to accidental injury. Uncovering such preexisting psychopathology not only helps the psychiatrist make clinical interventions with a variety of short-term therapeutic modalities but also may prevent the acute process from progressing to chronic invalidism [1].

The first task in the management of a disability syndrome associated with accidental injury is an accurate diagnosis. There are several disorders for which a careful interview will establish the diagnosis. These include major depressive disorder, posttraumatic stress disorder, and transient hypochondriacal states and other neurotic disorders [2]. Treatment of major depressive disorder in these patients is the same as treatment for primary major depressive disorder patients. The treatment of posttraumatic stress disorder involves multiple modalities. Psychotherapy is indicated because the accident has precipitated a crisis in a victim. The person may be searching for meaning in life through his/her accident or may be faced with the fragility of health and life for the first time. The person may be fearful of certain places or activities that reactivate memories of the accident [29]. Medical psychotherapy, behavioral modification techniques, and psychotropic medication are helpful for these symptoms. Antianxiety agents are most efficacious for posttraumatic stress disorder with predominant anxiety during the period immediately following an acute trauma. Antidepressant medications including imipramine are most useful for prolonged or delayed posttraumatic stress disorders, when symptoms more characteristic of depression are predominant. With patients for whom the disability represents a system problem in the family, a therapeutic intervention that includes family members may be necessary [2].

6.6 Conclusions

A variety of emotional factors and life stressors can be implicated as important causes of many accidents. Accidents result from the momentary convergence of psychological vulnerability, transient life stressors, and the physical opportunity for the accidents at one point in time. Victims of accidents often show resistance to and uncooperative attitude toward treatment because accidents work as a means of resolving their life problems. A detailed and investigative psychological interview will often elicit evidence indicating the psychological determinants and permit the consideration of various therapeutic options. Therefore, psychological understanding of accidents can prevent chronicity of disabilities after accidents and help treat patients. In addition, the general public should usually try to evaluate physical changes as well as psychological status suggesting stress in order to prevent accidents.

References

1. Rosenbaum JF, Groves JE. Accident proneness and accident victims. In: Cassem NH, editor. MGH handbook of general hospital psychiatry. St. Louis: Mosby Year Book; 1991.
2. Ford CV, Smith GR Jr. Somatoform disorders, factitious disorder, and disability syndromes. In: Stoudemire A, Fogel BS, editors. Principles of medical psychiatry. Orlando: Grune & Stratton; 1987.
3. Schulzigner MS. Accident syndrome – a clinical approach. Arch Indust Hyg Occup Med. 1954;10:426–33.
4. Freud S. In: Strachey J, editor. The psychopathology of everyday life, vol. 6. Standard ed. London: Hogarth Press; 1960.
5. Crancer A Jr, Quiring DL Jr. Driving records of persons hospitalized for suicidal gestures. Behav Res Highway Safety. 1970;1:33–43.
6. Selzer ML, Payne CE. Automobile accidents, suicide, and unconscious motivation. Am J Psychiatry. 1962;119:237–40.
7. Dunbar F. Mind and body. New York: Random House In; 1955.
8. Alexander F. The accident prone individual. Public Health Rep. 1949;64:357–62.
9. Farmer E, Chambers EG. A psychological study of individual differences in accident rates. London: Industrial Health Research Board Rep No.38; 1926.

10. Farmer E, Chambers EG. A study of personal qualities in accident proneness and proficiency. London: Industrial Health Research Board Rep No.55; 1929.
11. Selzer ML, Rogers JE, Kern S. Fatal accidents: the role of psychopathology, social stress and acute disturbance. Am J Psychiatry. 1968;124:1028–36.
12. Hirschfeld AH, Behan RC. The accident process: I. Etiological consideration of industrial injuries. JAMA. 1963;186:193–9.
13. McMurray L. Emotional stress and driving performance: the effect of divorce. Behav Res Highway Saf. 1970;1:100–14.
14. Selzer ML. Automobile accidents as an expression of psychopathology in an alcoholic population. Q J Stud Alcohol. 1967;28:505–16.
15. Tabachnick N, Litman RE, Osman M, et al. Comparative psychiatric study of accidental and suicidal death. Arch Gen Psychiatry. 1996;14:60–8.
16. Tomei G, Capozzella A, Rosati MV, et al. Stress and work-related injuries. Clin Ter. 2015;166:e7–e22.
17. Selzer ML. Alcoholism, mental illness, and stress in 96 drivers causing fatal accidents. Behav Sci. 1969;14:1–10.
18. Waller JA, Turkel HW. Alcoholism and traffic deaths. N Engl J Med. 1966;275:532–6.
19. Arbous AG, Kerrich JE. Accident statistics and the concept of accident proneness. Biometrics. 1951;7:340–432.
20. McLean AA. Accident proneness: a clinical approach to injury liability. Ind Med Surg. 1955;24:122–6.
21. Webb WB. Illusive phenomena in accident proneness. Public Health Rep. 1955;70:951–6.
22. Conger JJ. Psychological and psychophysiological factors in motor vehicle accidents. JAMA. 1959;169:1581–7.
23. Tillman WA, Hobbs GE. The accident-prone automobile driver: a study of the psychiatric and social background. Am J Psychiatry. 1949;106:321–31.
24. Tsuang MT, Boor M, Fleming J. Psychiatric aspects of traffic accidents. Am J Psychiatry. 1985;142:538–46.
25. Alexander F. Psychosomatic medicine. New York: WW Norton & Co; 1950.
26. Behan RC, Hirschfeld AH. The accident process: II. Toward more rational treatment of industrial injuries. JAMA. 1963;186:300–6.
27. Hirschfeld AH, Behan RC. The accident process: III. Disability—acceptable and unacceptable. JAMA. 1966;197:85–129.
28. Nemiah JC. Psychological complications in industrial injuries. Arch Environ Health. 1963;7:481–6.
29. Berger JC. Some psychological aspects of industrial injury. Illinois Med J. 1975;147:364–5.

Chapter 7
Cognitive Behavioral Approach to Stress

7.1 Introduction

Cognitive behavioral therapy (CBT) is a kind of psychotherapy which aims to modify cognitive distortions by using cognitive and behavioral techniques. This therapy has been known to be effective in patients with depressive and anxiety disorders [1]. In addition, CBT is likely to be effective in patients with psychological factors affecting other medical conditions (PFAOMC, previously called psychosomatic disorders) whose stress perception levels are lower than those of patients with emotional disorders such as depressive and anxiety disorders [2, 3].

CBT is a relatively short-term form of psychotherapy that is active, directive, and collaborative between patients and therapists. Two core elements of the approach are collaboration between patients and therapists and self-management. The goal of CBT is primarily to help the patient uncover his/her cognitive distortions but is ultimately to find out maladaptive assumptions and modify them. This approach is not to cure but rather to help the patient develop better coping strategies to deal with stress [4].

In this chapter are reviewed the rationale for application of cognitive behavioral approach to stress, theoretical backgrounds of cognitive behavioral approach, and its processes.

The original version of this chapter was revised. The correction to this chapter is available at https://doi.org/10.1007/978-3-030-02783-4_28

K. B. Koh, *Stress and Somatic Symptoms*,
https://doi.org/10.1007/978-3-030-02783-4_7

7.2 Rationale for Application of Cognitive Behavioral Approach to Stress

The rationale for application of cognitive behavioral approach in coping with stress is as follows:

First, an individual's cognitive pattern is important in the formation of stress experiences. It means one's subjective perception is more influential on the severity of stress than actual events [5]. What is meaningful to one person may not necessarily be meaningful to another person. The impact of a stressful life event depends on the meaning it has for the individual [5, 6].

Second, cognitive process that determines stress responses and helps cope with stress is important in the formation of stress experiences [7]. In other words, individuals' cognitive process can lead to either effective coping or ineffective coping, which eventually may result in health or illnesses.

7.3 Theoretical Background of Cognitive Behavioral Therapy

Both Beck and Ellis have played a central role in developing a cognitive model of psychotherapy [4]. Beck [8] has proposed a cognitive model of stress which deals with both the role of cognitions in the formulation of stress and the role of stress in the formulation of cognitions.

Linking Beck's conceptualization of the stress process to Lazarus and Folkman's notion of appraisal, cognitive techniques can be applied to maladaptive thought patterns [9]. In other words, primary appraisal (the judgment of whether a situation is stressful), secondary appraisal (evaluation of coping options), or reappraisal (new appraisal based on additional coping efforts or acquisition of new information) can be altered by these techniques [7].

CBT is a mixed form of therapy in which the importance of the internal dialogue has been introduced from the psychodynamic schools, whereas the scientific method and a variety of behavioral techniques and strategies have been mobilized from the behavioral school [4].

7.4 Differences Between Cognitive Therapy and Psychodynamic Therapy

Cognitive therapy is similar to psychodynamic therapy in terms of attempting to uncover dysfunctional thought patterns, often rooted in childhood experiences, which lead to faulty coping in adulthood [7]. However, there are some fundamental differences as well [4].

1. Cognitive therapy relies on active intervention rather than interpretation; cognitive therapy needs sufficient explanation, whereas psychodynamic therapy does not.
2. The cognitive therapist tries to remit symptoms by altering maladaptive thought patterns, but psychodynamic therapy tries to alter personality by understanding the patient's past conflicts.
3. Cognitive therapy is to help the patient alter his/her coping style, whereas psychodynamic therapy is to let the patient know his/her maladaptive coping style and defenses.

7.5 Principle of Cognitive Behavioral Approach

Stressed clients may have a poor conceptualization of what the problem at hand is and may only see one possible solution. Therefore, the clients have to be able to recognize their problems and be prepared to work on them [10]. In general, problem-solving is conceptualized as a form of self-control training, so that the client first learns to solve general problems and then apply knowledge of this skill to specific problems [7].

7.5.1 Cognitive Distortions and Maladaptive Assumptions

The main focus of CBT is negative cognitive distortions. The sources of these cognitive distortions are irrational beliefs (schema) or maladaptive assumptions (hypotheses). These schemas are often established early in childhood. Schema may be associated with individual, family, religion, society, culture, and law. Changes can be more lasting and more powerful in successful coping with the assumptions than in coping only with the cognitive distortions [4]. When an external event stimulates a particular schema, certain specific distortions can be seen. For example, in a patient who shows cognitive distortion, saying, "I am good for nothing" whenever he is blamed by his senior, his maladaptive assumption may be considered "I must always be perfect to get recognition."

7.5.2 Common Distorted Cognitions

Common distorted cognitions are as follows [4]:

1. All-or-nothing thinking: the tendency to evaluate performance or personal qualities in black-and-white categories.
2. Selective abstraction or attention: individuals selectively pay attention to the single or few pieces of evidence that support their negative ideas while ignoring all of the other available data.

3. Overgeneralization: individuals arbitrarily conclude that a single negative event will happen over and over again.
4. Catastrophizing: one's exaggeration of difficulty related to a disaster causes him/her to live in rather constant fear of the imminent end of the world.
5. Arbitrary inference: this involves jumping to an arbitrary, negative conclusion that is not justified by the facts.
6. Magnification: one magnifies imperfections, so the person is likely to end up thinking that he/she is inadequate and inferior to other people.
7. "Should" statements: these statements have the potential to generate guilt and resentment.
8. Labeling: personal labeling involves creating a negative identity that is based on one's errors and imperfections.
9. Emotional reasoning: this distortion involves taking one's emotions as evidence for the way things really are (e.g., "I feel inadequate. Therefore, I must be a worthless person").
10. Personalization: this involves taking events that have nothing to do with one and making them personally meaningful.

7.5.3 Format of Cognitive Behavioral Therapy

CBT is time-limited, usually 15–25 weeks and done at once-weekly meetings [11].

7.6 Process of Cognitive Behavioral Therapy

7.6.1 Cognitive Approach

The cognitive approach includes (1) identifying automatic thoughts and underlying maladaptive assumptions, (2) testing automatic thoughts and maladaptive assumptions, (3) cognitive challenge, (4) generating alternatives and reattribution, (5) self-instruction, and (6) application of new assumptions [11].

7.6.1.1 Identifying Automatic Thoughts and Underlying Maladaptive Assumptions

1. Identifying Automatic Thoughts

   The thought that women don't like him after a man was rejected by a woman can be an example. At this time, the client may be asked to collect specific data in the form of a diary (self-monitoring), frequency count, or a psychological tool such as sentence completion test (SCT) [12] in order to identify and quantify problematic thoughts.

2. Identifying Maladaptive Assumptions

   These assumptions are not conscious thoughts [13]. Examples of such assumptions or rules are "In order to be happy, I must be perfect" and "If anyone doesn't like me, I'm not lovable." Such rules inevitably lead to disappointments and failure and ultimately to depression [11].

3. Self-Monitoring

   Self-monitoring strategies are frequently used as homework assignments to identify and assess specific cognitions, particularly in conjunction with hypothesis testing [7]. Clients are taught to monitor their responses to stressors in their lives. The goal is to enable clients to identify patterns of covert and overt events that precede, accompany, and follow stressful transactions, then cognitive distortions, and maladaptive assumptions. Therapist should try to elicit detailed accounts of the client's responses to stressors, rather than global retrospective reports to make this therapeutic process effective. Therefore, the therapist needs to encourage the client to record their feelings, thoughts, and behavior prior to, during, and following stressful events. It is also helpful to have the clients imagine stressful situations and report their perceptions and experiences in order to elicit detailed information. As the client becomes familiar with this self-monitoring, the therapist assists the client in identifying relationships among situational variables, thoughts, and emotional, behavioral, and symptomatic responses [3].

Example of Self-Monitoring

The severity of emotion ranges from 1 to 100, and the degree of belief in his/her thought ranges from 1% to 100%.

Date: September 18

Situation (event): Suddenly another car passed by my car on an expressway.

Feeling: "This is crazy!" Anger (90)

Thought: "He will someday have a big accident" (90%)

Reaction or coping: "I will keep distance from other cars." Deep breath.

Outcome: Anger (30), initial thought (60%)

After his reaction or coping, his anger level was reduced from 90 to 30, and the degree of belief in his initial negative thought diminished from 90% to 60%.

7.6.1.2 Testing Automatic Thoughts and Maladaptive Assumptions

1. Testing Automatic Thoughts

   The goal is to encourage the patient to reject inaccurate or exaggerated automatic thoughts after careful examination [11]. For example, the therapist might propose the hypothesis, "Your automatic response to any encounter with another person is 'he likes me, he likes me not." The data collected will indicate whether the hypothesis should be confirmed, denied, or modified [7].

2. Testing Maladaptive Assumptions

   In order to test the accuracy of maladaptive assumptions, the therapist asks patients to defend the validity of their assumptions. For example, a patient may state that he/she should always work up to his/her potential, and a therapist may ask, "Why is that so important to you?" [11]. Then the client adopts and practices specific cognitive and behavioral responses to both anticipated and unexpected stressors [13].

7.6.1.3 Cognitive Challenges

Many potentially destructive cognitions, particularly absolutistic ones, can be challenged logically by providing evidence from the client's own history which contradicts the belief in question. The therapist may propose such challenges from his or her knowledge of the client ("You say that you have always been a failure, yet you told me last time you got promoted and your salary was raised") [7].

7.6.1.4 Generating Alternatives and Reattribution

1. Generating Alternatives

   Once automatic thoughts or irrational ideas are identified and challenged, the client needs to generate specific alternative thoughts which are reasonable and positive. Thereafter, the undesirable cognitions can be replaced by a more desirable cognition. For example, the idea that "I am a failure at everything that I do" may be replaced with the more desirable and less absolute "Although I did not do well in a certain situation, I have succeeded before and will probably succeed again" [7].
2. Reattribution

   Retraining in causal attribution may result in changes in cognitive and behavioral functioning [14, 15]. In general, it is desirable that reattribution focuses on encouraging clients to attribute problem cognition (e.g., "It's my fault that the team lost") or behaviors to causes which are personally controllable [7].

7.6.1.5 Self-Instruction

When cognitions are used to control and direct behavior in an adaptive fashion, these cognitions become self-instructions. Thus, the client may verbalize overtly or covertly directions about how to carry out the behavior in question and may simultaneously self-reinforce and adjust behavior on an ongoing basis [7].

7.6.1.6 Generalization and Application of New Assumptions

Therapy concludes with the generalization of new underlying assumptions and the application of these new assumptions to stressful circumstances [13].

7.6.2 *Examples of Interventions [11]*

1. Dichotomous thinking: his/her assumption is "Everything is either one extreme or another (black or white, good or bad)" At this time, the therapist asks him/her to demonstrate that events may be evaluated on a continuum.
2. Selective abstraction: his/her assumption is "the only events that matter are failures." The intervention needs to use logs to identify successes the client forgot.
3. Overgeneralization: his/her assumption is "If it's true in one case, it applies to any case that is even slightly similar." The therapist should expose faulty logic and establish criteria of which cases are similar to what degree. When distorted cognition is excessive responsibility, his or her assumption is "I am responsible for all bad things." For such assumption, reattribution technique can be helpful.
4. Catastrophizing: his/her assumption is "The worst thing is almost likely to happen to me." The therapist asks him/her to calculate real probabilities and focus on evidence that the worst did not happen.

7.6.3 *Techniques for Controlling Thoughts*

There are a number of cognitive and behavioral techniques which are designed simply to control or eliminate persistent undesirable thoughts. These techniques do not challenge or alter the identified thoughts. Such approaches may be useful for obsessive thoughts which may have already been challenged but which remain nevertheless. Some of the techniques for controlling or suppressing thoughts suggested by Shelton and Levy are as follows [16]:

1. Thought stopping: the client is asked to produce the unwanted thought voluntarily, usually out loud, and then the therapist yells, "Stop!," causing the verbalization to cease it. The client is then asked to say "stop" whenever the unwanted thought occurs [17].
2. Changing the environment: the client is asked to leave the room or change his or her activity when the thoughts occur.
3. Delaying the thoughts: the client is to put off thinking about the problem area for a specified period of time (e.g., to delay for 1.5 h before thinking about it).
4. Implosion (flooding in fantasy) of distressing thoughts: the client is required to experience the distressing thought over and over until such time as it no longer results in any emotional arousal. This may be done either by repeating the thought out loud or by describing the content of the thought. Repetition may be effective for primarily verbal thoughts; description may be more effective for recurring visual images.

In addition, punishment, aversive tasks, and redirecting thoughts to a certain place or to a particular time can help suppress thoughts.

7.6.4 Behavioral Approach

Among the behavioral techniques are scheduling activities, mastery and pleasure, graded task assignments, behavioral rehearsal, self-reliance training, role playing, and diversion techniques. To simplify the situation and allow mini-accomplishments, the therapist often breaks tasks into subtasks, as in graded task assignments, to show clients that they can succeed. In behavioral rehearsal, clients imagine and rehearse the various steps in meeting and mastering a challenge [11].

Relaxation methods can be used as a technique to manage anxiety as well as stress. The techniques for eliciting relaxation response consist of the following four basic elements [18]. First, there needs to be some constant stimulus, for example, a sound, a word, or a phrase repeated silently or audibly. Fixed gazing at an object is a suitable alternative. The purpose of this procedure is to focus attention away from the continuous flow of sensory distractions and intellectual preoccupations. Second, a passive attitude is helpful to disregard distracting thoughts during the aural or visual practice. Third, the subject should be in a comfortable position to minimize any muscular strain or tension. Finally, a quiet environment with decreased stimuli should be chosen. A quiet room where there is no concern about unexpected interruptions is usually suitable.

7.7 Advantages of Cognitive Behavioral Approach Against Biofeedback and Relaxation Approaches

Cognitive behavioral approach has the following potential advantages that biofeedback and relaxation approaches do not [3].

1. Cognitive behavioral approach can mobilize a variety of coping strategies, whereas biofeedback and relaxation training can provide only a single coping response such as relaxation. Relaxation may not be a sufficient method for coping with many of life stressors.
2. Cognitive behavioral approach appears better suited than biofeedback and relaxation therapies to combating the negative affect (e.g., depression) that can be both a precipitant and a consequence of physical symptoms. Especially in patients with chronic tension headache, cognitive therapy has been reported to be more effective than biofeedback treatment [19].
3. It has been suggested that cognitive therapy is more effective in long-term maintenance of therapeutic effect than biofeedback treatment [3, 20].

7.8 Problems in Cognitive Behavioral Approach

Although cognitive behavioral approach has many advantages, there remain unresolved questions about the mechanism and efficacy of change [7]:

1. It can be mental health which is a product of distorted or unrealistic perceptions [21]. Healthy cognitions tend to be characterized by overly positive self-evaluations and unrealistic optimism about one's own future. A realistic and accurate appraisal of one's own situation may well encourage rather than defeat depression [22].
2. It is difficult to hypothesize that cognitions always precede emotions in the relationship between cognitions and emotions. Attribution theorists suggest that physiological arousal is first perceived as emotion and then given cognitive meaning [23].
3. Being unfamiliar with self-evaluation can be an obstacle to application of cognitive behavioral approach [24]. Occasionally, someone reports that headaches are exacerbated by daily recording, because these individuals often have learned to minimize headache by deliberately not attending to their headache. However, it is usually desirable to explain that the information generated by daily recording is needed as more effective ways of controlling their headache [3].

7.9 Conclusions

The necessity for cognitive behavioral approach is emphasized because cognition (thought) is not only playing a central mediating role in coping with stressors but also cognitive distortions are associated with the onset and maintenance of psychopathology. The goal of cognitive behavioral approach is primarily to help the patient uncover his/her cognitive distortions but is ultimately to identify maladaptive assumptions and modify them. This approach is not to cure but rather to help the patient develop better coping strategies to deal with his life and work stress. Cognitive approach includes identifying automatic thoughts and underlying maladaptive assumptions, testing automatic thoughts and maladaptive assumptions, cognitive challenge, generating alternatives and reattribution, self-instruction, and application of new assumptions. In addition, there are a variety of behavioral techniques, such as scheduling activities, mastery and pleasure, graded task assignments, behavioral rehearsal, self-reliance training, role playing, and diversion techniques.

References

1. Beck AT, Rush AJ. Cognitive therapy. In: Kaplan HI, Sadock BJ, editors. Comprehensive textbook of psychiatry. Baltimore: Williams & Wilkins; 1989. p. 1541–50.
2. Koh KB. Stress perception of patients with psychosomatic disorders. J Korean Neuropsychiatr Assoc. 1988;27:514–23.
3. Holroyd KA, Appel MA, Andrasik F. A cognitive-behavioral approach to psychophysiological disorders. In: Meichenbaum D, Jaremko ME, editors. Stress reduction and prevention. New York: Plenum Press; 1983. p. 219–59.
4. Freeman A. Cognitive therapy: an overview. In: Freeman A, Greenwood V, editors. Cognitive therapy. New York: Human Science Press; 1987. p. 19–35.

5. Reiser MF. Mind, brain, body: toward a convergence of psychoanalysis and neurobiology. New York: Basic Books; 1984. p. 164–85.
6. Koh KB. Coping with job stress. New Med J. 1992;35:11–21.
7. Cotton DHG. Stress management: an integrated approach to therapy. New York: Brunner; 1990. p. 189–213.
8. Beck AT. Cognitive therapy and the emotional disorders. New York: Times-Mirror; 1976.
9. Lazarus RS, Folkman S. Stress, appraisal and coping. New York: Springer; 1984.
10. D'Zurilla TJ, Goldfried MR. Problem solving and behavior modification. J Abnorm Psychol. 1971;78:107–26.
11. Kaplan HI, Sadock BJ. Synopsis of psychiatry: behavioral sciences and clinical psychiatry. Philadelphia: Lippincott Williams & Wilkins; 2003. p. 956–60.
12. Koh KB. Stress and psychosomatic medicine. 2nd ed. Seoul: Ilchokak; 2011. p. 331–40.
13. Rush AJ. Cognitive therapy. In: Karasu TB, editor. The psychiatric therapies. Washington, DC: Am Psychiatric Assoc; 1984. p. 397–414.
14. Forsterling F. Attributional aspects of cognitive behavior modification: a theoretical approach and suggestions for technique. Cogn Ther Res. 1980;4:27–37.
15. Forsterling F. Attributional conceptions in clinical psychology. Am Psychol. 1986;41:275–85.
16. Shelton JL, Levy RL. Behavioral assignments and treatment compliance. Champaign: Research Press; 1981.
17. Stern RS. Treatment of a case of obsessional neurosis using thought-stopping technique. Br J Psychiatry. 1970;117:441–2.
18. Goldberg RJ. Anxiety in the medically ill. In: Stoudemire A, Fogel BS, editors. Principles of medical psychiatry. Orlando: Grune & Stratton; 1987.
19. Holroyd KA, Andrasik F, Westbrook T. Cognitive control of tension headache. Cogn Ther Res. 1977;1:121–33.
20. Lynn SJ, Freedman RR. Transfer and evaluation in biofeedback treatment. In: Goldstein AP, Kanfer F, editors. Maximizing treatment gains: transfer enhancement in psychotherapy. New York: Academic; 1979.
21. Taylor SE, Brown JD. Illusion and well-being: a social psychological perspective on mental health. Psychol Bull. 1988;103:193–210.
22. Beidel DC, Turner SM. A critique of the theoretical bases of cognitive-behavioral theories and therapies. Clin Psychol Rev. 1986;6:177–97.
23. Kendall PC. Cognitive processes and procedures in behavior therapy. In: Franks CM, Wilson A, Kendall PC, et al., editors. Annual review of behavior therapy, vol. 10. New York: Guilford Press; 1984. p. 123–63.
24. Koh KB. Stress and psychosomatic medicine. Seoul: Ilchokak; 2011. p. 263–85.

Part II
Somatization

Chapter 8
Changing Concept of Disorders with Somatic Symptoms in Psychiatry

8.1 Introduction

The history of disorders with somatic symptoms in psychiatry means the history of psychosomatic medicine. Psychosomatic medicine emphasizes the unity of mind and body and the interaction between the two [1]. Psychosomatic medicine mainly includes somatization and psychosomatic disorders. The latter term can be misunderstood as medical diseases caused by psychological factors. Thus, the term was changed to psychological factors affecting medical conditions (PFAMC) in the fourth edition of *Diagnostic and Statistical Manual of Mental Disorders* (DSM-IV-TR) [2]. Nevertheless, the term "psychosomatic disorder" has been widely used because of its brevity and convenience.

Somatization is the term that has been used to describe a subconscious process by which a patient translates emotional distress into bodily complaints [3]. The term 'somatization' was first used by Stekel [4]. Somatization is contrary to psychologization [5]. The latter term indicates that a patient uses psychological feelings as a way to explain a somatic symptom. Such an example is that a cardiac patient says, "My heart is anxious," when he/she complains of a somatic symptom.

Health is a positive value most people seek, but some choose illness as a way of life. Such choice is usually decided unconsciously, and they seek medical treatment repetitively as if they cannot live without illnesses [5]. Somatization is an unresolved issue in medicine and called borderland between medicine and psychiatry [6]. Somatization is not a disease entity, nor a diagnostic category. This is a general term used to describe experiential, cognitive, and behavioral characteristics seen in these patients [7].

In DSM-III-R [8] and DSM-IV [2], the disorders that have traditionally been labeled as somatization are classified largely in the categories of somatoform disorders, and some belong to the category of PFAMC. In the ICD-10 Draft [9], somatization syndromes are classified among the somatoform disorders, the dissociative (conversion) disorders, and neurasthenia, and a few are classified in the category

K. B. Koh, *Stress and Somatic Symptoms*,
https://doi.org/10.1007/978-3-030-02783-4_8

of behavioral syndromes and medical disorders associated with physiological dysfunction [3].

The relationship between classification of somatoform disorders and their terms was confusing. Such ambiguity in the concept of somatization arose from limited experimental data and the different backgrounds of their terms [10]. For example, the concept of conversion disorder was developed by psychoanalysis, and somatization was the term derived from phenomenological and descriptive approach. Pain disorder was recognized due to its clinical importance. In order to resolve such confusion, many controlled experimental data are needed [5].

In this chapter are reviewed the definition of somatization, the rationale for changing from somatoform disorders to somatic symptom and related disorders, major changes of disorders with somatic symptoms in DSM-5, and new problems in the DSM-5 diagnoses along with the difference between disease and illness, the concept of sick role, and illness behavior.

8.2 Disease and Illness

Disease refers to objective pathophysiological changes. Illness refers to the loss of health and a person's subjective experience of suffering and social disability. The extent of illness that a person experiences in response to a disease, and whether or not he/she becomes identified as a patient, is largely determined by factors unrelated to the disease process. The patient comes to the physician not so much because of disease as because of his/her perception or fear of illness [11].

8.3 Illness Behavior and Somatization

Illness behavior is the action, or lack of action, that a person takes in response to a symptom. Illness behavior is determined by the individual's personality, past experiences, current life events (stressors), and the presence or absence of social support. Somatization has been regarded as a unifying concept to bring together a variety of disorders characterized by abnormal illness behavior [11].

8.4 Sick Role and Somatization

Sick role is a privilege society gives a sick person; the sick person is released from the normal social obligations of society and absolved from blame for his condition. However, the sick person is expected to want to get well and to cooperate with such help in an effort to get well. The concept of the sick role is especially important in understanding somatization because its apparent goal is to obtain the status of a sick person [11].

8.5 Definition of Somatization

Although controversial, the definition of somatization was variously described [3]. Kleinman and Kleinman [12] defined somatization as the expression of personal and social distress in an idiom of bodily complaints with medical help-seeking. Ford [5, 11] defined it as the use of somatic symptoms for psychological purposes or for personal gain. Personal gains obtained by somatization include (1) the capacity to manipulate interpersonal relationships, (2) the intention to obtain release from duties and responsibilities, (3) financial gain, and (4) the seeking of attention or a closer relationship or sympathy from another person [11].

Lipowski [6] defined somatization as the experience and communication of psychological distress in the form of physical symptoms. Bass and Benjamin [13] viewed somatization as a process of one's denial of psychosocial problems along with his/her inappropriate preoccupation with somatic symptoms.

8.6 Misdiagnosed Somatoform Disorder

The term "somatoform disorders" was introduced in the third edition of the Diagnostic and Statistical Manual (DSM) in recognition that many patients present with somatic distress that does not fit in the rubric of physical diseases, anxiety, mood, or psychotic disorders [14]. Somatoform disorders represent heterogeneous subgroups, ranging from conversion disorder to hypochondriasis to somatization disorder to pain disorder [14]. The diagnosis of somatoform disorders relies on the presence of subjective distress in the absence of objective findings. As a result, there is always the possibility that a diagnosis will be missed or altered later. In addition, patients are sometimes misdiagnosed with somatoform disorders, because the doctor has simply missed the diagnosis by insufficient attention to the history, physical examination, or laboratory tests and by not relying on contemporary diagnostic techniques [14]. However, the rate of misdiagnosis for somatoform disorders (less than 10%) is not as high as expected, because it is in the range of misdiagnoses that are found for other mental disorders or physical diseases [15].

8.7 Limitations of Somatoform Disorders as Diagnoses

Many clinicians believe that the terminology "somatoform disorders" and classification system of the DSM-IV perform poorly in respect to the functions of diagnosis. First, the terminology is unacceptable to patients. Second, the category is inherently dualistic (medically explained and unexplained symptoms). Third, somatoform disorders do not form a coherent category; the overlap with other psychiatric disorders can be a potential cause of misdiagnosis. Fourth, somatoform disorders are incompatible with other cultures (e.g., Oriental society). Fifth, there is ambiguity in the stated exclusion criteria (e.g., irritable bowel syndrome). Sixth, somatoform disorders are unreliable. Seventh, somatoform disorders lack a clearly defined threshold (e.g., somatization disorder). Finally, somatoform disorders cause confusion in disputes over medical-legal and insurance entitlements [16].

8.8 Shortcomings of the Specific Somatoform Disorder Subcategories

Many of the diagnostic subcategories housed within the somatoform disorders either lacked validity as separate conditions or might be better housed elsewhere [16]. In somatization disorder, doubts were expressed about both its clinical value and conceptual basis [17] because it had substantial overlap with personality disorders, particularly borderline personality disorder [18]. Moreover, the diagnosis was based simply on counting the number of "unexplained" somatic symptoms. Such diagnosis merely represented an extreme of severity on what appeared to be a continuum of distress [19]. As such, the threshold of the criteria for somatization disorder was too high, and patients with this diagnosis were so rare. Therefore, somatization disorder had little clinical validity.

Hypochondriasis also remained controversial as a diagnostic category. Although there was good evidence of the co-occurrence of the triad of disease conviction, associated distress, and medical help-seeking, these symptoms were better conceived of as a form of anxiety that happened to focus on health matters and was closely related to other forms of anxiety disorder [20, 21].

Conversion disorder has long been a problem for diagnostic classification. DSM-III placed this disorder with other diagnoses in the somatoform section because of the shared characteristic of somatic symptoms that are not intentionally produced [22]. However, the DSM-IV workgroup recognized it has a close relationship with dissociative disorder [23].

The prevalence of undifferentiated somatoform disorder was high, ranging from 10% to 30% [24–26]. However, there were few studies on undifferentiated somatoform disorder. Its existence represented the need to have a diagnosis for a very large group of patients not easily classified elsewhere, even though this diagnosis was not widely used in clinical practice [16]. Despite revision of pain disorder between DSM-III and DSM-IV, there remained problems both in its definition and in establishing it as a separate disorder [27]. Body dysmorphic disorder might be better grouped with obsessive-compulsive disorder [28].

The heterogeneous classification of somatoform disorders according to the DSM-IV and the International Classification of Diseases (ICD-10) has been found to be insufficient to be used for therapeutic and scientific purposes [29–33]. Therefore, the identity of somatoform disorder was confusing, and there was an identity crisis related to the survival of somatoform disorders [34]. Some scientists have proposed that these diagnostic categories should be abolished and that a new term for somatic symptoms be adopted [16]. It was also emphasized that the diagnostic group should be made more homogeneous and its biopsychosociocultural characteristics should be elucidated in order to resolve the identity confusion [34].

8.9 Categories and Diagnostic Criteria of Disorders with Somatic Symptoms in the DSM-5

As mentioned earlier, the DSM-IV somatoform disorder category was controversial. Thus, the DSM-5 changed the term "somatoform disorders" to "somatic symptom and related disorders" and further modified diagnostic labels and criteria [35].

Somatic symptom and related disorders were categorized into the following five subgroups: (1) somatic symptom disorder, (2) illness anxiety disorder, (3) conversion disorder (functional neurological symptom disorder), (4) psychological factors affecting other medical conditions (PFAOMC), and (5) factitious disorder [36].

Diagnostic criteria of somatic symptom disorder are as follows:

Criterion A: one or more distressing somatic symptoms; the criterion is no longer limited to medically unexplained symptoms. In other words, medically explained symptoms are also included in this criterion.

Criterion B: excessive thoughts, feelings, and behaviors related to these somatic symptoms or associated health concerns. These positive psychological features are added to the diagnostic criteria [35].

8.10 Major Changes of Disorders with Somatic Symptoms in DSM-5

DSM-5 has broadened the scope of somatoform disorders and emphasizes the concept rather than simply counting symptoms [37]. First, in DSM-5, the terms somatization disorder, pain disorder, and undifferentiated somatoform disorder were removed. Second, PFAOMC and factitious disorder were added. Finally, hypochondriasis was renamed "illness anxiety disorder."

DSM-5 emphasizes a positive criterion, namely, maladaptive reaction to a somatic symptom, instead of the earlier negative criterion, namely, that the symptoms should be medically unexplained [35]. In other words, somatic symptom disorder deemphasizes the centrality of medically unexplained symptoms and defines the disorder on the basis of persistent somatic symptoms associated with disproportionate thoughts, feelings, and behaviors related to these symptoms [38].

One follow-up study reveals that mental functioning can be better predicted by the DSM-5 somatic symptom disorder than by DSM-IV somatoform disorders [39].

8.11 New Problems in the DSM-5 Diagnoses Related to Disorders with Somatic Symptoms

There have been some critical comments on somatic symptom disorder since its introduction in the DSM-5. There are two major ambiguities: (1) the use of the term "somatic symptoms" reflects an ill-defined concept of somatization and (2) abnormal illness behavior is included in all diagnostic rubrics, but it is never conceptually defined [40]. Somatic symptom disorder seems to neglect important features concerning abnormal illness behavior (e.g., illness denial or denial of psychosocial problems) [41]. This disorder risks mislabeling many people as mentally ill [42]. The term "somatic symptom disorder" may be misused as opposed to mental symptom disorder. For many known mechanisms, it is unclear whether their role can be applied to somatic symptom disorder [43].

In addition, one argues that the DSM-5 chapter on somatic symptom disorder is incoherent, contradicts the classification, and will be clinically unhelpful so that ICD-11 should attempt a more logical and consistent revision [44].

8.12 Common Features of Disorders with Somatic Symptoms

Somatic symptom and related disorders have some characteristics such as chronicity, social dysfunction, occupational difficulties, increased healthcare use, dissatisfaction for both the clinician and the patient [45], and resistance to psychiatric or psychological assessment and treatment [10, 46, 47].

8.13 Psychological Conceptualization of Disorders with Somatic Symptoms

The rationale for psychological intervention in disorders with somatic symptoms can be explained as follows:

1. Psychological intervention in disorders with somatic symptoms is based on a direct consequence of common psychological disorders (e.g., anxiety disorders, depressive disorders), such as autonomic arousal symptoms or somatic complaints [48].
2. Somatization is conceptualized as a way of responding to stress [3, 49, 50] or as a means of handling life stress [11].
3. Somatosensory amplification model [51] suggests that these somatizing patients are very sensitive to any bodily sensations by selecting out and amplifying weak sensations.

4. Biopsychosocial model [52] takes into consideration the interaction of the biopsychosocial factors in the perception and maintenance of the somatic symptoms.

8.14 Conclusions

The history of disorders with somatic symptoms in psychiatry means the history of psychosomatic medicine. Psychosomatic medicine mainly includes somatization and psychological factors affecting other medical conditions (PFAOMC). Somatization is the term that has been used to describe a subconscious process by which a patient translates emotional distress into bodily complaints. However, the heterogeneous classification of somatoform disorders according to the DSM-IV and the ICD-10 has been found to be insufficiently useful for therapeutic and scientific purposes. Thus, the DSM-5 changed the term "somatoform disorders" to "somatic symptom and related disorders." The DSM-5 has broadened the scope of somatoform disorders and emphasizes the concept rather than simply counting symptoms. The DSM-5 also emphasizes a positive criterion, namely, maladaptive reaction to a somatic symptom, instead of the earlier negative criterion. However, the somatic symptom disorder risks mislabeling many people as mentally ill. The term 'somatic symptom disorder' may be misused as opposed to mental symptom disorder. Therefore, these issues on the concept and definitions need more clarification through further studies in the future. In addition, the rationale for psychological intervention in disorders with somatic symptoms was described.

References

1. Sadock BJ, Sadock VA. Synopsis of psychiatry: behavioral sciences/clinical psychiatry. 9th ed. Philadelphia: Lippincott Williams & Wilkins; 2003. p. 822–50.
2. American Psychiatric Association. Diagnostic and statistical manual of mental disorders. 4th ed. Washington, DC: Am Psychiatric Association; 1994.
3. Kellner R. Psychosomatic syndromes and somatic symptoms. Washington, DC: American Psychiatric Press; 1991. p. 187–225.
4. Steckel W. The interpretation of dreams. New York: Liveright; 1943.
5. Ford CV. The somatizing disorders. Psychosomatics. 1986;27:327–37.
6. Lipowski ZJ. Somatization: medicine's unsolved problem. Psychosomatics. 1987;28:294–5.
7. Lipowski ZJ. Somatization: a borderland between medicine and psychiatry. Can Med Assoc J. 1986;135:609–14.
8. American Psychiatric Association (APA). Statistical and diagnostic manual of mental disorders. Revised 3rd ed. Washington, DC: Am Psychiatric Association; 1987.
9. World Health Organization (WHO). Draft of the 10th revision of the international classification of diseases. Geneva: WHO; 1988.
10. Barsky AJ. Somatoform disorders. In: Kaplan HI, Sodock BJ, editors. Comprehensive textbook of psychiatry. 5th ed. Baltimore: Williams & Wilkins; 1989. p. 1009–27.

11. Ford CV. The somatizing disorders: illness as a way of life. New York: Elsevier; 1984. p. 1–35, 243–59
12. Kleinman A, Kleinman J. Somatization: the interconnections among culture, depressive experiences, and the meaning of pain. In: Kleinman A, Good B, editors. Culture and depression. Berkeley: University of California Press; 1986. p. 429–90.
13. Bass C, Benjamin S. The management of chronic somatization. Brit J Psychiatry. 1993;162:472–80.
14. Dimsdale JE, Dantzer R. A biological substrate for somatoform disorders: importance of pathophysiology. Psychosom Med. 2007;69:850–4.
15. Rief W, Rojas G. Stability of somatoform symptoms – implications for classification. Psychosom Med. 2007;69:864–9.
16. Mayou R, Kirmayer LJ, Simon G, et al. Somatoform disorders: time for a new approach in DSM-V. Am J Psychiatry. 2005;162:847–55.
17. Bass CM, Murphy MR. Somatization disorder: critique of the concept and suggestions for further research. In: Bass CM, Cawley RH, editors. Somatization: physical symptoms and psychological illness. Oxford: Blackwell Scientific Publications; 1990.
18. Rost KM, Atkins RM, Brown FW, et al. The comorbidity of DSM-III-R personality disorders in somatization disorder. Gen Hosp Psychiatry. 2003;14:322–6.
19. Katon W, Lin E, Von Korff M, et al. Somatization: a spectrum of severity. Am J Psychiatry. 1991;148:34–40.
20. Barsky AJ, Wyshak G, Klerman GL. Hypochondriasis: an evaluation of the DSM-III criteria in medical outpatients. Arch Gen Psychiatry. 2003;43:493–500.
21. Salkovskis PM, Warwick HM. Morbid preoccupation, health anxiety and reassurance: a cognitive-behavioral approach to hypochondriasis. Behav Res Ther. 1986;24:597–602.
22. Hyler SE, Spitzer RL. Hysteria split asunder. Am J Psychiatry. 1978;135:1500–4.
23. Martin RL. Diagnostic issues for conversion disorder. Hosp Community Psychiatry. 1992;43:771–3.
24. De Waal MW, Arnold IA, Eekhof JA, et al. Somatoform disorders in general practice: prevalence, functional impairment and comorbidity with anxiety and depressive disorders. Br J Psychiatry. 2004;184:470–6.
25. Chang DF, Myers HF, Yeung A, et al. Shenjing shuairuo and the DSM-IV: diagnosis, distress, and disability in a Chinese primary care setting. Transcult Psychiatry. 2005;42:204–18.
26. LeiKeiknes KA, Finset A, Mount T, et al. Current somatoform disorders in Norway: prevalence, risk factors and comorbidity with anxiety, depression and musculoskeletal disorders. Soc Psychiatry Psychiatr Epidemiol. 2007;42:698–710.
27. Sullivan MD. DSM-IV pain disorder: a case against the diagnosis. Int Rev Psychiatry. 2000;12:91–8.
28. Phillips KA, McElroy SL, Hudson JI, et al. Body dysmorphic disorder: an obsessive-compulsive spectrum disorder, a form of affective spectrum disorder, or both? J Clin Psychiatry. 1995;56(Suppl 4):41–51.
29. Lowe B, Mundt M, Herzog W, et al. Validity of current somatoform disorder diagnoses: perspectives for classification in DSM-V and ICD-11. Psychopathology. 2008;41:4–9.
30. Kroenke K, Sharpe M, Sykes R, et al. Revising the classification of somatoform disorders: key questions and preliminary recommendations. Psychosomatics. 2007;48:277–85.
31. Janka A. Rethinking somatoform disorders. Curr Opin Psychiatry. 2005;18:65–71.
32. Creed F. Can DSM-V facilitate productive research into the somatoform disorders? J Psychosom Res. 2006;60:331–4.
33. Smith R, Gardiner J, Lyles J, et al. Exploration of DSM-IV criteria in primary care patients with medically unexplained symptoms. Psychosom Med. 2005;67:123–9.
34. Koh KB. Identity of somatoform disorders: comparison with depressive disorders and anxiety disorders. In: Koh KB, editor. Somatization and psychosomatic symptoms. New York: Springer; 2013. p. 3–15.

35. Van der Feltz-Cornelis CM, van Houdenhove B. DSM-5: from 'somatoform disorders' to 'somatic symptom and related disorders'. Tijdschr Psychiatr. 2014;56:182–6.
36. American Psychiatric Association (APA). Statistical and diagnostic manual of mental disorders. 5th ed. Washington, DC: Am Psychiatric Publishing; 2013.
37. Grover S, Ghosh A. Somatic symptom and related disorders in Asians and Asian Americans. Asian J Psychiatry. 2014;7:77–9.
38. Dimsdale JE, Creed F, Escobar J, et al. Somatic symptom disorder: an important change in DSM. J Psychosom Res. 2013;75:223–8.
39. Voigt K, Wollburg E, Weinmann N, et al. Predictive validity and clinical utility of DSM-5 Somatic Symptom Disorder: prospective 1-year follow-up study. J Psychosom Res. 2013;75:358–61.
40. Cosci F, Fava GA. The clinical inadequacy of the DSM-5 classification of somatic symptom and related disorders: an alternative trans-diagnostic model. CNS Spectr. 2016;21:310–7.
41. Sirri L, Fava GA. Diagnostic criteria for psychosomatic research and somatic symptom disorders. Int Rev Psychiatry. 2013;25:19–30.
42. Frances A. DSM-5 somatic symptom disorder mislabels medical illness as mental disorder. Aust Nez Psychiatry. 2013;47:483–4.
43. Rief W, Martin A. How to use the new DSM-5 somatic symptom disorder diagnosis in research and practice: a critical evaluation and a proposal for modifications. Ann Rev Clin Psychol. 2014;10:339–67.
44. Mayou R. Is the DSM-5 chapter on somatic symptom disorder any better than DSM-IV somatoform disorder? Br J Psychiatry. 2014;204:418–9.
45. Sharma MP, Manjula M. Behavioral and psychological management of somatic symptom disorders: an overview. Int Rev Psychiatry. 2013;25:116–24.
46. Nettleton S, Watt I, O'Malley L, et al. Understanding the narratives of people who live with medically unexplained illness. Patient Educ Couns. 2005;56:205–10.
47. Koh KB, Ki SW. A comparison of illness behavior among patients with somatoform disorders, depressive disorders and psychosomatic disorders. Kor J Psychosom Med. 1997;5:185–94.
48. Patel V, Sumathipala A. Psychological approaches to somatization in developing countries. Adv Psychiatr Treat. 2006;12:54–62.
49. Esler MD, Goulston KJ. Levels of anxiety in colonic disorders. N Engl J Med. 1973;288:16–20.
50. Anderson CD. Expression of affect and physiological response in psychosomatic patients. J Psychosom Res. 1981;25:143–9.
51. Barsky AJ. A comprehensive approach to the chronically somatizing patient. J Psychosom Res. 1998;45:301–6.
52. Sharpe M, Peveler R, Mayou R. The psychological treatment of patients with functional somatic symptoms: a practical guide. J Psychosom Res. 1992;36:515–29.

Chapter 9
Biological Mechanisms of Somatization

9.1 Introduction

A better understanding of the neurobiological underpinnings of somatizing disorders may not only help determine whether they are independent entities [1] but also help address the limitation of self-reporting when diagnosing somatizing patients. In the previous studies, physiological activities, alterations in blood flow and endocrine system, physiological arousal induced by stress, pain threshold, and gate control mechanism were examined. Recent studies include neural imaging, neural immune, and genetic studies in somatization.

9.2 Physiological Activities

Many of the symptoms of somatization are products of physiological activities accentuated by stress and emotion [2].

9.2.1 Contraction of Smooth Muscle

One of the most common causes of somatization is contraction of smooth muscle. For example, abnormal intestinal motility may cause functional or non-ulcer dyspepsia [3]. In addition, generalized colicky abdominal pain may be caused by contractions of the colon in irritable bowel syndrome [4].

K. B. Koh, *Stress and Somatic Symptoms*,
https://doi.org/10.1007/978-3-030-02783-4_9

9.2.2 Contraction of Striated Muscle

Activity of striated muscle increases during emotional arousal. For example, patients with tension headache showed greater levels of EMG activity in temporal muscle than healthy controls [5].

9.3 Alterations in Blood Flow and Endocrine System

Disturbances in blood flow without tissue pathology can be found in migraine headaches in which vasospasm is followed by vasodilation. Some of functional somatic symptoms are associated with alterations in blood flow during an arousal state, which are mediated by the endocrine and autonomic nervous system [2].

9.4 Physiological Arousal Induced by Stress

Individuals have a characteristic pattern of physiological responses to stress [6]. In some individuals, however, the response remains similar regardless of the kind of stressors used [7, 8]. Somatization may be the consequence of physiological activity that tends to be idiosyncratic. Moreover, physiological activity tends to become greater and somatization more severe at times of stress [2].

9.5 Low Pain Threshold

A lower pain threshold has been found in somatizing patients. For example, patients with irritable bowel syndrome have a low pain threshold to abdominal distension [9]. Patients with hypochondriasis and patients with disease phobia also have low pain thresholds [10]. In contrast, patients with silent myocardial ischemia tend to have high pain thresholds [11, 12]. Alterations in pain threshold may occur due to increases in muscular tension related to anxiety and depression. Muscular ischemia related to the release of pain-inducing substances, such as substance P and histamine, can alter pain threshold [13].

9.6 Gate Control Mechanism and Endorphin

It has been proposed that gate control mechanism situated in the dorsal horn of the spinal cord plays the role of a gate in controlling transmission of pain signals from the peripheral nerves to the central nervous system. In addition, endorphin deficiency seems to correlate with augmentation of incoming sensory stimuli [13].

9.7 Brain Imaging and Electroencephalogram (EEG)

Somatoform disorders (somatic symptom and related disorders in DSM-5) may involve a variety of neuronal pathways [13]. However, findings of brain imaging studies in somatizing patients were inconsistent. For example, in a single photon emission computed tomography (SPECT) study for somatization disorder patients, relative hypoactivity in the posterior parietal lobe [14] and hyperactivity in the right occipital lobe were reported [15]. In another SPECT study, undifferentiated somatoform disorder (somatic symptom disorder in DSM-5) patients showed hyperperfusion in the left hemisphere at the superior temporal gyrus, inferior parietal lobule, middle occipital gyrus, precentral gyrus, and postcentral gyrus and in the right hemisphere at the superior temporal gyrus, as compared to healthy controls. Hyperperfusion in the left superior temporal gyrus and hypoperfusion in the right parahippocampal gyrus were found in patients with undifferentiated somatoform disorder (somatic symptom disorder in DSM-5) and panic disorder when compared to healthy controls [16]. Together, these findings suggest that two disorders share neural activities.

A study using brain [18F]-fluorodeoxyglucose-PET with magnetic resonance imaging (MRI) reference reported that cerebral metabolism rates of glucose were lower in the caudate nuclei, left putamen, and right precentral gyrus in somatizing women compared with healthy volunteers [17]. The researchers, using brain MRI, also later reported bilateral enlargement of caudate nuclei volumes in somatoform disorder patients compared with healthy volunteers [18].

In a study using functional MRI, patients with somatoform pain disorder (somatic symptom disorder in DSM-5) showed increased activation in the amygdala, parahippocampal gyrus, anterior/mid-insula, primary and secondary somatosensory cortex, and inferior parietal cortex, in comparison to healthy controls [19]. The changes in pain memory observed in phantom and chronic pain conditions are also known to be modulated by fronto-medial, fronto-lateral, parietal, insular, and anterior cingulate activation which can influence pain perception [20–23]. Moreover, limbic connections may bind stress-regulating and pain-processing systems together, resulting in pain perception triggered by stress without specific noxious stimuli [24–26].

In addition, in patients with pain disorder (somatic symptom disorder in DSM-5), when compared with healthy controls, there was reduced gray matter in the anterior cingulate cortex, posterior cingulate cortex, lateral prefrontal cortex, ventromedial prefrontal cortex, and anterior insular cortex [27]. Another study reported increased activation of some prefrontal, temporal, and parietal regions during the first exposure to pain and of temporal and parietal areas during cognitive stress in patients with somatoform pain disorder (somatic symptom disorder in DSM-5) [28].

Synchrony between brain regions was examined in conversion disorder patients by using EEG, which found lower function in the dominant hemisphere system and dysfunctional hyperactivity in the nondominant hemisphere, suggesting abnormality in the relationship between the two hemispheres. Defects in dealing with intrinsic somatic signals and integrating sensory-motor signals are likely to be related to abnormalities in the dominant hemisphere system. Abnormal auditory-evoked potential was also found in patients with somatization disorder (somatic symptom disorder in DSM-5), which suggested functional disturbance in the cerebral cortex [9].

9.8 Abnormalities in Cerebral Hemispheres and Hemispheric Asymmetry

A study in which neuropsychological test was performed in hysteria (conversion disorder) patients and healthy controls revealed that hysteria patients exhibited bifrontal impairment and a greater global dysfunction of the nondominant hemisphere, when compared to healthy controls [29].

It has been suggested that failure to integrate emotion and language by functional commissurotomy, that is, failure to translate emotion of the right hemisphere into language of the left hemisphere (rationality), may be related to somatization [30].

Symptoms of somatization disorder tend to be asymmetric [31]. Symptoms of conversion disorder more often appear on the left of the body than on the right. Pain complaints tend to be more predominant on the left except trigeminal neuralgia [32], which suggests that the right hemisphere is more likely to be linked to the reticular activating system than is the left hemisphere [33].

9.9 Disturbances in Wakefulness and Concentration

It has been proposed that disturbances of the reticular activating system related to wakefulness and concentration might be a cause of conversion disorder and hypochondriacal disorder (illness anxiety disorder in DSM-5) [34, 35].

9.10 Serotonin

Serotonin is probably a major neurotransmitter in the descending inhibitory pathway [13]. Effective responses to selective serotonin reuptake inhibitors (SSRIs) in patients with pain disorder (somatic symptom disorder in DSM-5) suggest the possibility of serotonin's involvement in the pathophysiology of somatization [9]. In addition, serotonergic amino acids were decreased in patients with multiple unexplained symptoms, even when no depression was present [36].

9.11 Immunity

Studies that have examined immune activity in patients with somatoform disorder (somatic symptom and related disorders in DSM-5) are sparse in comparison with those in depressive disorder [37–40] and anxiety disorder patients [41–45]. One study showed reduced lymphocyte proliferation in patients with undifferentiated somatoform disorder (somatic symptom disorder in DSM-5) compared with healthy controls [46]. In another study [47], somatizing patients had significantly lower levels of serum IL-6 than depressed patients and normal controls.

It has been reported that the activity of cytokines, such as interleukins, tumor necrosis factor, and interferon, is likely to be altered in somatization disorder (somatic symptom disorder in DSM-5) [48]. In particular, proinflammatory cytokines may not only regulate the mounting of the adaptive immune responses that involve T and B lymphocytes but also trigger a brain-cytokine system that organizes the sickness response. Therefore, alteration of proinflammatory cytokines as well as T cells can be anticipated in patients with somatoform disorders (somatic symptom and related disorders in DSM-5) who often show sickness behavior [49]. However, another study did not find any significant differences in T-cell mitogen-stimulated cytokine production, such as IL-2, IL-4, IL-5, IL-6, IL-10, TNF-α, and IFN-γ between patients with medically unexplained symptoms and healthy controls [50].

9.12 Brain-Immune Interaction

In a study on the relationship between immunity and neural activity in patients with undifferentiated somatoform disorder (somatic symptom disorder in DSM-5), Koh et al. [46] reported that hypoperfusion was significant at the left inferior parietal lobule and the left supramarginal gyrus in the more immune-suppressed subgroup compared to the less immune-suppressed subgroup. These results suggest that the left inferior parietal lobule and left supramarginal gyrus might play an immunomodulating role in patients with undifferentiated somatoform disorder (somatic symptom disorder in DSM-5) (Fig. 9.1). These findings also suggest that the left cerebral activation may play a role in enhanced immune function in patients with undifferentiated somatoform disorder (somatic symptom disorder in DSM-5). In previous studies, it was reported that cerebral asymmetry was associated with immunity in healthy individuals [51, 52]. In addition, an animal experiment found that relative right-sided activation caused by partial ablation of the left frontoparietal cerebral cortex decreased immune responses [53].

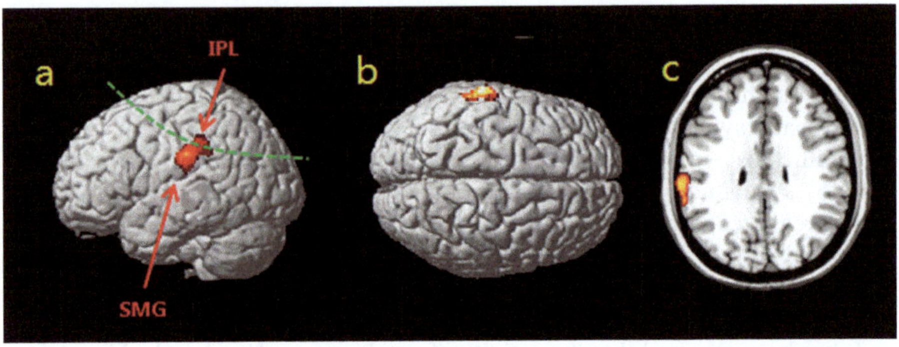

Fig. 9.1 Hypoperfused brain areas in more immune-suppressed group compared with less immune-suppressed group in surface projection (**a, b**) and transaxial plane (**c**). Hypoperfusion was significant at the left inferior parietal lobule (IPL) and the left supramarginal gyrus (SMG) in more immune-suppressed group compared with less immune-suppressed group (FDR, $p < 0.05$). *FDR* false discovery rate. (From Koh et al. [46])

9.13 Genetic Factors

Adoption studies also suggested that somatization was genetically related [54]. However, genetic factors did not play a great role in formation of somatic symptoms in a twin study for adolescents [55], nor was it clear how much genetic factors were involved in somatization in twin studies for adult psychiatric patients [56]. It was suggested that somatization disorder (somatic symptom disorder in DSM-5) and antisocial personality disorder were likely to have a common background genetically because the prevalence of antisocial personality was unexpectedly high in patients with somatization disorder (somatic symptom disorder in DSM-5) [9].

Recently, one study examined serotonin-related gene polymorphisms in patients with undifferentiated somatoform disorder (somatic symptom disorder in DSM-5) and healthy controls. However, no significant differences were found in serotonin-related gene polymorphisms between the two groups. Therefore, serotonin-related gene pathways are unlikely to be genetic risk factors for undifferentiated somatoform disorder (somatic symptom disorder in DSM-5) [57].

On the other hand, it has been reported that aggression in major depressive disorder patients is more susceptible to an excess of TPH1 CC homozygote than in patients with undifferentiated somatoform disorder (somatic symptom disorder in DSM-5), although the two disorders are high risk groups for aggression [58].

Therefore, some of somatization patients are likely to be genetically related, whereas others are likely to be environmentally related [2].

9.14 Future Directions

An overview of psychobiological studies focused on heritability, polymorphisms in special candidate genes, immune activation, hypothalamic-pituitary-adrenal (HPA) axis reactivity, serotonergic pathways, monoamino acids, and fatty acid concentrations in patients with depression and/or somatization-associated syndromes. Many psychobiological pathways were found to act differently in depression and somatization, suggesting that these differences in psychobiology favor the distinction of these syndromes in classification approaches [59].

Some of biological mechanisms may help differentiate between somatizing disorders and other mental disorders, such as depressive disorders and anxiety disorders. In particular, somatizing disorders are biologically more similar to anxiety disorders than to depressive disorders, especially major depressive disorder in terms of brain imaging findings [60]. Further studies are needed to elucidate the brain-immune and genetic-immune interactions in these disorders.

9.15 Conclusions

Biological mechanisms of somatization include physiological activities, alterations in blood flow and endocrine system, physiological arousal induced by stress, pain threshold, gate control mechanism, brain imaging and electroencephalogram (EEG), abnormalities in cerebral hemispheres and hemispheric asymmetry, disturbances in wakefulness and concentration, serotonin, immunity, and genetic factors. Some of biological mechanisms may help differentiate between somatizing disorders and other mental disorders, such as depressive disorders and anxiety disorders. Further studies are needed to elucidate the brain-immune and genetic-immune interactions in these disorders.

References

1. Nutt DJ, Stein DJ. Understanding the neurobiology of comorbidity in anxiety disorders. CNS Spectr. 2006;11:13–20.
2. Kellner R. Psychosomatic syndromes and somatic symptoms. Washington, DC: American Psychiatric Press; 1991. p. 187–225.
3. Toouli J. Sphincter of Oddi motility. Br J Surg. 1984;71:251–6.
4. Holdstock DJ, Misiewicz JJ, Waller SL. Observation on the mechanism of abdominal pain. Gut. 1969;10:19–31.
5. Fujii S, Kachi T, Sobue I. Chronic headache: its psychosomatic aspect. Jpn J Psychosom Med. 1981;21:411–9.

6. Anderson CD. Expression of affect and physiological response in psychosomatic patients. J Psychosom Res. 1981;25:143–9.
7. Lacey JI, Lacey BC. Verification and extension of the principle of autonomic response-stereotype. Am J Psychol. 1958;71:50–73.
8. Lacey JI, Bateman DE, Van Lehn R. Autonomic response specificity: an experimental study. Psychosom Med. 1953;15:8–21.
9. Merskey H, Spear FG. Pain: psychological and psychiatric aspects. London: Ballire, Tindall and Cassell; 1967.
10. Bianchi GN. Origins of disease phobia. Aust NZJ Psychiatry. 1971;5:241–57.
11. Droste C, Roskamm H. Experimental pain measurement in patients with asymptomatic myocardial ischemia. J Am Coll Cardiol. 1983;1:940–5.
12. Glazier JJ, Chierchia S, Brown MJ, et al. Importance of generalized defective perception of painful stimuli as a cause of silent myocardial ischemia in chronic stable angina pectoris. Am J Cardiol. 1986;58:667–72.
13. Guggenheim FG. Somatoform disorder. In: Sadock BJ, Sadock VA, editors. Comprehensive textbook of psychiatry. 7th ed. Baltimore: Lippincott Williams & Wilkins; 2000.
14. Lazarus A, Cotterell KP. SPECT scan reveals abnormality in somatization disorder patient. J Clin Psychiatry. 1989;50:475–6.
15. James L, Singer A, Zurynski Y, et al. Evoked potentials and regional cerebral blood flow in somatization disorder. Psychother Psychosom. 1987;47:190–6.
16. Koh KB, Kang JI, Lee JD, et al. Shared neural activity in panic disorder and undifferentiated somatoform disorder compared with healthy controls. J Clin Psychiatry. 2010;71:1576–81.
17. Hakala M, Karlsson H, Ruotsalainen U, et al. Somatization in women is associated with altered brain glucose metabolism. Psychol Med. 2002;32:1379–85.
18. Hakala M, Karlsson H, Kurki T, et al. Volumes of the caudate nuclei in women with somatization disorder and healthy women. Psychiatry Res Neuroimaging. 2004;131:71–8.
19. Gundel H, Valet M, Sorg C, et al. Altered cerebral response to noxious heat stimulation in patients with somatoform pain disorder. Pain. 2008;137:413–21.
20. Rainville P, Duncan GH, Price DD, et al. Pain affect encoded in human anterior cingulate but not somatosensory cortex. Science. 1997;277:968–71.
21. Wager TD, Rilling JK, Smith EE, et al. Placebo-induced changes in FMRI in the anticipation and experience of pain. Science. 2004;303:1162–7.
22. Schreckenberger M, Siessmeier T, Viertmann A, et al. The unpleasantness of tonic pain is encoded by the insular cortex. Neurology. 2005;64:1175–83.
23. Treede RD. Assessment of pain as an emotion in animals and in humans. Exp Neurol. 2006;197:1–3.
24. LeDoux JE. Emotion circuits in the brain. Annu Rev Neurosci. 2000;23:155–84.
25. Price DD. Psychological and neural mechanisms of the affective dimension of pain. Science. 2000;288:1769–72.
26. Sandkuhler J. Learning and memory in pain pathways. Pain. 2000;88:113–8.
27. Valet M, Gundel H, Sprenger T, et al. Patients with pain disorder show gray-matter loss in pain-processing structures: a voxel-based morphometric study. Psychosom Med. 2009;71:49–56.
28. Stoeter P, Bauermann T, Nickel R, et al. Cerebral activation in patients with somatoform pain disorder exposed to pain and stress: an fMRI study. NeuroImage. 2007;36:418–30.
29. Flor-Henry P, Fromm-Auch D, Tapper M, et al. A neuropsychological study of the stable syndrome of hysteria. Biol Psychiatry. 1981;16:601–26.
30. Hoppe KD. Split brains and psychoanalysis. Psychoanal Q. 1977;46:220–44.
31. Galin D, Diamond R, Braff D. Lateralization of conversion symptoms: more frequent on the left. Am J Psychiatry. 1997;134:578–80.
32. Mersky H, Watson GD. The lateralization of pain. Pain. 7:271–80.
33. Heilman KM. Neglect and related disorders. In: Heilman KM, Balenstein E, editors. Clinical neuropsychology. New York: Oxford University Press; 1979.
34. Whitlock F. The aetiology of hysteria. Acta Psychiatr Scand. 1967;43:144–62.

35. Miller L. Neuropsychological concepts of somatoform disorders. Int J Psychiatry Med. 1984;14:31–46.
36. Rief W, Pilger F, Ihle D, et al. Psychobiological aspects of somatoform disorders: contributions of monoaminergic transmitter systems. Neuropsychobiology. 2004;49:24–9.
37. Kronfol A, Silva J, Gredin J, et al. Impaired lymphocyte function in depressive illness. Life Sci. 1983;33:241–7.
38. Kronfol Z, House JD. Depression, cortisol, and immune function. Lancet. 1984;1:1026–7.
39. Krueger RB, Levy EM, Cathcart ES. Lymphocyte subsets in patients with major depression: preliminary findings. Advances. 1984;1:5–9.
40. Andreoil A, Keller SE, Taban C, et al. Immune function in major depressive disorder: relation to panic disorder comorbidity. Biol Psychiatry. 1990;27(Suppl):9A–95A.
41. Brambilla F, Bellodi L, Perna G, et al. Psychoimmunoendocrine aspects of panic disorder. Neuropsychobiology. 1992;26:12–22.
42. La Via MF, Munno I, Lydiard RB, et al. The influence of stress intrusion on immunodepression in generalized anxiety disorder patients and controls. Psychosom Med. 1996;58:138–42.
43. Koh KB, Lee BK. Reduced lymphocyte proliferation and interleukin-2 production in anxiety disorders. Psychosom Med. 1998;60:479–83.
44. Rapaport MH. Circulating lymphocyte phenotypic surface markers in anxiety disorder patients and normal volunteers. Biol Psychiatry. 1998;43:458–63.
45. Koh KB, Lee Y. Reduced anxiety level by therapeutic interventions and cell-mediated immunity in panic disorder patients. Psychother Psychosom. 2004;73:286–92.
46. Koh KB, Sohn S-H, Kang JI, et al. Relationship between neural activity and immunity in patients with undifferentiated somatoform disorder. Psychiatry Res Neuroimaging. 2012;202:252–6.
47. Rief W, Pilger F, Ihle D, et al. Immunological differences between patients with major depression and somatization syndrome. Psychiatry Res. 2001;105:165–74.
48. Kaplan HI, Sadock BJ. Synopsis of psychiatry. 8th ed. Baltimore: Williams & Wilkins; 1998.
49. Dantzer R. Somatization: a psychoneuroimmune perspective. Psychoneuroendocrinology. 2005;30:947–52.
50. Houtveen JH, Kavelaars A, Heijnen CJ, et al. Heterogeneous medically unexplained symptoms and immune function. Brain Behav Immun. 2007;21:1075–82.
51. Kang D-H, Davidson RJ, Coe CL, et al. Frontal brain asymmetry and immune function. Behav Neurosci. 1991;105:860–9.
52. Davidson RJ, Coe CC, Dolski I, et al. Individual differences in prefrontal activation asymmetry predict natural killer cell activity at rest and in response to challenge. Brain. Behav Immun. 1999;13:93–108.
53. Renoux G, Biziere K, Renoux M, et al. A balanced brain asymmetry modulates T cell-mediated events. J Neuroimmunol. 1983;5:227–38.
54. Cadoret RJ. Psychopathology in adopted-away offspring of biologic parents with antisocial behavior. Arch Gen Psychiatry. 1978;35:176–84.
55. Gottesman II. Differential inheritance of the psychoneuroses. Eugenics Q. 1962;9:223–67.
56. Torgersen S. Genetics of somatoform disorders. Arch Gen Psychiatry. 1986;43:502–5.
57. Koh KB, Choi EH, Lee Y, et al. Serotonin-related gene pathways associated with undifferentiated somatoform disorder. Psychiatry Res. 2011;189:246–50.
58. Koh KB, Kim CH, Choi EH, et al. Effect of tryptophan hydroxylase gene polymorphism on aggression in major depressive disorder and undifferentiated somatoform disorder. J Clin Psychiatry. 2012;73:e574–9.
59. Rief W, Hennings A, Riemer S, et al. Psychobiological differences between depression and somatization. J Psychosom Res. 2010;68:495–502.
60. Koh KB. Identity of somatoform disorders: comparison with depressive disorders and anxiety disorders. In: Koh KB, editor. Somatization and psychosomatic symptoms. New York: Springer; 2013.

Chapter 10
Psychosociocultural Mechanisms of Somatization

10.1 Introduction

Somatization is a broad term describing a person's belief that a physical disease is present. It is also a kind of communication of emotional distress, consciously or unconsciously coded in the language of the body [1]. Somatization represents a powerful method of coping with psychosocial distress in all cultures [2].

Patients with somatization report fewer normalizing symptom attributions than nonclinical subjects [3]. Somatization patients have more organic attributions than depressed patients [3, 4], but they usually do not have monocausal simplistic explanations [3]. Somatoform disorders (somatic symptom and related disorders in DSM-5) are similar to anxiety disorders in the severity of somatic symptoms and depression, but the two disorders are different from depressive disorders in the levels of depression [5].

Increased health-care use is a main characteristic of somatization [3, 6]. In other illness behaviors, such as body scanning and expression of symptoms, there were also significant differences between somatization patients and controls [7]. In addition, chronic pain syndromes are associated with reassurance-seeking behavior [8].

There have been a variety of theories on mechanisms of somatization. They can largely be divided into biological and psychosociocultural mechanisms. This chapter focuses on psychosociocultural mechanisms which include psychological, behavioral, social, and cultural factors.

K. B. Koh, *Stress and Somatic Symptoms*,
https://doi.org/10.1007/978-3-030-02783-4_10

10.2 Psychological Factors

10.2.1 Personality Development and Personality Traits

Psychological pain underlying physical pain revealed that the sufferer had a problem with his/her parents who did not care for him/her sufficiently, reflecting his/her unmet hunger or sense of emptiness [9]. Some personality traits, such as neuroticism [10], are associated with a high prevalence of somatic symptoms [11].

10.2.2 Anxiety

In a number of studies, anxiety is usually accompanied by somatic symptoms. Generalized anxiety disorder and panic disorder are also described as main causes of somatization [12]. In patients with panic disorder referred to psychiatry for consultation, somatic symptoms, such as chest pain, palpitation, irregular heartbeat, epigastric distress, headache, dizziness, and paresthesia, are frequently noted. Some panic disorder patients only have somatic symptoms [13]. Patients with anxiety disorders are known to have higher levels of illness anxiety than patients with somatoform disorders (somatic symptom and related disorders in DSM-5) [14].

10.2.3 Depression

Many studies have found that there are significant correlations between depression and somatization. Depressed patients tend to have more somatic symptoms than do nondepressed patients, whereas somatizing patients tend to be more depressed than patients with physical diseases [15–18]. In addition, patients with depressive disorders have more somatic symptoms than patients with somatoform disorders (somatic symptom and related disorders in DSM-5) [14]. Depression is known to enhance physical suffering and lower the threshold for perceiving somatic symptoms, thereby intensifying subjective symptoms [19]. Depression occasionally coexists with somatization.

10.2.4 Anger and Anger Management Style

Anger, especially anger suppression, is known as a crucial factor in somatization [20–22]. Patients with somatoform disorder (somatic symptom and related disorders in DSM-5) scored significantly higher on the Stress Response Inventory (SRI) anger subscale than normal controls. However, somatoform disorder or anxiety disorder patients are less likely to have high levels of anger than depressive disorder patients [23].

Somatic symptoms in patients with somatoform disorders (Fig. 10.1) and anxiety disorders (Fig. 10.2) are associated with anger suppression [24], whereas somatic symptoms in depressive disorder patients are more associated with anger expression (Fig. 10.3) [5, 22]. Therefore, in terms of anger levels and the relationship between anger management style and somatic symptoms, somatoform disorders (somatic symptom and related disorders in DSM-5) are similar to anxiety disorders but are different from depressive disorders [5].

10.2.5 Illness Anxiety

Health anxiety level is elevated in somatization and hypochondriasis groups as compared to mixed clinical controls [25]. However, the content of worry may be different in somatization versus hypochondriasis [26]. Different chronic pain syndromes share health anxiety as a common feature [8].

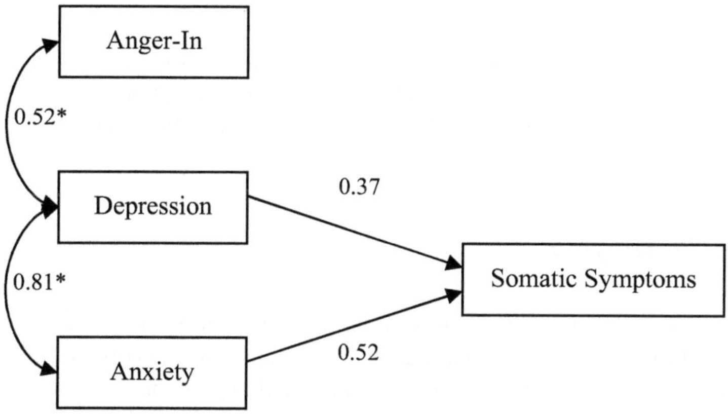

Fig. 10.1 The relation between anger management style, mood, and somatic symptoms in somatoform disorders (somatic symptom and related disorders in DSM-5). Bentler's comparative fit index: 1.00; $R^2 = 0.71$. * Indicates coefficients of Pearson correlation. (From Koh et al. [24])

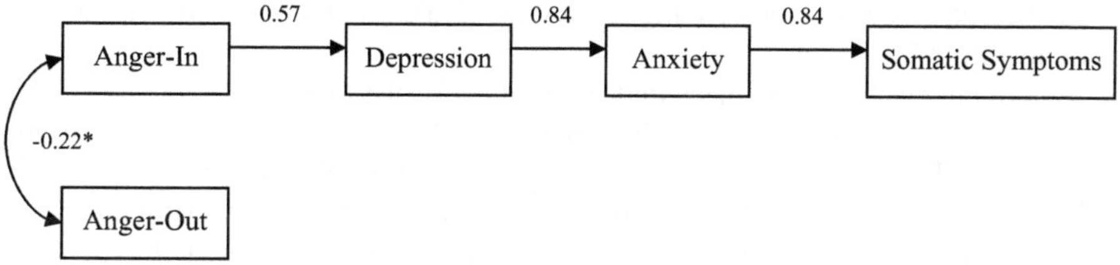

Fig. 10.2 The relation between anger management style, mood, and somatic symptoms in anxiety disorders. Bentler's comparative fit index: 0.93; $R^2 = 0.70$. * Indicates coefficients of Pearson correlation. (From Koh et al. [24])

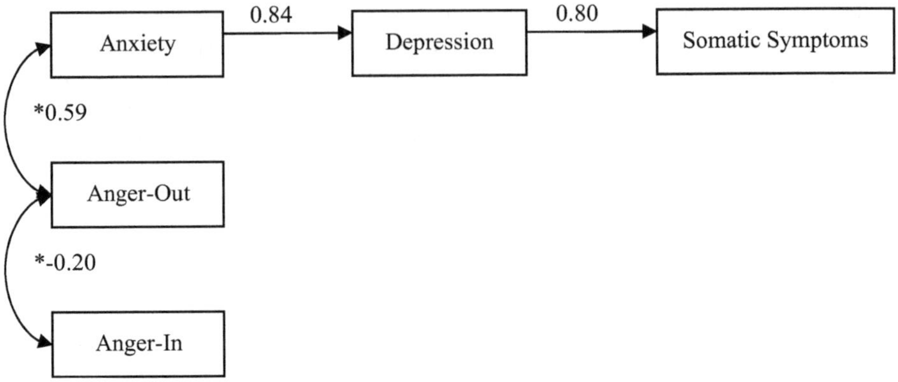

Fig. 10.3 The relation between anger management style, mood, and somatic symptoms in depressive disorders. Bentler's comparative fit index: 0.93; $R^2 = 0.65$. * Indicates coefficients of Pearson correlation. (From Koh [5])

10.2.6 Inhibition of Emotion

Denial of, repression of, and lack of confiding about distressful events and emotion are known to be associated with somatization [27, 28]. Talking about a major traumatic event was found to be associated with fewer symptoms and illness episodes [29].

10.2.7 Alexithymia

Alexithymic patients have difficulties in expressing emotions in words, and they do not have fantasies expressive of feelings; their thought content is dominated by details of events [30]. They also show a deficit in nonverbal expression of emotion [31].

Alexithymia was once regarded as characteristic of psychosomatic disorders (psychological factors affecting other medical conditions (PFAOMC) in DSM-5), but later it has been proposed that alexithymia is likely to be one of the features of specific psychosomatic disorders (e.g., tension headache) rather than nonspecific psychosomatic disorders [32]. Additionally, patients with hypertension and those with ulcerative colitis showed higher levels of alexithymia than other medical patients [33–35].

Emotional awareness as measured by the Levels of Emotional Awareness Scale (LEAS) was lower in patients with somatoform disorders (somatic symptom and related disorders in DSM-5) compared with healthy controls [36]. In another study [37], the levels of alexithymia, as measured by each of the Toronto Alexithymia Scale (TAS-20) and the Affect Consciousness Interview (ACI), were found to be higher in ICD-10 somatoform disorders (somatic symptom and related disorders in DSM-5) than in healthy controls. Adolescents with persistent somatoform pain disorder (somatic symptom disorder in DSM-5) also have higher levels of alexithymia than healthy adolescent controls [38]. In addition, alexithymia was negatively correlated with quality of life in patients with somatoform pain disorder (somatic symptom disorder in DSM-5) [39].

However, it remains controversial whether alexithymia is either a cause or consequence of somatization.

10.2.8 Communication and Defense

Somatization is often used as a means of communication when direct expression is blocked, as seen in patients with conversion disorder [40]. Somatization may be explained as defense mechanisms, such as denial, displacement, or rationalization (e.g., attributing one's failure to bodily symptoms), or an attempt to resolve conflicts [41, 42]. However, somatizing patients deny acknowledging their psychological conflicts consciously [4].

10.2.9 Amplification of Somatic Sensation

Increased somatic symptom reports are associated with higher somatosensory amplification [3, 43]. Amplification of somatic sensation means a tendency to experience somatic sensation intensely, which is a kind of abnormal illness behavior. Such amplification phenomenon is often seen in somatization. Somatizing patients usually amplify their psychological suffering and depression into unpleasant somatic sensations [44].

Somatization patients overinterpret minor physical symptoms as possible signs of illnesses and have a self-concept of being "weak." The catastrophizing of physical symptoms is specific to somatization and hypochondriasis but is not seen in patients with depressive and anxiety disorders. The self-concept of being "weak" distinguishes between patients with somatoform disorders and patients with other mental disorders [25].

However, there are contradictory results regarding the specificity of somatosensory amplification in somatoform disorders, especially concerning the differentiation from patients with anxiety disorders and depressive disorders [3].

10.3 Behavioral Factors

10.3.1 Learning

Somatization has been described as learned abnormal perceptions or cognitive style. Thus, childhood experiences may act as predisposing factors of somatization [45]. Children's symptoms are often a copy of symptoms occurring in other members of the family [46]. On the other hand, adult somatization is associated with parental attention to symptoms during the patient's childhood [11]. Somatizing patients learn that there are compensations for their illnesses and that physical illnesses are more acceptable to their society than psychological disorders [41].

10.3.2 Gain

Somatic symptoms can be used for an individual's need or gain, such as sick role, economic compensation, interpersonal control, and dealing with difficult work or avoiding it. Patients who receive such gain, especially economic gain (e.g., pensions or disability compensation), showed somatic symptoms or physical disabilities for longer period of time, even with diseases of similar severity than those without such gain [47].

10.4 Social Factors

10.4.1 Sick Role

Sick role can be a main motivation for somatization. The sick role can be used to solve life problems, but society does not accept emotional disorders or difficulties as sick role. People with such problems can get transient relief from their overburdened stress by translating them into socially acceptable somatic complaints (e.g., backache) which give them the sick role [41].

10.4.2 Doctor-Patient Relationship

Illness is a way of life for somatizing patients. In their devotion to the treatment of illness, physicians have also made illness a way of life. Therefore, physicians and somatizing patients have many similarities. Physicians frequently experience their own or their family members' illnesses during their childhood and have dependency conflict, marital problems, and difficulties in interpersonal relationship. In addition, they are usually obsessive-compulsive and emotionally constricted. All of these characteristics are also commonly seen in somatizing patients [41].

Physicians often use reaction formation and counterphobic mechanisms. Thus, they maintain fantasies of omniscience and omnipotence rather than feeling weak and helpless. In an effort to defend against anxiety, the physicians may not want to hear of their patients' problems such as depressive symptoms, dependent need, and marital conflicts, subtly rejecting them. To the contrary, as a way of denying uncomfortable feelings, the physicians may overcompensate and unwittingly reinforce somatizing behavior [41].

10.4.3 Stigma of Psychiatric Diagnoses

Social stigma of psychiatric diagnoses may cause somatizing patients to avoid psychiatry and to be a motivation for visiting other departments and rationalizing their somatic complaints [19]. Public officials, military officers, politicians, and senior officers are afraid of disadvantages by such stigma and often translate their psychological problems into somatic symptoms. From a religious perspective, psychiatric illnesses may be regarded as an act of evil. Therefore, these religious people cannot help but complain of somatic symptoms because such religion has the doctrine in which depression is a sin and true believers must be full of joy [48].

10.5 Cultural Factors

Somatic symptoms are prominent in various "culture-bound syndromes." In particular, the relationship between the number of somatic symptoms and illness worry is similar in different cultures. Despite these similarities, however, there are differences in somatic symptoms among cultures and ethnic groups. The description of somatic symptoms varies with linguistic and other local cultural factors. These somatic presentations have been described as idioms of distress because somatic symptoms may have special meanings and shape patient-clinician interactions in the particular cultural contexts. Burnout, the sensation of heaviness, too much heat in the body, or burning in the head are examples of symptoms that are common in some cultures or ethnic groups but rare in others [49].

There is a high tendency of somatization in Koreans [50]. Under the influence of traditional philosophies including Confucianism and the traditional patriarchal authoritative culture, people have been taught to suppress anger and not to jeopardize social or familial harmony with authority figures, such as fathers, teachers, and kings. Therefore, the socially weak, especially women, have adopted somatization or hwabyung as a way for nonverbal communication of their suffering [51]. In other words, sociocultural restraints may contribute to the presentation of a variety of somatic symptoms by blocking emotionally charged feelings or ideas from being expressed [52]. Hwabyung is a representative somatic syndrome (also known as an anger syndrome) specific to Korean culture and characterized by a variety of somatic symptoms (e.g., a feeling of a mass in epigastrium, hot sensation, palpitation, dyspnea, fatigue) resulting from long-standing anger suppression [53–56]. Such a syndrome can be a good means for obtaining a sick role which saves their faces in the Korean cultural context [51].

Korean depressives tended to somatize their depression. In particular, visceral symptoms, such as indigestion, abdominal discomfort, heart pounding, and respiratory stuffiness, were thought to be a predominant manifestation of their somatized depression [57]. Chinese culture was also known to inhibit emotional expression [58]. In China, a physical term such as neurasthenia is used instead of major depressive disorder, although it corresponds to the diagnostic criteria of major depressive disorder [48]. In the past, somatization was known to be more prevalent in non-Western cultures than Western cultures [59–62]. However, epidemiological data have not shown cross-national differences in the somatization of depression [63, 64]. Thus, somatization is now considered a universal psychopathology [65, 66].

10.6 Conclusions

Psychosociocultural mechanisms of somatization can largely be grouped into psychological, behavioral, social, and cultural factors. Psychological factors include personality development, anxiety, depression, anger and anger management style, illness anxiety, inhibition of emotion, alexithymia, communication and defense, and amplification of somatic sensation. Behavioral factors include learning and gain. Social factors include sick role, doctor-patient relationship, and stigma of psychiatric diagnoses. Cultural factors include inhibition of emotional expression in Korean and Chinese cultures. Furthermore, multifactorial interactions should be considered a motivation for somatization.

References

1. Brodsky CM. Sociocultural and interactional influences on somatization. Psychosomatics. 1984;25:673–80.
2. Katon W, Kleinman A, Rosen G. Depression and somatization: a review, part 1. Am J Med. 1982;72:127–35.
3. Duddu V, Isaac MK, Chaturvedi SK, et al. Somatization, somatosensory amplification, attribution styles and illness behavior: a review. Int Rev Psychiatry. 2006;18:25–33.
4. Koh KB, Ki SW. A comparison of illness behavior among patients with somatoform disorders, depressive disorders and psychosomatic disorders. Kor J Psychosom Med. 1997;5:185–94.
5. Koh KB. Identity of somatoform disorders: comparison with depressive disorders and anxiety disorders. In: Koh KB, editor. Somatization and psychosomatic symptoms. New York: Springer; 2013. p. 3–15.
6. Kolk AM, Schagen S, Hanewald GJ. Multiple medically unexplained physical symptoms and health care utilization: outcome of psychological intervention and patient-related predictors of change. J Psychosom Res. 2004;57:379–89.
7. Rief W, Martin A, Klaiberg A, et al. Specific effects of depression, panic, and somatic symptoms on illness behavior. Psychosom Med. 2005;67:596–601.
8. Aggarwal VR, McBeth J, Zakrzewska JM, et al. The epidemiology of chronic syndromes that are frequently unexplained: do they have common associated factors? Int J Epidemiol. 2006;35:468–76.
9. Giovacchini PL. Characterological problems: the need to be helped. Arch Gen Psychiatry. 1970;22:245–51.
10. Kellner R, Sheffield BF. A self-rating scale of distress. Psychol Med. 1973;3:88–100.
11. Pennebaker JW. The psychology of physical symptoms. New York: Springer-Verlag; 1982.
12. Kellner R. Somatic sensations, and bodily complaints. In: Noyes R, Roth M, Burrows GD, editors. Handbook of anxiety, vol 2: classification, etiological factors, and associated disturbances. New York: Elsevier; 1988. p. 213–37.

13. Beitman BD, Basha I, Flaker G. Non-fearful panic disorder: panic attacks without fear. Behav Res Ther. 1987;25:487–92.
14. Hanel G, Henningsen P, Herzog W, et al. Depression, anxiety, and somatoform disorders: vague or distinct categories in primary care? Results from a large cross-sectional study. J Psychosom Res. 2009;67:189–97.
15. Kleinman A, Kleinman J. Somatization: the interconnections among culture, depressive experiences, and the meaning of pain. In: Kleinman A, Good B, editors. Culture and depression. Berkeley: University of California Press; 1986. p. 429–90.
16. Kellner R. Somatization and hypochondriasis. New York: Praeger-Greenwood; 1986.
17. Cadoret RJ, Widmer RB, Troughton EP. Somatic complaints: harbinger of depression in primary care. J Affect Disord. 1980;2:61–70.
18. Lloyd GG. Psychiatric syndromes with a somatic presentation. J Psychosom Res. 1986;30:113–20.
19. Lipowski ZJ. Somatization and depression. Psychosomatics. 1990;31:13–21.
20. Kellner R. Psychosomatic syndromes and somatic symptoms. Washington, DC: American Psychiatric Press; 1991. p. 187–225.
21. Koh KB. Stress and psychosomatic medicine. Seoul: Ilchokak; 2002. p. 231–49.
22. Koh KB, Kim DK, Kim SY, et al. The relation between anger expression, depression, and somatic symptoms in depressive disorders and somatoform disorders. J Clin Psychiatry. 2005;66:485–91.
23. Koh KB, Kim CH, Park JK. Predominance of anger in depressive disorder compared to anxiety disorder and somatoform disorder. J Clin Psychiatry. 2002;63:486–92.
24. Koh KB, Kim DK, Kim SY, et al. The relation between anger management style, mood, and somatic symptoms in anxiety disorders and somatoform disorders. Psychiatry Res. 2008;160:372–9.
25. Rief W, Hiller W, Margraf J. Cognitive aspects of hypochondriasis and the somatization syndrome. J Abnorm Psychol. 1998;107:587–95.
26. Noyes R, Stuart S, Watson DB, et al. Distinguishing between hypochondriasis and somatization disorder: a review of the existing literature. Psychother Psychosom. 2006;75:270–81.
27. Pennebaker JW. Traumatic experience and psychosomatic disease: exploring the roles of behavioral inhibition, obsession, and confiding. Can J Psychol. 1985;26:82–95.
28. Pennebaker JW. Confession, inhibition and disease. Adv Exp Soc Psychol. 1989;22:211–44.
29. Pennebaker JW, OHeeron RC. Confiding in others and illness rate among spouse of suicide and accidental-death victims. J Abnorm Psychol. 1984;93:473–6.
30. Nemiah JC. Alexithymia: theoretical considerations. Psychother Psychosom. 1977;28:199–206.
31. McDonald PW, Prkachin KM. The expression and perception of facial emotion in alexithymia: a pilot study. Psychosom Med. 1990;52:199–210.
32. Koh KB. Comparison of alexithymia among patients with psychosomatic disorders, anxiety disorders and depressive disorders. Kor J Psychosom Med. 1994;2:59–68.
33. Fava GA, Pavan L. Large bowel disorders: II. Psychopathology and alexithymia. Psychother Psychosom. 1976/1977;27:100–5.
34. Fava GA, Baldaro B, Osti RMA. Towards a self-rating scale for alexithymia. Psychother Psychosom. 1980;34:34–9.
35. Smith GR. Alexithymia in medical patients referred to a consultation/liaison service. Am J Psychiatry. 1983;140:99–101.
36. Subic-Wrana C, Beutel ME, Knebel A, et al. Theory of mind and emotional awareness deficits in patients with somatoform disorders. Psychosom Med. 2010;72:404–11.
37. Waller E, Scheidt CE. Somatoform disorders as disorders of affect regulation: a study comparing the TAS-20 with non-self-report measures of alexithymia. J Psychosom Res. 2004;57:239–47.
38. Burba B, Oswald R, Grigaliunien V, et al. A controlled study of alexithymia in adolescent patients with persistent somatoform pain disorder. Can J Psychiatry. 2006;51:468–71.
39. Nunez G, Rufer M, Leenen K, et al. Quality of life and alexithymia in somatoform pain disorder. Schmerz. 2010;24:62–8.

40. Ford CV, Folks DG. Conversion disorder: an overview. Psychosomatics. 1985;26:371–83.
41. Ford CV. The somatizing disorders: illness as a way of life. New York: Elsevier; 1984. p. 1–35, 243–59
42. Raskin M, Talbott JA, Meyerson AT. Diagnosed conversion reactions: predictive value of psychiatric criteria. JAMA. 1966;197:530–4.
43. Rief W, Broadbent E. Explaining medically unexplained symptoms-models and mechanisms. Clin Psychol Rev. 2007;27:821–41.
44. Barsky AJ. Amplification, somatization, and the somatoform disorders. Psychosomatics. 1992;33:28–34.
45. Kellner R. Functional somatic symptoms and hypochondriasis: a survey of empirical studies. Arch Gen Psychiatry. 1985;42:821–33.
46. Apley J, Keith RM, Meadow R. The child and his symptoms: a comprehensive approach. Oxford: Blackwell Scientific Publications; 1978.
47. Better SR, Fine PR, Simison D. Disability benefits as disincentives to rehabilitation. Health Soc. 1979;57:412–27.
48. Ford CV. The somatizing disorders. Psychosomatics. 1986;27:327–37.
49. American Psychiatric Association (APA). Statistical and diagnostic manual of mental disorders. 5th ed. Washington, DC: Am Psychiatric Publishing; 2013.
50. Lee HY, Namgoong K, Lee MH, et al. The psychiatric epidemiological study of Kanghwa Island (III). The prevalence of major psychiatric disorders. J Kor Neuropsychiatr Assoc. 1989;28:984–99.
51. Min SK. Culture and somatic symptoms: hwabyung, a culture-related anger syndrome. In: Koh KB, editor. Somatization and psychosomatic symptoms. New York: Springer; 2013.
52. Guggenheim FG. Somatoform disorder. In: Sadock BJ, Sadock VA, editors. Comprehensive textbook of psychiatry. 7th ed. Baltimore: Lippincott Williams & Wilkins; 2000.
53. Lin K. Hwa-pyung: a Korean culture-bound syndrome? Am J Psychiatry. 1983;142:798–805.
54. Lee SH. A study on hwa-byung. Kor Hosp J. 1977;1:63–9.
55. Mezzich JE, Lin K, Hughes CC. Acute and transient psychotic disorders and culture-bound syndromes. In: Sadock BJ, Sadock VA, editors. Comprehensive textbook of psychiatry. 7th ed. Baltimore: Lippincott Williams & Wilkins; 2000.
56. Min SK, Lee MH, Shin JH, et al. A diagnostic study of hwa-byung. J Kor Med Assoc. 1986;29:653–61.
57. Min SK, Kim KH. Somatic symptoms in depression. J Kor Neuropsychiatr Assoc. 1988;17:149–54.
58. White GM. The role of cultural explanations in somatization and psychologization. Soc Sci Med. 1982;16:1519–30.
59. Kleinman A. Neurasthenia and depression: a study on somatization and culture in China. Cult Med Psychiatry. 1982;6:117–90.
60. Pfeiffer W. The symptomatology of depression viewed transculturally. Transcult Psychiatry Res Rev. 1968;5:121–4.
61. Mezzich JE, Raab ES. Depressive symptomatology across the Americas. Arch Gen Psychiatry. 1980;37:818–23.
62. Bhatt A, Tomenson B, Benjamin S. Transcultural patterns of somatization in primary care: a preliminary report. J Psychosom Res. 1989;33:671–80.
63. Parker G, Cheah YC, Roy K. Do the Chinese somatize depression? – A cross-cultural study. Soc Psychiatry Psychiatr Epidemiol. 2001;36:287–93.
64. Simon GE, VonKorff M, Piccinelli M, et al. An international study of the relation between somatic symptoms and depression. New Engl J Med. 1999;341:1329–35.
65. Kim K-I. Culture and somatization. Kor J Psychosom Med. 2003;11:3–14.
66. Becker AE, Kleinman A. Anthropology and psychiatry. In: Sadock BJ, Sadock VA, editors. Comprehensive textbook of psychiatry. 7th ed. Baltimore: Lippincott Williams & Wilkins; 2000.

Chapter 11
Interview Techniques for Assessment and Management of Somatization

11.1 Introduction

Somatization is a process in which there is inappropriate focus on physical symptoms and psychosocial problems are denied [1]. Somatizing patients have more organic attributions than depressed patients [2, 3] and are more likely to over-interpret and catastrophize physical symptoms than patients with depressive or anxiety disorders [4].

Somatization is highly prevalent in primary care where 20–30% of patients fulfill criteria for somatoform disorders (somatic symptom and related disorders in DSM-5) [5–7]. In a general medical clinic in the United States, 84% of presentations of common physical symptoms had no identified organic cause [8], and over half of new referrals to a Dutch medical out-patient clinic had symptoms that remained medically unexplained [9].

Despite its high prevalence, somatization often goes unrecognized [6, 10]. Somatizing patients are called "medical orphans" [11], because they go "doctor shopping" but cannot find a willing physician. They suffer distress for a long time and seek treatment that results in disappointment because a correct diagnosis is not made by physicians. They often make the complaint that their symptoms are genuine, but everything is coming back negative [12].

Sophisticated technologies may facilitate diagnosis, but they also serve to reinforce the boundary between medically explained and medically unexplained symptoms [13]. The default use of biomedical approaches may cause iatrogenic harm and disable somatizing patients [14, 15].

K. B. Koh, *Stress and Somatic Symptoms*,
https://doi.org/10.1007/978-3-030-02783-4_11

11.2 Rationale for Using Special Interview Technique in Somatizing Patients

Treatment of somatization is challenging because it cannot be treated according to the existing biomedical model and somatizing patients are usually resistant to psychosocial approach [16]. Physicians may be less skilled in providing support and care against a background of diagnostic uncertainty [13]. Somatic symptoms persist despite treatment [8], and patients are dissatisfied with their management. This may be because clinicians do not effectively address patients' needs other than the management of pathology [17].

Somatizing patients often express concern that physicians presume their symptoms are "all in the mind" and show resistance to psychological explanations [12]. Therefore, normal test results present major problems for patients and physicians. Such concerns further amplify their marginalization from medical care [12]. However, there is no evidence that somatization helps the patient deny the presence of psychiatric disorder [18].

Research done in primary and secondary care in the United Kingdom has shown that patients' main expectations are for explanations and understanding, which are more important than expectations for support, testing, and diagnosis [19, 20]. Therefore, specific assessment skills and treatment techniques are required to approach them effectively [1]. In this regard, it is important for health professionals and medical students to learn about the biopsychosocial approach to patient-centered care.

11.3 Interview Techniques for Physicians

There are some important interview techniques for physicians to learn for effective assessment and management of somatization.

11.3.1 Empathetic Listening and Patience

Empathetic listening is critical to effective patient-centered care. Practitioners can help by listening to patients' accounts of their symptoms and their attempts to overcome them [12]. Management of somatizing patients often requires patience from physicians because patients may be angry and dissatisfied, feeling that they are not being taken seriously [17]. At the same time, some physicians cannot tolerate patients' frequent complaints and demands, showing anger toward such patients not only because their illness behavior is different from other patients but also their symptoms are not medically explained. This counter-transference can be frequently observed during the management of somatizing patients [21, 22], which leads to the breaking down of the doctor-patient relationship.

11.3.2 Accept Patient's Suffering

People who suffer from an undiagnosed illness want their symptoms to be acknowledged as "genuine," and they also want to feel that practitioners will work with them to suggest and negotiate strategies that may help alleviate their symptoms and better "manage" their situation. Therefore, their suffering should be accepted by physicians as legitimate. In addition, physicians should avoid a strict mind/body dualism while explaining symptoms. However, attempts to integrate the mind and body may be challenging because such separation remains so culturally ingrained [12].

11.3.3 Biopsychosocial Assessment

There is no dichotomy between physical and psychological disorders. Rather, the proportion of physical or psychological etiology varies across a continuum [23]. Psychological factors such as health anxiety and symptom attributions may influence the genesis and presentation of physical symptoms, even in the absence of psychiatric disorders. Therefore, from the beginning of assessment, equal attention should be devoted to understanding biopsychosocial factors, such as somatic, psychological, environmental, dietary, and physiotherapeutic aspects in somatizing patients [17]. When taking the patient's history, physicians should be aware of psychosocial cues and then should be consistent and unambiguous in their management of the patients [1]. In particular, physicians should assess patients' anger because anger – especially anger suppression – may play an important role in somatization as seen in cases of Hwabyung or somatoform disorders (somatic symptom and related disorders in DSM-5) [24]. Hwabyung is anger syndrome specific to Korean culture, which is characterized by a variety of somatic symptoms (e.g., a feeling of a mass in epigastrium, hot sensation, etc.), associated with long-term anger suppression [25–28]. Thus, physicians need to assess and understand cultural aspects for effective management of somatization, in Asians, especially in Koreans.

11.3.3.1 Understand Patient's Illness Experience

Physicians need to understand the problems faced by people with undiagnosed illness. One way of helping somatizing patients might be for physicians to adopt patient-centered care. Physicians trained in biomedical models of care may be able to satisfactorily identify and treat a disease but may be less at ease with providing care and support. In contrast, patient-centered care, with an emphasis not just on the disease but also the illness experience, may provide a framework for physicians to provide enhanced care and support [29].

Patient-centered care also stresses the importance of finding common ground with the patient. In relation to an undiagnosed illness, it may be particularly helpful for physicians and patients to reach a mutual understanding and agreement of the problems. If a full biomedical explanation is not possible, then partial explanations that are consistent with the patient's point of view may be valuable to patients' outcomes [30].

11.3.3.2 Learn Communication Skills

Once somatizing patients have been identified by physicians, these physicians need to develop the following skills:

1. Let the patient know his/her potential diagnosis and its prognosis by explaining test results and the nature of the illness.
2. Use general terms such as "tension" and "stress," and avoid using professional (or psychological) terms to minimize patients' resistance [16].
3. Explain the mechanisms of somatization by giving an example of common somatic symptoms, such as palpitation, headache, and backache [1, 31].
4. Make sure patients will improve when they receive treatment from specialists, such as psychiatrists.
5. Administer the appropriate treatment, which may or may not involve psychiatric referral [1].

11.3.3.3 How to Refer the Patient for Psychiatric or Psychological Assessment

Physicians should learn how to refer somatizing patients for psychiatric or psychological assessment [1] because these patients show resistance to psychological explanations [12]. First, physicians should inform patients about their negative test results and provide explanations for the symptoms [1]. Second, medical students and physicians should be trained to give the patient positive messages based on positive experiences of the therapeutic process for somatizing patients during their clinical clerkship and based on physicians' clinical experiences. For example, such statements may include "I've seen many patients get better after they were referred to specialists and received treatment." Finally, they should develop their skills for referral by practicing this experience or using role-playing.

The abovementioned effective approach to somatizing patients for physicians is presented in the Fig. 11.1 [32].

11.4 Education for Medical Students and Primary Care Physicians

Depression, anxiety, and somatization are the most common mental disorders encountered in primary care [5]. General practitioners (GPs) are usually the first contact person for patients suffering from psychological and physical problems and

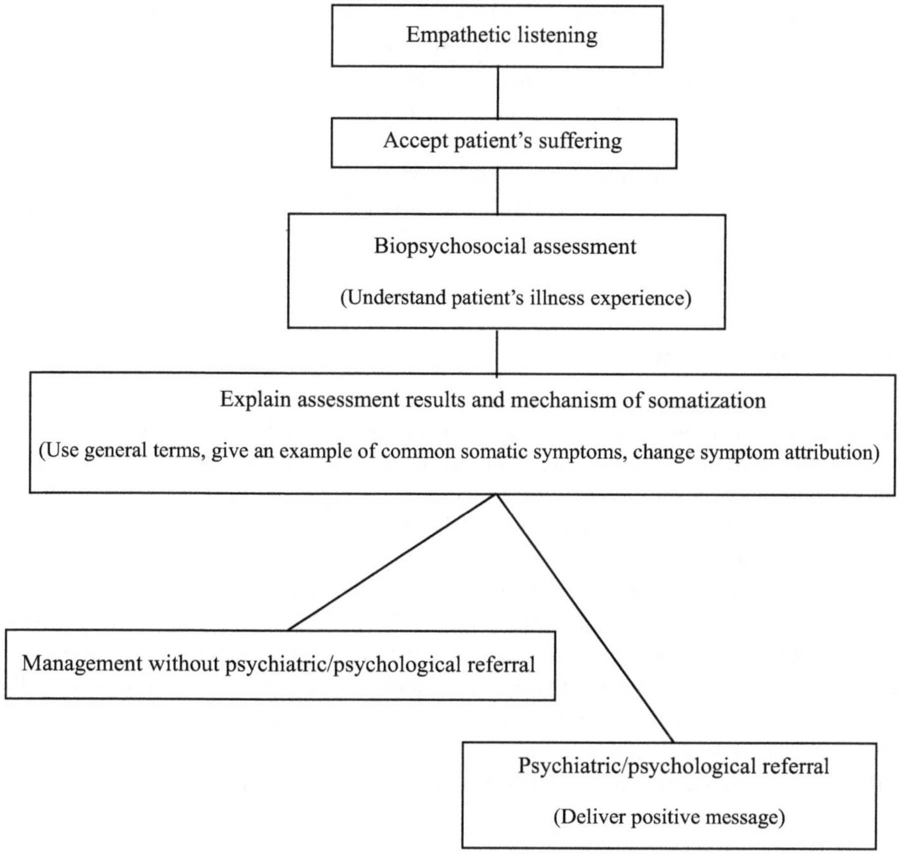

Fig. 11.1 An effective approach to somatization assessment and management for physicians. (From Koh [32])

therefore play a central role in the detection, prevention, and management of mental disorders. Adequate detection and management of these disorders pose a challenge to the health-care system [33–36].

Somatizing patients are good candidates for medical students and primary care physicians to learn about the biopsychosocial approach for patient-centered care because their symptoms cannot be biomedically explained. Primary care physicians feel that effective management strategies are lacking [37, 38]. Therefore, psychological skills should be taught to medical students during their clinical rotations and to GPs during GP training period [1]. During these training periods, psychiatrists play an important role in helping other physicians develop the skills to identify and manage patients with somatization [1].

Educational programs should include information about somatization such as diagnostic criteria for somatization [39]; the role of stress, anger, and mood in the disorder [1, 24]; skills training in biopsychosocial history taking; a general treatment model for somatization; and advice on the management of chronic cases [39].

Several teaching techniques, particularly modeling, role-playing, and video feedback, are known to be effective in teaching psychological skills both to psychiatrists [40] and to GPs [41, 42]. The importance of interview techniques has been stressed in identifying somatizing patients in a few studies [43, 44]. These techniques are often employed when physicians try to reattribute patients' symptoms [43]. Actually most GPs recognize that helping a patient with a psychiatric illness reattribute his or her somatic symptoms to a psychological rather than a physical etiology is an important, but difficult, task [45].

11.5 Conclusions

Interviewing techniques are essential for the identification and management of somatizing patients. Somatizing patients need explanations and understanding, above expectations for support and for tests and diagnosis. In this regard, nonpsychiatric physicians should avoid mind-body dualism. Instead, from the beginning of assessment, equal attention should be devoted to each of biopsychosocial factors. Physicians need to adopt patient-centered care with an emphasis on illness experience as a way of helping somatizing patients. Medical students and primary physicians should learn how to refer a somatizing patient for psychiatric or psychological assessment. Role-playing is known to be effective in teaching psychological skills (e.g., interview techniques) both to psychiatrists and general practitioners. A positive explanation of possible causes, combined with an optimistic prognosis, may be effective in management as well as referral of somatizing patients.

References

1. Bass C, Benjamin S. The management of chronic somatization. Brit J Psychiatry. 1993;162:472–80.
2. Duddu V, Isaac MK, Chaturvedi SK, et al. Somatization, somatosensory amplification, attribution styles and illness behavior: a review. Int Rev Psychiatry. 2006;18:25–33.
3. Koh KB, Ki SW. A comparison of illness behavior among patients with somatoform disorders, depressive disorders and psychosomatic disorders. Kor J Psychosom Med. 1997;5:185–94.
4. Rief W, Hiller W, Margraf J. Cognitive aspects of hypochondriasis and the somatization syndrome. J Abnorm Psychol. 1998;107:587–95.
5. Toft T, Fink P, Oernboel E, et al. Mental disorders in primary care: prevalence and co-morbidity among disorders. Results from the functional illness in primary care (FIP) study. Psychol Med. 2005;35:1175–84.
6. Fink P, Sorensen L, Engberg M, et al. Somatization in primary care. Prevalence, health care utilization, and general practitioner recognition. Psychosomatics. 1999;40:330–8.
7. Arnold IA, de Waal MW, Eekhof JA, et al. Somatoform disorder in primary care: course and the need for cognitive-behavioral treatment. Psychosomatics. 2006;47:498–503.
8. Kroenke K, Mangelsdorff D. Common symptoms in ambulatory care: incidence, evaluation, therapy and outcome. Am J Med. 1989;86:262–6.

9. van Hemert AM, Hengeveld MW, Bolk JH, et al. Psychiatric disorders in relation to medical illness among patients of a general medical out-patient clinic. Psychol Med. 1993;23:167–73.
10. Goldberg D, Bridges K. Screening for psychiatric illness in general practice: the general practitioner versus the screening questionnaire. J R Coll Gen Pract. 1987;37:15–8.
11. Aronowitz RA. When do symptoms become a disease? Ann Intern Med. 2001;134:803–8.
12. Nettleton S, Watt I, O'Malley L, et al. Understanding the narratives of people who live with medically unexplained illness. Patient Educ Couns. 2005;56:205–10.
13. Rhodes LA, McPhillips-Tangum CA, Markham C, et al. The power of the visible: the meaning of diagnostic tests in chronic back pain. Soc Sci Med. 1999;48:1189–203.
14. Fink P. Surgery and medical treatment in persistent somatizing patients. J Psychosom Res. 1992;36:439–47.
15. Smith GR Jr, Monson RA, Ray DC. Patients with multiple unexplained symptoms. Their characteristics, functional health, and health care utilization. Arch Intern Med. 1986;146:69–72.
16. Koh KB. Stress and psychosomatic medicine. Seoul: Ilchokak; 2011. p. 263–85.
17. Price JR. Managing physical symptoms: the clinical assessment as treatment. J Psychosom Res. 2000;48:1–10.
18. Hotopf M, Wadsworth M, Wessely S. Is "somatisation" a defense against the acknowledgment of psychiatric disorder? J Psychosom Res. 2001;50:119–24.
19. Williams S, Weinman J, Dale J, et al. Patient expectations: what do primary care patients want from the GP and how far does meeting expectations affect patient satisfaction? Fam Pract. 1995;12:193–201.
20. Matthews DA, Sledge WH, Lieberman PB, et al. Evaluation of intern performance by medical inpatients. Am J Med. 1987;35:936–44.
21. Gorlin R, Zucker HD. Physician's reactions to patients: a key to teaching humanistic medicine. N Engl J Med. 1983;308:1059–63.
22. Groves JE. Taking care of the hateful patient. N Engl J Med. 1978;298:883–7.
23. Mayou RA, Bass C, Sharpe M. Treatment of functional somatic symptoms. Oxford: Oxford University Press; 1995.
24. Koh KB, Kim DK, Kim SY, et al. The relation between anger management style, mood, and somatic symptoms in anxiety disorders and somatoform disorders. Psychiatry Res. 2008;160:372–9.
25. Lin K. Hwa-byung: a Korean culture-bound syndrome? Am J Psychiatry. 1983;142:798–805.
26. Lee SH. A study on hwa-byung. Kor Hosp J. 1977;1:63–9.
27. Mezzich JE, Lin K, Hughes CC. Acute and transient psychotic disorders and culture-bound syndromes. In: Sadock BJ, Sadock VA, editors. Comprehensive textbook of psychiatry. 7th ed. Baltimore: Lippincott Williams & Wilkins; 2000.
28. Min SK, Lee MH, Shin JH, et al. A diagnostic study of hwa-byung. J Kor Med Assoc. 1986;29:653–61.
29. Stewart M, Brown J, Weston W, et al. Patient-centered medicine transforming the clinical method. Oxford: Radcliffe Medical Press; 2003.
30. Salmon P. Patients who present with physical symptoms in the absence of physical pathology: a challenge to existing models of doctor-patient interaction. Patient Educ Couns. 2000;39:105–13.
31. Sharpe M, Bass C. Pathophysiological mechanisms in somatization. Int Rev Psychiatry. 1992;4:81–97.
32. Koh KB. An effective approach to somatization assessment and management. In: Koh KB, editor. Somatization and psychosomatic symptoms. New York: Springer; 2013. p. 99–111.
33. Henningsen P, Zipfel S, Herzog W. Management of functional somatic syndromes. Lancet. 2007;369:946–55.
34. Aragones E, Pinol JL, Labad A. Depression and physical comorbidity in primary care. J Psychosom Res. 2007;63:107–11.
35. de Waal MW, Arnold IA, Eekhof JA, et al. Follow-up study on health care use of patients with somatoform, anxiety and depressive disorders in primary care. BMC Fam Pract. 2008;9:5.

36. Gask L, Sibbald B, Creed F. Evaluating models of working at the interface between mental health services and primary care. Br J Psychiatry. 1997;170:6–11.
37. Kerwick S, Jones R, Mann A, et al. Mental health care training priorities in general practice. Br J Gen Pract. 1997;47:225–7.
38. Reid S, Whooley D, Crayford T, et al. Medically unexplained symptoms – GPs' attitudes towards their cause and management. Fam Pract. 2001;18:519–23.
39. Fink P, Rosendal M, Toft T. Assessment and treatment of functional disorders in general practice: the extended reattribution and management model – an advanced educational program for nonpsychiatric doctors. Psychosomatics. 2002;43:93–131.
40. Maguire GP, Goldberg DP, Hobson RF, et al. Evaluating the teaching of a method of psychotherapy. Br J Psychiatry. 1984;144:575–80.
41. Goldberg DP, Smith C, Steele JJ, et al. Training family doctors to recognize psychiatric illness with increased accuracy. Lancet. 1980;ii:521–3.
42. Gask L, Goldberg DP, Lesser AL, et al. Improving the psychiatric skills of the general practice trainee: an evaluation of a group training course. Med Educ. 1988;22:132–8.
43. Gask L, Goldberg D, Porter R, et al. The treatment of somatization: evaluation of a teaching package with general practice trainees. J Psychosom Res. 1989;33:697–703.
44. Craig TKJ, Boardman AP. Somatization in primary care settings. In: Bass C, editor. Somatization: physical symptoms and psychological illness. Oxford: Blackwell; 1990.
45. Grol R. To heal or to harm. The prevention of somatic fixation in general practice. London: Royal College of General Practitioners; 1988.

Chapter 12
General Management of Somatization

12.1 Introduction

The number of patients who seek help at primary and secondary care for somatic symptoms which cannot be explained by any known medical condition is enormous. A number of psychological and behavioral interventions for somatic symptoms have been carried out at primary, secondary, and tertiary care settings, and there have recently been more attempts to involve the primary care physicians in the psychological interventions [1].

The basic premise of any psychological intervention in somatizing disorders is that somatization is a universal phenomenon and is a direct consequence of common emotional symptoms such as anxiety or depression (i.e., autonomic arousal symptoms or somatic complaints) [2].

The perception, appraisal, and interpretation of the bodily sensations are known to be influenced by personal factors such as cognitions about health and contextual cues [3]. The following cognitive consequences of symptoms maintain the symptoms: (a) preoccupation and selective attention leading to an increase in worrying and awareness of physical symptoms and (b) catastrophic thinking about the potentially harmful origin of bodily sensations (e.g., fear) and resulting in new symptoms or a lower threshold for symptom perception [1].

Psychological interventions can be broadly classified into delivery or referral by physicians and management by trained physicians or psychiatrists using cognitive behavioral techniques [1]. Herein this chapter focuses on the latter rather than the former. However, overemphasis on psychosocial causation of somatic symptoms further alienates these patients. Such somatic symptoms are not only a source of

"Whenever I see difficult somatizing patients, I think their personal needs and their views on illness should be understood and respected. On one hand, management for these patients requires empathetic patience from therapists. On the other hand, love and care from their important person involved may be a panacea for their illness in some cases."

K. B. Koh, *Stress and Somatic Symptoms*,
https://doi.org/10.1007/978-3-030-02783-4_12

distress and dissatisfaction for patients but also a challenge for professionals. On the other hand, they are grossly neglected by psychiatrists [4–7].

Sharpe et al. [3] proposed a biopsychosocial model to understand unexplained physical symptoms, which takes all the biopsychosocial aspects into consideration and lends itself to the utilization of cognitive behavioral techniques. In addition, psychiatric consultation and psychopharmacotherapy can be used in somatizing patients.

12.2 Cognitive Behavioral Therapy (CBT)

CBT is known to be effective in patients with somatic symptom and related disorders [8]. The central idea of this approach is to focus on consequences rather than the causes of symptoms, providing an opportunity to treat physical symptoms without fruitless discussions of causes. This approach takes into consideration the interaction of the biopsychosocial factors in the perception and maintenance of the somatic symptoms [3].

CBT components are as follows [1]:

1. Relaxation techniques to reduce physiological arousal symptoms
2. Inclusion of pleasurable and meaningful activities to increase activity levels, pacing the activities to reduce strain or overwork
3. Making the link between emotions and the intensity of symptoms by increasing the awareness of emotions and enhancing the communication of thoughts and emotions
4. Modification of dysfunctional beliefs through cognitive restructuring
5. Behavioral experiments to refute the symptom-related catastrophic beliefs
6. Reducing reinforcement of illness behavior

Some of the other components included are problem-solving training, assertiveness training, visualization, graded increases in activity level, coping skills training, biofeedback, exercise, and breathing training [1].

12.2.1 Cognitive Therapy in Medical Care

Cognitive factors may contribute to the genesis of all physical symptoms and to associated distress, disability, and health-care use. A physical symptom has two essential components: the awareness of a bodily sensation and the attribution of abnormality to the sensation. In particular, attributions influence the sufferer's response to the sensation. Therefore, cognitions such as symptom attributions clearly have a role in the presentation of physical symptoms to medical care [9].

Cognitive therapy is a psychological treatment that, in the treatment of persistent and troubling physical symptoms, aims to change symptom attributions and thereby improve outcomes. This therapy is usually conducted individually in ten or more weekly sessions of about 1 h each. Patients are actively involved in testing out and modifying their dysfunctional beliefs about their physical symptoms. Cognitive therapy is time-consuming and expensive [9].

The twin obstacles of availability and acceptability of cognitive therapy can be overcome by integrating aspects of cognitive therapy into medical care [9]. Cognitive therapy of medically unexplained physical symptoms and hypochondriasis includes identifying and challenging patients' evidence for their misinterpretations of bodily sensations [3, 10]. In a general hospital clinic, the clinician may act as a cognitive therapist by eliciting the patient's beliefs, explaining his or her view about the cause of the symptoms, and presenting evidence from the assessment to support his or her view and, if appropriate, challenge the patient's view. Therefore, the clinical assessment, such as history taking, physical examination, and testing, may modify cognitive factors such as symptom attribution and consequently improve outcomes [9].

A cognitive-educational intervention suffices without performing an investigation. There is some randomized evidence to support the therapeutic effect of explanation supported only by history taking and consultation. Perhaps clinicians can evoke similar therapeutic effects by using history taking and clinical examinations as well [11]. In sum, assessment is a vital and powerful part of treatment rather than being merely its subordinate and prelude [9]. Observational studies in patients with headache and bowel symptoms suggest that the consultation itself may improve outcomes [12, 13]. Thus, discussion of the problem and its cause appears to be therapeutic. Changes in symptom attributions are probably the mediator of the therapeutic effects arising from such discussions [9].

The potential power of this cognitive approach in the treatment of physical symptoms is evidenced in trials of cognitive therapy for a range of disorders that present to a general hospital. However, it is not possible to offer formal cognitive therapy to every patient presenting with physical symptoms, and such an approach would not be acceptable to many patients. Simple cognitive approaches may be able to reframe cognitions and result in meaningful improvements in outcomes. These may help patients understand the cause and prognosis of his/her symptoms. History taking, a physical examination, and testing may contribute to evidence that can be used to confirm or refute patients' beliefs. If symptoms remain medically unexplained, a positive explanation of possible causes, combined with an optimistic prognosis, may be effective [9].

12.2.2 Mindfulness-Based Cognitive Therapy (MBCT)

MBCT is a psychological therapy designed to prevent the relapse of depression [14]. It uses a combination of cognitive behavioral therapy (CBT) methods and psychological strategies such as mindfulness and mindfulness meditation. Cognitive methods include educating the participant about depression [15]. Mindfulness and mindfulness meditation focus on becoming aware of all incoming thoughts and feelings and accepting them, but not attaching or reacting to them [16]. The goal of MBCT is to interrupt recurring automatic cognitive processes and teach the participants to focus less on reacting to incoming stimuli and instead accepting and observing them without judgment [17].

One meta-analysis indicated a small to moderate positive effect of mindfulness-based therapy (MBT) (compared to waitlist or support group controls) in reducing pain, symptom severity, depression, and anxiety associated with somatizing disorders (e.g., fibromyalgia, chronic fatigue syndrome, irritable bowel syndrome) and improving the quality of life in patients with these disorders. Mindfulness-based stress reduction (MBSR) and MBCT were found to be more effective than eclectic/unspecified MBT [18].

MBCT can help improve mental functioning (e.g., vitality and social functioning) in patients with persistent and medically unexplained symptoms, although it may not improve physical functioning [19]. Change of unhelpful behavioral patterns and increased self-care and self-compassion can also result from this process [20]. In particular, the fact that patients increased their use of mental health care after MBCT indicates that somatizing patients become more willing to receive mental health care. In this respect, MBCT can be considered a meaningful therapy for patients with somatizing disorders [21].

12.3 Psychiatric Consultation as Therapeutic Strategy

Psychiatric consultation was known to be one of the most effective interventions for patients with somatoform disorders (somatic symptom and related disorders in DSM-5) [22]. Psychiatric consultation followed by a management planning letter has been found to offer only modest benefit in the health status or the satisfaction of the patients [23]. At that time, psychiatric consultation can effectively be used as a moderator in transition from primary physicians to psychiatrists so that patients' resistance to direct psychiatric approach can be minimized. In particular, education for patients and primary physicians and joint visit (conjoint interviews by a psychiatrist and a primary physician) are known to lower the morbidity of mental disorders such as depressive disorders rather than individual short-term intervention by a psychiatrist without collaboration with primary physicians [24].

12.4 Psychopharmacotherapy

Psychopharmacotherapy is essential for management of somatization due to the following reasons [25]:

1. A high proportion of patients with somatic symptom and related disorders have comorbid anxiety and depressive disorders which are often underdetected and inadequately treated. Sometimes somatic presentation could be an underlying depressive or anxiety disorder itself.

2. Medications are more acceptable to patients as they may feel relieved when there is something wrong and treatment is available.
3. Pharmacotherapy is cost-effective and simple.
4. Physicians are at ease in prescribing medication rather than focusing on finding a psychosocial cause of somatic symptoms which is speculative rather than a proof.
5. Selective serotonin reuptake inhibitors (SSRIs) and serotonin and noradrenalin reuptake inhibitors (SNRIs) act both peripherally and centrally in reducing the perception of pain and other heightened perceptions, a common presenting symptom in patients with somatization [26, 27]. The common side effects such as somnolence and increased appetite of some of the antidepressants can be a therapeutic advantage as many patients have poor sleep and appetite.

In clinical practice, all classes of psychotropics such as tricyclic antidepressants, SSRIs, SNRIs, anxiolytics, atypical antipsychotics, and herbal medication are effective in a wide range of disorders. In particular, antidepressants seem to be effective against somatizing disorders [25].

12.4.1 Antidepressants

Antidepressants are the most commonly used class of drugs for somatization. There is merit in using antidepressants for a number of reasons: pain is often a common presenting symptom in patients with somatization, and antidepressants have analgesic property. In addition, somatic symptoms may be a presentation of undiagnosed anxiety and depressive disorder [26–28].

Antidepressants with dual action of serotonin and noradrenaline such as SNRIs (e.g., venlafaxine, duloxetine) seem more effective than other antidepressants if pain is the main symptom, and SSRIs (e.g., fluoxetine, paroxetine) seem to be more effective in hypochondriasis [25].

12.4.2 Practical Issues for Psychopharmacotherapy

The following factors are important in planning psychopharmacological treatment for somatization [25].

1. Provide symptomatic treatment until a definite etiology and intervention are identified.
2. Prepare patients for psychopharmacotherapy by explaining the rationale, expected outcome, and common side effects before initiation of medication.
3. Focus on care rather than cause or cure.
4. Aim at improving the quality of life.
5. Focus on relief, coping, and return to function.

6. Give adequate trial for at least 12 weeks before declaring any drug as ineffective and explain it to patients so that they will expect improvement over several weeks or months.
7. Emphasize that different treatments may act synergistically. Psychological treatments are not a substitute for pharmacological treatment, and different treatments are complementary.
8. Start at a low dose and titrate gradually over weeks as these patients are usually sensitive to side effects. Compliance can be an issue if the medication is titrated upward too quickly.

12.5 Integrated Therapy

None of the therapeutic methods on their own has provided a satisfactory outcome [8, 29]. A paradigm shift is required in conceptualization and management of somatization. There is urgent need to explore interventions beyond psychological interventions to retain responsibility for this group of patients [25]. Considering the limitations of time for physicians, an integrated brief therapy is recommended for such patients. This form of therapy should be multimodal by combining the effective components of therapy from different therapeutic models [1]. Particularly, it is desirable to integrate the psychiatric consultation, CBT, and psychopharmacotherapy for somatizing patients.

12.6 Primary Care Treatment for Somatization

Primary care treatment for somatization has taken two main directions. One approach is shared care, where mental health specialists offer patient assessment and treatment guidelines [30]. Another approach is the education for primary care physicians to improve their management of somatization within their own setting by using the reattribution model [30, 31].

Some of the skills described in this chapter and Chap. 11 have been successfully taught to general practice trainees using videotaped learning packages [32]. Another education program including the reattribution model for primary care physicians has been tested in a 3-month, pre-post study and has reported positive effects on patients' physical functioning, psychiatric disorder symptoms [30], illness attributions, and satisfaction [31]. However, the training of primary care physicians was not found to have a significant effect on clinical outcomes and may not result in any significant improvement in patient satisfaction with care for those scoring high for somatization in a few areas such as doctor-patient relationship, medical-technical care, and information and support [33]. This research suggests that physicians will have to receive long-term training from specialists such as psychiatrists in order to manage these somatizing patients effectively. Otherwise, physicians should focus on referral process rather than management.

12.7 Conclusions

Cognitive behavioral therapy (CBT) is known to be effective in patients with somatic symptom and related disorders. History taking, physical examination, and investigations can be used to confirm or refute the patients' beliefs. Mindfulness-based cognitive therapy (MBCT) can help improve mental functioning (e.g., vitality and social functioning) in somatizing patients and change unhelpful behavioral patterns and increase self-care. In particular, MBCT can be considered a meaningful therapy for patients with somatizing disorders because it encourages them more willing to receive mental health care. Psychiatric consultation can be used as therapeutic strategy. In addition, psychopharmacotherapy is essential for management of somatization. Considering the limitations of time for physicians, an integrated brief therapy is recommended for such patients. This form of therapy should be multimodal by combining psychiatric consultation, CBT, and psychopharmacotherapy.

References

1. Sharma MP, Manjula M. Behavioral and psychological management of somatic symptom disorders: an overview. Int Rev Psychiatry. 2013;25:116–24.
2. Patel V, Sumathipala A. Psychological approaches to somatization in developing countries. Adv Psychiatry Treat. 2006;12:54–62.
3. Sharpe M, Peveler R, Mayou R. The psychological treatment of patients with functional somatic symptoms: a practical guide. J Psychosom Res. 1992;36:515–29.
4. Bass C, Benjamin S. The management of chronic somatization. Brit J Psychiatry. 1993;162:472–80.
5. Bass C, Peveler R, House A. Somatoform disorder: severe psychiatric illnesses neglected by psychiatrists. Brit J Psychiatry. 2001;179:11–4.
6. Fink P, Rosenthal M. Recent developments in the understanding and management of functional somatic symptoms in primary care. Curr Opin Psychiatry. 2008;21:182–8.
7. Kroenke K. Patients presenting with somatic complaints: epidemiology, psychiatric comorbidity and management. Int J Methods Psychiatr Res. 2003;12:34–43.
8. Kroenke K. Efficacy of treatment for somatoform disorders: a review of randomized controlled trials. Psychosom Med. 2007;69:881–8.
9. Price JR. Managing physical symptoms: the clinical assessment as treatment. J Psychosom Res. 2000;48:1–10.
10. Salkovskis PM. Somatic problems. In: Hawton K, Salkovskis PM, Kirk J, et al., editors. Cognitive behavior therapy for psychiatric problems. A practical guide. Oxford: Oxford University Press; 1989.
11. Thomas KB. General practice consultations: is there any point in being positive? BMJ. 1987;294:1200–2.
12. Fitzpatrick RM, Hopkins A. Referrals to neurologists for headaches not due to structural disease. J Neurol Neurosurg Psychiatry. 1981;44:1061–7.
13. van Dulmen A, Fennis JF, Mokkink HG, et al. Doctor-dependent changes in complaint-related cognitions and anxiety during medical consultations in functional abdominal complaints. Psychol Med. 1995;25:1011–8.
14. Piet J, Hougaard E. The effect of mindfulness-based cognitive therapy for prevention of relapse in recurrent major depressive disorder: a systematic review and meta-analysis. Clin Psychol Rev. 2011;31:1032–40.

15. Manicavasgar V, Parker G, Perich T. Mindfulness-based cognitive therapy vs cognitive behavior therapy as a treatment for non-melancholic depression. J Affect Disord. 2011;130:138–44.
16. Hofmann SG, Sawyer AT, Fang A. The empirical status of the new wave of cognitive behavioral therapy. Psychiatr Clin N Am. 2010;33:701–10.
17. Felder JN, Dimidjian S, Segal Z. Collaboration in mindfulness-based cognitive therapy. J Clin Psychol. 2012;68:179–86.
18. Lakhan SE, Schhofield KL. Mindfulness-based therapies in the treatment of somatization disorders: a systematic review and meta-analysis. PLoS One. 2013;8:e71834.
19. van Ravesteijn H, Lucassen P, Bor H, et al. Mindfulness-based cognitive therapy for patients with medically unexplained symptoms: a randomized controlled trial. Psychother Psychosom. 2013;82:299–310.
20. van Ravesteijn H, Suijkerbuijk YB, Langbroek JA, et al. Mindfulness-based cognitive therapy for patients with medically unexplained symptoms: process of change. J Psychosom Res. 2014;77:27–33.
21. van Ravesteijn H. Mindfulness-based cognitive therapy for patients with somatoform disorders. Tijdschr Psychiatry. 2016;58:198–206.
22. Smith GR Jr. Effectiveness of treatment for somatoform disorder patients. Psychiatry Med. 1991;9:545–58.
23. van der Feltz-Cornelis CM, van Oppen P, Ader HJ, et al. Randomized controlled trial of a collaborative care model with psychiatric consultation for persistent medically unexplained symptoms in general practice. Psychother Psychosom. 2006;75:282–9.
24. Strain JJ. Consultation-liaison psychiatry. In: Sadock BJ, Sadock VA, editors. Comprehensive textbook of psychiatry. 7th ed. Baltimore: Lippincott Williams & Wilkins; 2000.
25. Somashekar B, Jainer A, Wuntakal B. Psychopharmacotherapy of somatic symptoms disorders. Int Rev Psychiatry. 2013;25:107–15.
26. Linch ME. Antidepressants as analgesics: a review of randomized controlled trials. J Psychiatry Neurosci. 2001;26:30–6.
27. Sussman N. SNRIs versus SSRIs: mechanisms of action in treating depressions and painful physical symptoms. Primary Care Companion J Clin Psychiatry. 2003;5:19–26.
28. Fishbain DA, Cutler RB, Rosomoff HL. Do antidepressants have an analgesic effect in psychogenic pain and somatoform pain disorder? A meta-analysis. Psychosom Med. 1998;60:503–9.
29. Noyes R Jr, Holt CS, Kathol RG. Somatization: diagnosis and management. Arch Fam Med. 1995;4:790–5.
30. Morriss R, Gask L, Ronalds C, et al. Clinical and patient satisfaction outcomes of a new treatment for somatized mental disorder taught to general practitioners. Br J Gen Pract. 1999;49:262–7.
31. Morriss RK, Gask L. Treatment of patients with somatized mental disorder: effects of reattribution training on outcomes under the direct control of the family doctor. Psychosomatics. 2002;43:394–9.
32. Gask L, Goldberg D, Porter R, et al. The treatment of somatization: evaluation of a teaching package with general practice trainees. J Psychosom Res. 1989;33:697–703.
33. Rosendal M, Olesen F, Fink P, et al. A randomized controlled trial of brief training in the assessment and treatment of somatization in primary care: effects on patient outcome. Gen Hosp Psychiatry. 2007;29:364–73.

Chapter 13
Approach to Somatic Symptom and Related Disorders

13.1 Introduction

The DSM-5 changed the term "somatoform disorders" to "somatic symptom and related disorders" and further modified diagnostic labels and criteria [1]. This new category includes the diagnoses of somatic symptom disorder, illness anxiety disorder, conversion disorder (functional neurological symptom disorder), psychological factors affecting other medical conditions (PFAOMC), and factitious disorder [2]. DSM-5 emphasizes a positive criterion, namely, maladaptive reaction to a somatic symptom, instead of the earlier negative criterion, namely, that the symptoms should be medically unexplained [1].

Somatic symptom and related disorders have some characteristics such as chronicity, social dysfunction, occupational difficulties, increased healthcare use, dissatisfaction for both the clinician and the patient [3], and resistance to psychiatric assessment and treatment [4–6].

Individuals with these disorders are commonly encountered in primary care and other medical settings but are less commonly encountered in psychiatric and other mental health settings. Therefore, these reconceptualized diagnoses are more useful for primary care and other medical (nonpsychiatric) clinicians [2].

13.2 Etiological Factors of Somatic Symptom and Related Disorders

A number of factors may contribute to somatic symptom and related disorders. These include genetic and biological vulnerability (e.g., increased sensitivity to pain), early traumatic experiences (e.g., abuse, deprivation), and learning (e.g., attention obtained from illness), as well as social/cultural norms that stigmatize psychological suffering as compared with physical suffering. In addition, variations

K. B. Koh, *Stress and Somatic Symptoms*,
https://doi.org/10.1007/978-3-030-02783-4_13

in symptom presentation are likely the result of the interaction of multiple factors within cultural contexts that affect how individuals identify and classify bodily sensations, perceive illness, and seek medical attention for them. Thus, somatic presentations can be viewed as expressions of personal suffering inserted in a social and cultural context [2].

13.3 Somatic Symptom Disorder

Patients with somatic symptom disorder may include individuals who were considered in the past for a diagnosis of somatization disorder, pain disorder, and undifferentiated somatoform disorder. This disorder is characterized by excessive thoughts, feelings, and behaviors as reactions to somatic symptoms. These patients are often unresponsive to medical interventions. Some patients with the disorder seem unusually sensitive to medication side effects [2].

Management of patients with somatic symptom disorder is described in detail in other chapters such as interview techniques for somatizing patients and general management of somatization as well as approach to chronic pain.

13.4 Illness Anxiety Disorder

In DSM-5, hypochondriasis was renamed “illness anxiety disorder.” This disorder refers to preoccupation with and fear of having a serious physical disorder over a period of 6 months despite no abnormal findings and reassurance after a thorough medical evaluation [2]. The terms “hypochondriasis” and “illness anxiety disorder” are used interchangeably here.

Patients with hypochondriasis repeatedly visit their physicians with a variety of concerns, often interpreting them as indicative of a serious disease. They often seek medical care because they are concerned or anxious about having a specific disease, rather than because they are troubled by a specific symptom. Usually these patients can be reassured only temporarily by hearing that the symptom is not a reflection of serious organic pathology [7].

13.4.1 Risk Factors

Their child home was frequently without emotional warmth except when someone was ill. They are often emotionally constricted and have difficulty in communicating to others except through physical complaints [8–10].

Some psychodynamic theories of the mechanisms of hypochondriasis have been proposed. Schmale [11] postulates that focusing anxiety on bodily functions is a defense against acting out a forbidden wish. Sullivan proposes that hypochondriasis is a defense against low self-esteem, while Engel [12] and Lipsitt [13] propose that it is a defense against guilt or innate badness. Barsky and Klerman [14] have suggested hypochondriasis is a kind of amplification of somatic symptoms.

Illness anxiety disorder may sometimes be precipitated by a major life stressor or a serious but ultimately benign threat to the individual's health. A history of childhood abuse or of a serious childhood illness may predispose to development of the disorder in adulthood. Hypochondriacal symptoms may be the presentation of somatized depression [15, 16].

13.4.2 Management

First, the goal of management for hypochondriacal patients is to avoid unnecessary diagnostic testing and to obviate overly aggressive medical and surgical intervention. Second, the physicians help the patient cope with and tolerate his/her symptoms, rather than trying to eliminate them completely. And third, the physicians should try to build a durable relationship with the patient, based on their interest in the patient as a person and not just in his/her symptoms. The primary physician needs to appreciate that these patients have psychosocial reasons for being symptomatic and that no medical intervention can cure their need to feel sick [17].

Hypochondriacs are more often harmed by overaggressive than underaggressive medical management. Therefore, the best medical interventions should be modest, simple, and benign (e.g., frequent physical examinations and vitamins). The most successful psychiatric interventions with these patients are probably cognitive, educational, and supportive, as opposed to insight-oriented psychotherapy [17]. Some clinicians feel that these patients tend to do better in group therapy than in individual therapy [18]. Behavioral therapy and hypnosis may be useful. Psychopharmacotherapy alleviates hypochondriacal symptoms only when a patient has an underlying drug-responsive condition, such as anxiety disorder or major depressive disorder [19].

Case

A middle-aged woman visited the department of internal medicine, being afraid of having a serious disease such as stomach cancer despite mild digestive disturbance. However, no abnormalities were found on gastroscopy. She was therefore transferred to the department of psychiatry. Her neighbor had suffered from indigestion and died several days after she was diagnosed with stomach cancer. The patient was shocked, because she experienced similar symptoms such as indigestion and abdominal discomfort. Thereafter, she began to show intolerable anxiety, guessing she might have stomach cancer, and visited a number of internists for gastric examinations, which revealed no abnormalities. Despite the physicians' reassurance, she did not accept their explanation. Rather, she was suspicious that the physicians were trying to hide the diagnosis of stomach cancer from her. She continued to be anxious for a considerable period of time after she was transferred to the department of psychiatry and treated with medication such as antianxiety and antidepressant agents as well as with supportive psychotherapy.

13.5 Conversion Disorder

In DSM-5, conversion disorder is called functional neurological symptom disorder. This disorder refers to neurological symptoms or deficits. However, the manifestations are incompatible with known pathophysiologic mechanisms or anatomic pathways [2].

The most frequent symptoms include paralysis, anesthesia, movement disorders, or sensory changes (e.g., vision, hearing) [7]. Episodes of abnormal generalized limb shaking with apparent loss of consciousness may resemble epileptic seizures (also called psychogenic or non-epileptic seizures) [2].

Although the diagnosis requires that the symptom is not explained by neurological disease, it should not be made simply because results from investigations are normal or because the symptom is bizarre. There must be clinical findings that show clear evidence of incompatibility with neurological disease [2].

Conversion disorder may coexist with neurological disease [2]. However, the differentiation of conversion disorder from neurologic disease is often very difficult because conversion symptoms appear to occur more frequently when there is an underlying neurologic disease [20, 21] or a history of head trauma. A significant number of patients who have persistent conversion symptoms will later develop an organic disease that, in retrospect, will explain the original symptoms [22]. While assessment of stress and trauma is important, the diagnosis should not be withheld if none is found [2].

13.5.1 Risk Factors

The potential etiological relevance of stress or trauma may be suggested by a close temporal relationship [2]. Three major theories have been proposed to explain the etiology of conversion phenomena: neurophysiologic, behavioral, and psychoanalytic theories [23]. Neurophysiologic theories suggest that there is an inherent defect or weakness in certain brain functions. Ludwig [24] proposed a theoretical model of hysteria which suggested that the disorder is basically a dysfunction of attention and recent memory due to corticofugal inhibition of afferent stimulation. In addition, bifrontal impairment and a greater global dysfunction of the nondominant hemisphere were exhibited in these patients, when compared to normal controls [25].

Behavioral theories of conversion phenomena suggest that the patient has learned methods to communicate feelings of helplessness and to elicit environmental changes through his/her symptoms. Thus, learned helplessness during childhood can be used in adulthood to manipulate and control one's interpersonal relationships, including relationships with physicians [26, 27]. It is also possible that certain physiologic responses are learned through prior experiences and then evoked as conversion disorders in responses to certain stimuli [28].

Psychoanalytic theories stress the importance of the symbolic communication of the conversion phenomenon and assert that the symptoms provide a compromise between the instinctual drives and their prohibitions [8, 29, 30]. Engel [31] suggests that the conversion symptom has four unconsciously determined aims. They are (1) to permit expression of the forbidden wish but disguised in such a manner as not to be recognized by the person with the symptom nor by the person for whom it was intended, (2) to impose punishment through suffering and disability for having such a wish, (3) to remove the person from a threatening or disturbing life situation, and (4) to provide a new method of relating to others, the sick role.

The various explanations are not mutually exclusive because a mixture of factors may be operative for any one patient or different factors in different patients [8].

13.5.2 Management

Most conversion symptoms are transient and may remit spontaneously or respond to a wide variety of therapeutic interventions, such as suggestive therapies (e.g., hypnosis), psychotherapy, or environmental manipulation [32]. Often the key element in the therapeutic approach is to allow the patient the opportunity to discard the symptom in a face-saving manner [7].

Some persistent symptoms are perpetuated by positive reinforcers in the environment, such as family attention or financial benefits from disability. Patients with persistent symptoms often require intensive diagnostic and therapeutic interventions, such as inpatient psychiatric hospitalization and utilization of behavioral modification techniques, to extinguish this form of abnormal illness behavior [7].

With patients who are resistant to the idea of psychotherapy, physicians can suggest that the psychotherapy will focus on issues of stress and coping. Hypnosis, anxiolytics, and behavioral relaxation exercises are effective in some cases. Parenteral lorazepam may be helpful in obtaining additional historic information, especially when a patient has recently experienced a traumatic event [19].

Suggesting that the conversion symptom will improve ordinarily begins with the reassuring news that tests of the involved body system show no damage and therefore recovery is certain. However, confrontation is seldom helpful. If the conversion symptom persists, if precipitating stress is chronic, or if there is massive secondary gain, then resolution of the situation becomes a target of the intervention [17].

Psychodynamic approaches such as psychoanalysis and insight-oriented psychotherapy may be used for patients with conversion disorder in order to explore their intrapsychic conflicts and the symbolism of the conversion symptoms [19].

Since the stressors are often social, couple or family therapy may be instrumental in achieving final resolution. In general, a favorable outcome depends more on the patient's psychological strengths and on the absence of other psychopathology than on the specific nature of the conversion symptom itself [17]. The longer the duration of the patients' sick role and the more they have regressed, the more difficult the treatment [19].

Case
A 45-year-old woman was admitted to the department of psychiatry with aphonia after no organic abnormalities were found during examinations at the ear, nose, and throat (ENT) department. At first, she was defensive, denying any stressful events. She had, however, recently learned about her husband's extramarital affair with another woman. From that moment, she was not able to pronounce anything she was trying to say. However, her symptoms rapidly improved after treatment, including supportive psychotherapy and medication such as antianxiety and antidepressant agents.

13.6 Psychological Factors Affecting Other Medical Conditions (PFAOMC)

In DSM-5, PFAOMC (previously called psychosomatic disorders) is also included in somatic symptom-related disorders. Its essential feature is the presence of one or more clinically significant psychological or behavioral factors that adversely affect the course or outcome of a medical condition. Psychological or behavioral factors include psychological distress, patterns of interpersonal interaction, coping styles, and maladaptive health behaviors, such as denial of symptoms or poor adherence to medical recommendations [2].

13.6.1 Management

In the treatment of PFAOMC, reassurance and the process of improving patients' life situations are needed. Patients with PFAOMC are usually more reluctant to deal with their emotional problems than patients with other psychiatric problems. Therefore, psychiatrists must focus therapy on understanding the motivations and mechanisms of disturbed functioning and helping patients realize the nature of their illness and the implications of its costly adaptive patterns. These insights can lead to changed and healthier patterns of behavior [19].

Group therapy and family therapy are helpful in patients with PFAOMC. Family therapy offers hope of a change in the relationship between family members who are often mentally stressed and reactively hostile to the sick member. In addition, relaxation techniques, hypnosis, and biofeedback can be tried for these patients [19].

Management of PFAOMC is described in other chapters which address individual physical diseases and functional physical disorders.

13.7 Factitious Disorder

Factitious disorder is an illness in which patients artificially produce symptoms themselves in the absence of obvious external rewards and try to seek sick roles. In the majority of reported cases of factitious disorder, individuals present with somatic symptoms. In DSM-5, factitious disorder is included among the somatic symptom-related disorders [2].

Onset is usually in early adulthood, often after hospitalization for a medical condition or a mental disorder [7]. Malingering is differentiated from factitious disorder by the intentional reporting of symptoms for external gains (e.g., to obtain disability or compensation payments or to avoid conscription into military service) [2]. The motivation of factitious disorder is believed to be determined by intrapsychic or interpersonal reasons [7].

13.7.1 Management

No specific psychiatric therapy has been effective in factitious disorder patients. Thus, treatment is best focused on management rather than on cure. In general, working in concert with the patient's primary care physician is more effective than working with the patient in isolation. The staff should remain aware that even though the patient's illness is factitious, the patient is ill. At the same time, the therapist needs to be mindful of countertransference whenever he/she suspects factitious disorder [19].

The therapeutic approach to factitious disorder begins with confronting the patient with the physician's knowledge of the behavior. This can be done in a supportive manner that conveys the physician's concern for the patient and willingness to be helpful [33]. For those who accept psychiatric treatment, the techniques of psychotherapy are those that would be appropriate for treatment of borderline personality [34]. Occasionally some patients with factitious disorder have an underlying depression. These patients' prognosis is better because depression is a treatable disorder [7]. Psychopharmacotherapy of factitious disorder is of limited use. Selective serotonin reuptake inhibitors (SSRIs) may be useful in decreasing impulsive behavior in acting-out factitious behavior [19].

On the other hand, for patients with malingering whose symptoms are not so distinct to differentiate from conversion disorder, suggestions that the etiology of the symptom is known and that improvement is expected may have remarkable therapeutic effects [35]. This may be more effective if done in a face-saving manner for the patient rather than by direct confrontation [7].

Case 1
A 65-year-old woman was admitted to the eye department of a general hospital with sudden loss of vision, but physical and neurological examinations did not reveal any abnormalities. She was therefore transferred to the department of psychiatry. She did not complain of anything except her loss of vision. However, she seemed indifferent and defensive, not expressing her feelings for a considerable period of time. Later, one of her family members revealed that she had experienced a serious conflict with her son-in-law due to economic problems. When he asked her to lend him money, she refused. Thereafter, he avoided her eyes whenever he met her while they were living in the same house. Supportive psychotherapy and medication, including the antianxiety agent ethyl loflazepate and the antidepressant amitriptyline, did not improve her symptoms. After being discharged from the hospital without improvement, the patient continued to complain of her loss of vision when visiting the outpatient department; she was not able to see the knob in front of the door when leaving the room after the interview was finished. However, at home she was found picking up hair in her room by a family member.

Case 2
A 20-year-old military serviceman was admitted to the department of psychiatry at a military hospital, via the emergency room, with a generalized convulsion. According to a colleague, he suddenly lost consciousness and started convulsing while undergoing hard physical training. Soon after he was transferred to the psychiatric ward, he knelt down and confessed that he had feigned the seizure attack in order to avoid the hard physical training.

The first of these two cases was initially considered conversion disorder, but later diagnosed as factitious disorder. The latter case was categorized as malingering.

13.8 Conclusions

The DSM-5 changed the term "somatoform disorders" to "somatic symptom and related disorders." This new category includes the diagnoses of somatic symptom disorder, illness anxiety disorder, conversion disorder (functional neurological symptom disorder), psychological factors affecting other medical conditions (PFAOMC), and factitious disorder. DSM-5 emphasizes a positive criterion, namely, maladaptive reaction to a somatic symptom, instead of the earlier negative criterion, namely, that the symptoms should be medically unexplained. Assessment and management of each of these disorders along with risk factors were addressed. In addition, case examples related to each of somatic symptom and related disorders, particularly illness anxiety disorder, conversion disorder, and factitious disorder, were presented. Somatic symptom disorder was described in more detail in Chap. 14.

References

1. Van der Feltz-Cornelis CM, van Houdenhove B. DSM-5: from ‘somatoform disorders’ to ‘somatic symptom and related disorders.’. Tijdschr Psychiatr. 2014;56:182–6.
2. American Psychiatric Association (APA). Statistical and diagnostic manual of mental disorders. 5th ed. Washington, DC: Am Psychiatric Publishing; 2013.
3. Sharma MP, Manjula M. Behavioral and psychological management of somatic symptom disorders: an overview. Int Rev Psychiatry. 2013;25:116–24.
4. Barsky AJ. Somatoform disorders. In: Kaplan HI, Sodock BJ, editors. Comprehensive textbook of psychiatry. 5th ed. Baltimore: Williams & Wilkins; 1989. p. 1009–27.
5. Nettleton S, Watt I, O’Malley L, et al. Understanding the narratives of people who live with medically unexplained illness. Patient Educ Couns. 2005;56:205–10.
6. Koh KB, Ki SW. A comparison of illness behavior among patients with somatoform disorders, depressive disorders and psychosomatic disorders. Korean J Psychosom Med. 1997;5:185–94.
7. Ford CV, Smith GR Jr. Somatoform disorders, factitious disorder, and disability syndromes. In: Stoudemire A, Fogel BS, editors. Principles of medical psychiatry. Orlando: Grune & Stratton; 1987.
8. Ford CV. The somatizing disorders: illness as a way of life. New York: Elsevier; 1983.
9. Kenyon FE. Hypochondriasis: a survey of some historical, clinical and social aspects. Br J Med Psychol. 1965;38:117–33.
10. Pilowsky I. Primary and secondary hypochondriasis. Acta Psychiatr Scand. 1970;47:484–509.
11. Schmale AH. Somatic expressions and consequences of conversion reactions. NY State Med J. 1969;69:1878–84.
12. Engel GC. Psychogenic pain and the pain prone patient. Am J Med. 1959;26:899–918.
13. Lipsitt DR. Medical and psychological characteristics of crocks. Psychiatry Med. 1970;1:15–25.
14. Barsky AJ, Klerman GL. Hypochondriasis, bodily complaints, and somatic styles. Am J Psychiatry. 1983;140:273–83.
15. Katon W, Kleinman A, Rosen G. Depression and somatization: a review (part 1). Am J Med. 1982;72:127–35.
16. Katon W, Kleinman A, Rosen G. Depression and somatization: a review (part 2). Am J Med. 1982;72:241–7.
17. Cassem NH, Barsky AJ. Functional somatic symptoms and somatoform disorders. In: Cassem NH, editor. MGH handbook of general hospital psychiatry. 3rd ed. St Louis: Mosby Year Book; 1991.
18. Barsky AJ, Geringer E, Wool CA. A cognitive-educational treatment for hypochondriasis. Gen Hosp Psychiatry. 1988;10:322–7.
19. Sadock BJ, Sadock VA. Synopsis of psychiatry – behavioral sciences/clinical psychiatry. 9th ed. Philadelphia: Lippincott Williams & Wilkins; 2003.
20. Caplan LR, Nadelson T. Multiple sclerosis and hysteria: lessons learned from their association. JAMA. 1980;243:2418–21.
21. Merskey H, Buhrich NA. Hysteria and organic brain disease. Br J Med Psychol. 1975;48:359–66.
22. Watson CG, Buranen C. The frequency and identification of false positive conversion reactions. J Nerv Ment Dis. 1979;167:243–7.
23. Jones MM. Conversion reaction: Anachronism or evolutionary form: a review of the neurologic, behavioral, and psychoanalytic literature. Psychol Bull. 1980;87:427–41.
24. Ludwig AM. Hysteria: a neurobiological theory. Arch Gen Psychiatry. 1972;27:771–7.
25. Flor-Henry P, Fromm-Auch D, Tapper M, et al. A neuropsychological study of the stable syndrome of hysteria. Biol Psychiatry. 1981;16:601–26.
26. Halleck SL. Hysterical personality traits. Arch Gen Psychiatry. 1967;16:750–7.
27. Celani D. An interpersonal approach to hysteria. Am J Psychiatry. 1976;133:1414–8.
28. Barr R, Abernethy V. Single case study: conversion reaction: differential diagnosis in the light of biofeedback research. J Nerv Ment Dis. 1977;164:287–92.

29. Hollender MH. Conversion hysteria: a post-Freudian reinterpretation of 19th century psychosocial data. Arch Gen Psychiatry. 1972;26:311–4.
30. Hollender MH. Hysteria: the culture-bound syndromes. P N G Med J. 1976;19:24–9.
31. Engel GL. Conversion symptoms. In: Macbryde CM, Blacklow RS, editors. Sign and symptoms: applied pathologic physiology and clinical interpretation. 5th ed. Philadelphia: Lippincott; 1970.
32. Folks DG, Ford CV, Regan WM. Conversion symptoms in a general hospital. Psychosomatics. 1984;25:285–95.
33. Hollander MH, Hersh SP. Impossible consultation made possible. Arch Gen Psychiatry. 1970;23:343–5.
34. Stone MH. Factitious illness: psychological findings and treatment recommendations. Bull Menninger Clin. 1977;3:239–54.
35. Krammer KK, LaPiana FG, Appleton B. Ocular malingering and hysteria: diagnosis and management. Surv Ophthalmol. 1979;24:89–96.

Chapter 14
Approach to Chronic Pain

14.1 Introduction

In the past (DSM-IV), pain disorder refers to preoccupation with pain for more than 6 months despite the absence of either organic pathology or pathophysiological mechanism [1]. In the DSM-5, however, pain disorder was excluded and instead included in "somatic symptom disorder" [2].

Patients with pain cite it as the source of all their misery. Such patients often deny any other sources of emotional dysphoria and insist that their lives are blissful except for their pain [3]. Pain patients go "doctor shopping" due to their persistent pain. They believe that their pain arises from physical problems so that they look for physicians who will relieve pain by using specific treatment method [4].

In particular, pain causes not only emotional problems such as anxiety and depression but also makes patients difficult to adapt to their occupational and social life, leading to familial conflicts and even familial disintegration. In addition, they may abuse drugs, undergo unnecessary examinations and surgery, and commit suicide due to a sense of hopelessness and helplessness. They are often absent from work and leave their jobs, resulting in a huge economic loss for individuals and their society.

The problem in the treatment of such patients is that physicians are trying to treat pain patients based on biological model. Their symptoms are likely to be prolonged as their underlying psychosocial problems are not addressed. Therefore, biopsychosocial aspects of pain are emphasized in regard to the assessment and treatment of pain.

K. B. Koh, *Stress and Somatic Symptoms*,
https://doi.org/10.1007/978-3-030-02783-4_14

14.2 Etiology

14.2.1 Biological Factors

There are some neurophysiological theories on pain perception: gate control theory, specific theory, and pattern theory [5]. Gate control theory is a hypothesis that gate control mechanism situated in substantia gelatinosa of the dorsal horn of the spinal cord plays the role of a gate in controlling transmission of pain signals from the peripheral nerves to the central nervous system [1]. Nerve fibers with large diameter have inhibitory effects on this mechanism to reduce the transmission of impulses to the brain, while nerve fibers with small diameter have stimulative effects. According to this theory, phantom pain can be explained based on disinhibitory effects. That is, the loss of nerve fibers with large diameter often seen in amputated organs keeps the gate control mechanism open so that patients are vulnerable to pain perception. How acupuncture stimulating inhibitory nerve fibers with large diameter relieves pain can also be explained by this theory. However, the existence of this mechanism is still controversial [5].

Specific theory is a hypothesis that there is a specific pain receptor from which pain is transmitted to a specific nucleus of the thalamus. This theory is appropriate for explaining acute pain mechanism, but not for explaining chronic pain. Moreover, on the basis of this theory, it is difficult to explain phantom pain phenomenon in which there is no stimulus to specific pain receptor [5].

Pattern theory is a hypothesis that the brain perceives pain by mobilizing specific firing pattern of the reflex circuit in the spinal cord nuclei regardless of specific stimuli. This theory can explain phantom pain phenomenon but has a limitation in providing the evidences that there are reflex circuits causing or maintaining pain [5].

In addition, serotonin is likely to work for pain because antidepressants such as SSRIs are effective in the management of pain. Endorphin also plays a role in the central nervous system modulation of pain. Endorphin deficiency seems to correlate with augmentation of incoming sensory stimuli [3, 6].

Genetic inheritance is possibly involved in the transmission of pain disorder. First-degree relatives of patients with pain disorder have an increased likelihood of having the same disorder [3].

14.2.2 Psychological Factors

Psychological factors such as emotion, personality, psychodynamic factor, interpersonal factor, and behavioral factor play an important role in pain [3]. In addition, pain is greatly affected by a variety of factors including individuals' characteristics such as anticipation, suggestion, previous pain experiences, and sociocultural environment [5].

14.2.2.1 Emotion and Personality

Pain is not only caused by emotion such as anxiety and depression but also is revealed as a manifestation of mental disorders [7, 8]. Increased anxiety enhances pain response, but decreased anxiety reduces pain response [5]. Pain is also a common symptom of depression, accounting for 60–100% of patients with depressive disorders [9]. Therefore, chronic pain without organic disorders can be seen as a form of depression. This hypothesis is supported by some evidence that patients with chronic pain have symptoms of depression and have the family history of depression, and that chronic pain is well responsive to antidepressants. In a depressive state, physical sensation such as minimal distress can be amplified to severe pain. Like this, depression may exacerbate pain, and then pain elicits depression, leading to a vicious cycle of depression-pain. Therefore, antidepressants can be effectively used to stop such a vicious cycle, when depression is comorbid with pain [10].

In addition, pain is associated with anger and aggression. Anger exacerbates pain, whereas pain may trigger aggression [11]. However, patients with persistent pain are likely to suppress hostilities instead of expressing them overtly [12].

Personality of pain patients can make a great influence on responses to pain, whereas prolonged and severe intensity of pain can also affect their personality. For example, extrovert people tend to have higher levels of pain tolerance but are more likely to exaggerate pain experience than introvert people [13].

Anticipation for pain can play an important role in pain experiences. People who were told to anticipate severe pain in an experimental pain situation showed higher levels of pain tolerance than those who were not [14].

14.2.2.2 Psychodynamic Factors

Patients who experience pains without identifiable physical causes may be symbolically expressing an intrapsychic conflict through the body. By displacing the conflict to the body, they may feel that they have a legitimate claim to the fulfillment of their dependency needs [3].

In addition, pain can function as a method of obtaining love, a punishment for wrongdoing, and a way of expiating guilt [3]. According to Engel [15], the first pain often occurs during a period of adolescence and is associated with the sense of guilt about sexual impulses. Pain can be a response to either actual or imaginary loss, and it may be caused by the sense of guilt about forbidden aggressive or sexual impulses.

Identification plays a part when a patient takes on the role of an ambivalent love object (e.g., a parent) who has pain [3]. The sites of their pain are similar to those experienced by people close to them and can be determined by symbols associated with guilt about their conscious and unconscious wish for pain to be experienced by another person [15].

14.2.2.3 Interpersonal Factors

Intractable pain has been conceptualized as a means for manipulation and gaining advantage in interpersonal relationships. For example, pain can be used to ensure the devotion of a family member or stabilize their insecure marital status [3]. In this case, pain is used as a means to reunite the patient with a person with whom he/she would like to be close [4].

14.2.2.4 Behavioral Factors

Pain behavior refers to all behaviors shown to represent that they have pain [7]. Pain behaviors are reinforced when rewarded and are inhibited when ignored or punished. For example, moderate pain symptoms may become intense when followed by the attentive behavior of others (e.g., spouse, close family members), by monetary gain, or by the successful avoidance of aversive environment and distasteful activities at work [3].

14.3 Psychosocial Characteristics of Pain Patients

Lower pain thresholds were found for women, blacks, Orientals, and older persons [16]. Chronic pain increases anxiety levels regardless of organicity or functionality [17]. Depression also can occur due to chronic and severe pain caused by tissue damage [18].

Most of pain patients show depression, a sense of guilt, dependence, masochism, and preoccupation with somatic distress, although they deny depression [19]. On the Minnesota Multiphasic Personality Inventory (MMPI), elevated scores were noted on the neurotic triad of hypochondriasis, hysteria, and depression in patients with chronic pain [20–22]. In addition, interpersonal isolation was observed as a main characteristic of patients with chronic pain, when they were randomly investigated by using a variety of personality tests [23].

Pain patients are known to be narcissistic. They mistrust and ignore others, whereas they seek self-pride and compliments from others. They are vulnerable to helplessness and anxiety after accidents, although they were healthy before the accidents. After narcissistic injury, these patients may show anger toward their family and therapeutic team members including physicians [24].

Patients' complaints of severe pain despite no objective organic pathology was interpreted as their attempt to express their hard life. Thus, they do not give up their proclamation of pain easily. The more exaggerated their subjective pain was on evaluation, the more pain-focused their life was, and the more greatly their ordinary life was affected by pain [23].

Patients with self-esteem-related pain have more difficulty coping with pain psychologically than those with physical pain, because patients with injury to self-esteem project their problems externally [7].

14.4 Assessment

Assessment of pain patients is to make sure if stressful situations made an influence on the onset and exacerbation of pain. Intensive physical evaluation of pain is necessary, because it helps differentiate organic from functional pain [7]. Physical pain fluctuates in intensity and is highly sensitive to emotional, cognitive, attentional, and situational influences. Pain that does not vary and is insensitive to any of these factors (e.g., distraction or analgesics) is likely to be psychogenic [3].

Assessment of patients with chronic pain is to evaluate how psychological factors play roles in pain. The interaction between psychological factors and chronic pain is revealed as psychophysiological mechanism, operant mechanism, and comorbid psychiatric disorders as mentioned below [25].

14.4.1 Psychophysiological Mechanism

Pain as seen in patients with tension headache, migraine, and irritable bowel syndrome is associated with psychophysiological mechanism. However, these patients are often unaware of stressful events. This is called "alexithymia" [26]. Therefore, specific psychiatric interview techniques are required to elicit important psychological information from pain patients [25].

1. The psychiatrist needs to review the history of present illness, past history, family history, and personal history and then examine mental status. At this time, physicians should not try to explore the patients' psychological problems.
2. Physicians have to check if there are relationships between stressors and the exacerbation of pain.
3. Patients are encouraged to keep their diaries of events along with pain rating (0–10). This diary not only provides a baseline for therapeutic plans but may also illuminate the relationship between life events and symptoms.
4. Their family members need to be interviewed in order to ascertain the assessment of the patients' problems.

14.4.2 Operant Mechanism

Operant factors such as compensation and sick role can cause pain behavior to be perpetuated beyond the normal course of the actual painful experience. Patients' ordinary daily life activities and the impact of pain on their life should be checked to evaluate operant factors (e.g., economic, familial, and legal problems) in patients with chronic pain [25].

14.4.3 *Psychiatric Disorders Related to Pain*

The development of a psychiatric disorder significantly affects the progress of chronic pain. Psychiatric assessment of chronic pain patients requires evaluation for anxiety disorders, depressive disorders, somatoform disorders (somatic symptom and related disorders in DSM-5), and substance abuse [25].

14.4.3.1 Anxiety Disorders

About 30% of patients with intractable pain showed anxiety disorders such as generalized anxiety disorder and panic disorder [7].

14.4.3.2 Depressive Disorders

More than half of pain patients have symptoms of depressive disorders [8, 27, 28]. Among these depressive disorders, some are secondary to the pain itself, (e.g., adjustment disorders, psychological factors affecting other medical conditions: PFAOMC), and others are major depressive disorder [3, 8]. Patients with chronic pain may commit suicide, especially within 10 days after administration of antidepressants. About 44% of patients with pain deny emotions, particularly, anger [29]. However, it was reported that patients with major depressive disorder showed lower sensitivity to painful stimuli than healthy controls [9, 30, 31]. Therefore, the hypothesis that depression can increase pain is challenged.

14.4.3.3 Somatoform Disorders (Somatic Symptom and Related Disorder in DSM-5)

Somatoform disorder group accounts for about 5–15% of treated patients with chronic pain [7].

14.4.3.4 Factitious Disorder and Malingering

In factitious disorder patients, the most commonly recognized presentation is abdominal pain. The absence of some external gain or the evidence of an intrapsychic need to maintain a sick role suggests factitious disorder. Malingering refers to feigning somatic symptoms in order to obtain an external gain (e.g., obtaining money or drugs, avoiding work, exemption from military service) [7].

14.5 Treatment

14.5.1 General Principle

In general, a variety of therapeutic interventions are needed because the causes of pain are multiple [32]. First, the patients must be stabilized by pharmacotherapy. Then behavioral therapy is considered to minimize the levels of pain. Family assessment and therapy are also needed to sustain improvement at home. Finally, for some patients, a more growth-oriented psychotherapy is the final step in total rehabilitation. However, not all patients are required to go through all these stages [25].

Physicians should acknowledge that pain is true, even though some psychological factors may be involved in pain. For this purpose, physicians should mobilize all possible therapeutic modalities. These include relaxation therapy, education about pain, and massage as well as medication [7].

An important principle of management is to assure patients that treatment will continue even if there is no immediate improvement. One of the fears expressed by many chronic pain patients is of abandonment, that is, giving up treatment and referring them to someone else. It is important for physicians to maintain an optimistic attitude toward treatment in which there may be some ways to reduce pain or distress, although cure is not possible. Physicians should guard against being affected by the patients' sense of discouragement and helplessness. Therefore, great patience is required for the physicians who treat pain patients [7].

Patients with chronic pain suffer not only physical discomfort but also damaged self-esteem. Therefore, the techniques for interviewing these chronic pain patients are necessary for establishing a diagnostic working relationship and developing an effective treatment plan [7].

Pain patients should be encouraged to express their emotion. However, forcing patients to express their emotion too much may prevent them from expressing their true feelings. Too much support may not only bypass the patients' psychological problems but may actually increase conflicts related to suppression, control, and dependency. Therefore, the physician's kindness should not reach a point where it becomes an obstacle to patient treatment [33].

It is desirable not to hospitalize patients with chronic pain if possible, because hospitalization may foster regressive behaviors [6]. Effective treatment of chronic pain means not only relief of pain but also improvement of the quality of life. In most cases, treatment can lead to improving distress and functional disturbance, although it cannot remove pain completely. The threshold of perceived pain is known to be increased up to about 40% by using biofeedback, positive emotional state, relaxation, guided imagery, suggestion, hypnosis, placebo, and analgesics [6].

14.5.2 Pharmacotherapy

Analgesics and psychotropics are used for patients with chronic pain. Too little analgesia eventually leads to excessive amounts of analgesics in order to elicit pain relief. In particular, these drugs are frequently used as needed (prn) in acute pain cases, considering possible risks of drug dependency. However, such a risk seems to be extremely rare [5]. It is better to use analgesics at fixed regular intervals rather than as prn because of the following reasons [33]:

1. Administration of analgesics based on their half-life can relieve anxiety about pain by preventing the occurrence of pain before administration of the next dose.
2. The dose administered as needed (prn) can be much more required until the recurrence of pain occurs than the dose administered at fixed regular intervals.
3. If analgesics are used as needed, patients are put on a dependent state whenever asking for medication. Therefore, they are likely to be excessively preoccupied with those drugs or feel self-shame.
4. Elderly patients or those with cognitive impairment may have troubles in calling nurses for more medication.

Cases in which prn administration is exceptionally better are patients with liver diseases prolonging half-life of drugs, elderly patients (over 80 years old) with impaired liver metabolism, and patients with nocturnal pain [34].

Oral analgesics are better recommended than parenteral analgesics, because oral administration is simpler and more economical [35]. However, parenteral analgesics are more recommended in cases with tolerance to drugs and with difficulty in swallowing oral medication [25].

It is not desirable to use benzodiazepine antianxiety agents for patients with chronic pain, because they require long-term use of these drugs so that they are at high risk for drug dependency. It has been suggested that the role of serotonergic pathways in inhibiting pain is important. Many studies found that antidepressants including amitriptyline and imipramine are more effective than placebo in chronic pain patients [32, 36, 37]. In particular, imipramine has been found to be effective for chest pain unaccompanied by coronary heart disease [38]. If the agent is not effective after a few days, it should be considered to change to another antidepressant. However, pain symptoms in patients with major depressive disorder require 2–4 weeks of treatment with antidepressants as depression does [25, 37]. Selective serotonin receptor uptake inhibitors (SSRIs) such as clomipramine and fluoxetine are known to be effective in relieving pain in pain patients [6]. However, SSRIs were not found to be more effective than tricyclic antidepressants in chronic pain patients [39].

Antipsychotic agents such as chlorpromazine and haloperidol are sometimes used in patients with acute pain or severe preterminal cancer pain, because these drugs potentiate actions of narcotic analgesics. However, these drugs should be avoided because of the potential for tardive dyskinesia [40]. In addition, antiepileptics acting as mood stabilizers are often used in patients with chronic pain. For example, carbamazepine is effective in relieving pain caused by diabetic neuropathy

[41]. However, physicians need to pay attention to a potential serious side effect such as Stevens-Johnson syndrome, a type of severe skin reaction, while using this medication. Gabapentin is known to partially relieve neuropathic pain in patients with multiple sclerosis [42] and in those with pain in the head and neck [43].

14.5.3 Placebo Therapy

General effects caused by patients' contact with a medical system can be called placebo effect. In particular, positive placebo effect refers to obtaining pain relief from saline or some other inert substance. Placebo is a potent therapeutic tool equivalent to 1/2–2/3 of morphine in relieving severe pain [44].

The mechanism for the placebo response is probably related to the endorphin pain-inhibiting system, but it is influenced by both psychological and neurological factors [7]. As a psychological mechanism of placebo effect, sufficing dependency needs can play a role. In one study, placebo analgesic effect was reported to be related to naloxone [45].

The most frequent misuse of placebo is for a diagnostic purpose. However, placebo should not be used for such a purpose because it is impossible to differentiate organic from functional pain [46]. For example, relief of pain caused by injection of saline should not be regarded as functional, because even patients with organic abnormalities who complain of severe pain may actually respond well to placebo.

Placebo can cause side effects such as nausea, tachycardia, febrile sensation, and so on. Side effects related to interpersonal relationship in a medical environment can occur. For example, if patients realize that placebo was used to treat their persistent pain, they may feel tricked and become angry, eventually leading to a disruption in doctor-patient relationship [5].

14.5.4 Psychosocial Treatment

The necessity of nonphysical treatments such as psychotherapy and behavioral therapy is emphasized because pain treatment by medication has a limitation. Most patients with chronic pain have a vicious cycle such as repetition of pain and psychosocial problems. In order to disconnect this cycle, they need psychosocial approach [6].

14.5.4.1 Psychotherapy

The first step in psychotherapy is to develop a solid psychotherapeutic alliance by empathizing with the patient's suffering. Clinicians should not confront somatizing patients with comments such as "This is all in your head." For the patient, pain is real and clinicians must acknowledge the reality of the pain, even as they understand that it is largely intrapsychic in origin. A useful entry point into the emotional aspects of the pain is to examine its interpersonal ramifications of the patient's life [3].

The first contact with patients with chronic pain also constitutes an important part of the whole treatment. Physicians should not give patients the promise that they can cure pain completely. In contrast, patients should be told in advance that treatment of pain is not only done by physicians but requires their own effort and that they must not expect immediate results. Therefore, it should be emphasized that it is not possible to cure pain and that rather the patients should learn to live with pain to some extent. In such cases, some pain patients who expect cure go "doctor shopping" for precise diagnosis and best treatment. However, they recognize that there are no magical ways to cure chronic pain and then give up doctor shopping and return to work [47].

Clinicians should discuss the issue of psychological factors early in treatment [3]: for example, "Pain itself may be caused by psychological problems" and "Treatment should be integrative including the body and mind to be effective for pain" [4].

14.5.4.2 Behavioral Therapy

Behavioral therapy plays an important role in the treatment of chronic pain. It is not primarily for pain itself but rather for the behaviors associated with pain [23]. That is, the goal of this therapy is to remove pain behavior and then shape new behavior incompatible with pain. It helps therapists recognize the nature of pain behavior by having patients write their diaries for 2 weeks. From these diaries, the therapists find out some behavioral patterns, set the goal of treatment with the patients and their families, and introduce therapeutic techniques fit for the goal. For example, there are behaviors to be modified for each individual: reduced activity, protection-inducing pain behaviors, excessive dependency on analgesics, and decreased social activities [48].

Behavioral therapy is subdivided into self-management techniques and operant techniques [49]. Self-management techniques include biofeedback, exercise, and cognitive therapy. Operant techniques refer to treatment paradigms in which desired behavior is rewarded and undesired behavior is ignored. Biofeedback treatment is a technique whereby the patient is taught to relax muscle in conjunction with electromyography (EMG) training through feedbacks such as sound and light. This technique is known to be effective in tension headache [50], migraine [51], chronic backache, and phantom limb pain [49].

Mindfulness-based stress reduction (MBSR) is a mindfulness-based program which uses a combination of mindfulness meditation, body awareness, and yoga to help people become more mindful [52]. MBSR aims to help participants develop nonjudgmental awareness of moment-to-moment experience [53]. This MBSR program is known to reduce pain intensity and pain-related distress in patients with chronic pain (e.g., backache, joint pain) [54]. Fibromyalgia patients also benefited modestly from a MBSR intervention. In addition, health-related quality of life was significantly improved in the MBSR group [53].

Operant approach is based on the notion that behaviors are controlled by their consequences. If a behavior is followed by reward (positive reinforcement), such a behavior is likely to persist. Therefore, pain behavior (e.g., complaints of pain, grimacing) increases when there is positive reinforcement for it [25]. For example, when nurses withheld positive reinforcement for pain behaviors (e.g., complaints of pain) but provided attention for well behaviors (e.g., increased activity) in chronic pain patients, they showed significant improvement. In addition, administration of analgesics at fixed regular intervals rather than as needed produced marked improvement [55]. It is also more effective for therapists to have supportive sessions at regular intervals regardless of pain than whenever they complain of pain [6].

In general, operant approaches are used when physical abnormalities are either absent or minimal and when there is a high level of pain behavior. In contrast, self-management techniques are used when there is more evidence of tissue damage, shorter duration of symptoms, or less evidence that positive reinforcement will be effective [25].

14.5.4.3 Cognitive Behavioral Therapy (CBT)

Patients are taught to imagine pleasant events, to focus on distracting some elements in the environment, or to concentrate on other sensations as a way to combat their pain. These approaches are often combined with other techniques including assertiveness training. CBT is a way to enhance self-esteem and control his/her own behaviors [25].

In a number of studies, CBT provided a small incremental benefit over control interventions in reducing pain, negative mood, and disability at the end of treatment and at long-term follow-up in children, adolescent, and adults with fibromyalgia [56]. Randomized controlled trials that assessed the use of CBT in adults with sub-acute and chronic neck pain also found that CBT was more effective for short-term pain reduction when compared to no treatment [57]. In addition, noncardiac chest pain that is common both in patients with coronary heart disease and in patients whose cardiac workup is negative responds to CBT [38].

One study based on an analysis of fMRI scans revealed that CBT led to increased activations in the ventrolateral prefrontal/lateral orbitofrontal cortex, regions associated with executive cognitive control. These findings suggest that CBT changes the brain's processing of pain through an altered cerebral loop between pain signals, emotions, and cognitions, leading to increased access to executive regions for reappraisal of pain [58].

14.5.4.4 Traditional Psychotherapy and Group Therapy

Traditional psychotherapy is another technique for treating patients with chronic pain. However, this psychotherapy is not an effective treatment modality in terms of cost-effect except when individuals' conflicts are prominent and little changes in behavior are noted [4].

Group therapy is known to be more effective in treatment for patients with chronic pain than individual therapy. It was reported that patients with chronic pain admitted at the pain center responded well to brief group therapy unexpectedly [19]. Group therapy was noted to help patients have more self-confidence in social activities and more active life regardless of the presence or absence of pain experience [4].

14.6 Comprehensive Approach

In chronic pain patients, treatment should focus on sick role. Comprehensive approach is required for diagnosis and treatment of chronic pain. It is desirable for pain patients to be placed in a comprehensive pain control program or clinic where multidisciplinary modalities are available, including cognitive, behavioral, group therapy as well as physical therapy, exercise, and vocational rehabilitation. Under such therapeutic environment, the possibility of manipulation by patients and their noncompliance can be reduced. In addition, pain patients are likely to accept psychological intervention in terms of integrative approach at this clinic rather than their physicians' recommendation for psychiatric treatment [3, 4].

Because it may not be possible to remove the pain, the therapeutic goal in chronic pain should be rehabilitation rather than cure [4]. Therapists should consider termination of treatment, when no improvement was noted 6 months after the above treatment modalities were used [1].

Case 1
A 20-year-old male patient with end-stage renal failure was several times admitted to the department of nephrology of a general hospital to receive long-term hemodialysis. During hospitalization, he often complained of paroxysmal and severe abdominal pain. His pain was rarely relieved by either analgesics or tricyclic antidepressants. His family members could not afford to visit him, not only because they were busy working but also because they were tired of taking care of him due to his chronic illness. He was therefore left alone most of the time. The nurses injected him with analgesics whenever he complained of paroxysmal abdominal pain, but he would soon complain again. He was referred to the department of psychiatry for consultation and thoroughly interviewed by a psychiatrist, who found out that the patient was afraid of coping with his illness alone, without being in his family members' care. Thereafter, the patient was interviewed for about 30 min twice every week, and his complaints of paroxysmal pain became less frequent.

This case illustrates that supportive psychotherapy can be more effective in patients with abdominal pain than medication such as analgesics and antidepressants.

Case 2
A 40-year-old male patient suffered from abdominal pain for 7 months and then underwent a variety of laboratory examinations including gastroendoscopy.

However, no abnormalities were found except for signs of mild gastritis. When an internist recommended him to see a psychiatrist, the patient cast doubt on their ability to evaluate his symptoms and thereby went "doctor shopping." No abnormal findings were found on additional physical and laboratory examinations. The patient would often lie down in his office due to severe abdominal pain, and occasionally he was absent from work. Tricyclic antidepressants were prescribed, but he continued to complain of abdominal pain, often with a grimace on his face. His pain barely improved, even after the dose of the antidepressants was increased.

During an interview, the patient denied experiencing any stressors. His wife labeled him as being "egotistic" but could also not point to any significant stressors. He had been brought up by his mother as an only son, and his mother, while living with him, had never put any burden on him.

After several months, he admitted during an interview, "I get very anxious because I cannot compete with new younger employees who are good at using computers, while I am very poor at using them." He also said, "it was a huge burden for me to attend those long-term teaching programs. I was not confident of getting good results in the post-education examinations." After this interview, the patient gave up on getting promoted and decided to be more concerned with his own health. Since then, the intensity of his pain was markedly reduced, although he sometimes still complained of abdominal pain.

In this case, psychological factors associated with pain were revealed after having received psychiatric treatment for a considerable period of time. Therapists therefore need to be patient and wait until patients reveal such issues in the treatment of chronic pain patients, even if no psychological factors can be found at an earlier time.

14.7 Conclusions

The onset and exacerbation of pain are affected by psychosocial factors as well as physical factors. As secondary responses to pain, anxiety and depression can occur and pain may be expressed as one of manifestations of a mental disorder. In addition, chronic pain may reflect hardship in life. Therefore, the assessment and treatment of pain require biopsychosocial approaches. Therapists need to mobilize a variety of therapeutic modalities such as psychopharmacotherapy, relaxation therapy, and cognitive behavioral therapy. It is more effective to administer analgesics at fixed regular times than as needed (prn). It is dangerous to use a placebo in order to differentiate between organic and functional pain. In particular, treatment of patients with chronic pain requires multidisciplinary and integrative approach. It is desirable for therapists to focus on rehabilitation rather than on cure as a therapeutic goal for patients with chronic pain. Special therapeutic techniques are required for treatment of pain, because patients' denial of psychological problems is likely to develop resistance to psychological approach.

References

1. Guggenheim FG, Smith GR. Somatoform disorders. In: Kaplan HI, Sadock BJ, editors. Comprehensive textbook of psychiatry. 6th ed. Baltimore: Williams & Wilkins; 1995.
2. American Psychiatric Association (APA). Statistical and diagnostic manual of mental disorders. 5th ed. Washington, DC: Am Psychiatric Publishing; 2013.
3. Sadock BJ, Sadock VA. Synopsis of psychiatry – behavioral sciences/clinical psychiatry. 9th ed. Philadelphia: Lippincott Williams & Wilkins; 2003. p. 643–60.
4. Ford CV. The somatizing disorders: illness as a way of life. New York: Elsevier Biomedical; 1984. p. 98–126.
5. Leigh H, Reiser MF. The patient: biological, psychological and social dimensions of medical practice. 2nd ed. New York: Plenum Medical Book; 1985. p. 209–40.
6. Kaplan HI, Sadock BJ. Synopsis of psychiatry: behavioral sciences & clinical psychiatry. 7th ed. Baltimore: Williams & Wilkins; 1994. p. 628–30, 764–5
7. Bouckoms A, Hackett TP. The pain patient: evaluation and treatment. In: Cassem NH, editor. MGH handbook of general hospital psychiatry. 3rd ed. St. Louis: Mosby Year Book; 1991.
8. Reich J, Tupin J, Abramowitz S. Psychiatric diagnosis of chronic pain patients. Am J Psychiatry. 1983;140:1495–8.
9. von Knorring L. The experience of pain in depressed patients. Neuropsychobiology. 1975;1:155–65.
10. Blumer D, Heilbronn M. Chronic pain as a variant of depressive disease. J Nerv Ment Dis. 1982;170:381–406.
11. Sternbach RA. Pain: a psychophysiological analysis. New York: Academic; 1968.
12. Ulrich RE, Hutchinson RR, Azrin NH. Pain-elicited aggression. Psychol Rev. 1965;15:111–26.
13. Lynn R, Eysenck HJ. Tolerance for pain, extraversion, and neuroticism. Percept Motor Skills. 1961;12:161–2.
14. Kanfer FH, Goldfoot DA. Self-control and tolerance of noxious stimulation. Psychol Rev. 1966;18:79–85.
15. Engel GL. Psychogenic pain and the pain-prone patient. Am J Med. 1959;36:899–918.
16. Woodrow KM, Friedman CD, Sielgelaub AB. Pain tolerance: differences according to age, sex, and race. Psychosom Med. 1972;34:548–56.
17. Bond MR. The relation of pain to the Eysenck personality inventory, Cornell medical index, and Whitely index of hypochondria. Br J Psychiatry. 1971;119:671.
18. Robinson H, Kirk RF, Frye RF. A psychological study of patients with rheumatoid arthritis and other painful diseases. J Psychosom Res. 1972;16:53–6.
19. Pinsky JJ. Chronic, intractable, benign pain: a syndrome and its treatment with intensive short-term group psychotherapy. J Hum Stress. 1978;4:1721.
20. Blumetti AE, Modesti LM. Psychological predictors of success or failure of surgical intervention for intractable back pain. In: Bonica JJ, Albe-Fessard D, editors. Advances in pain research and therapy, vol. 2. New York: Raven Press; 1976.
21. Strassberg DS, Reimherr F, Ward M, et al. The MMPI and chronic pain. J Consult Clin Psychol. 1981;49:220–6.
22. Sternbach RA, Wolf SR, Murphy RW, et al. Traits of pain patients: the low-back 'loser.'. Psychosomatics. 1973;14:226–9.
23. Timmermans G, Sternbach RA. Factors of human chronic pain: an analysis of personality and pain reaction variables. Science. 1974;184:806–8.
24. Blazer DG. Narcissism and the development of chronic pain. Int J Psychiatry Med. 1980;10:69–79.
25. Houpt JL. Chronic pain management. In: Soudemire A, Fogel BS, editors. Principles of medical psychiatry. Orlando: Grune & Stratton; 1987.
26. Postone N. Alexithymia in chronic pain patients. Gen Hosp Psychiatry. 1986;8:163–7.

27. Bradley JJ. Severe localized pain associated with the depression syndrome. Br J Psychiatry. 1963;109:741–5.
28. Lyndsay P, Wyckoff M. The depression-pain syndrome and its response to antidepressants. Psychosomatics. 1981;22:571–3.
29. Antczak-Bouckoms A, Bouckoms AJ. Affective disturbances and denial of problems in dental patients with pain. Int J Psychosom. 1985;32:9–11.
30. Davis GC, Bucsbuum MS, Bunney WE. Analgesia to painful stimuli in affective illness. Am J Psychiatry. 1979;136:1148.
31. Kim JC, Kim MJ. Pain threshold in major depressive disorder. J Korean Neuropsychiatr Assoc. 1985;24:227–35.
32. Magni G. The use of antidepressants in the treatment of chronic pain: a review of the current evidence. Drugs. 1991;42:730–48.
33. Pilowsky I. Pain as abnormal illness behavior. J Hum Stress. 1978;4:22–7.
34. Twycross RG, Lack SA. Therapeutics in terminal cancer. London: Pitman Publishing; 1984.
35. Beaver WT. Management of cancer pain with parenteral medication. J Am Med Assoc. 1980;244:2653–7.
36. Onghena P, Van Houdenlove B. Antidepressant induced analgesic in chronic nonmalignant pain: a meta-analysis of 39 placebo controlled studies. Pain. 1992;29:205–19.
37. Moore DP. Treatment of chronic pain with tricyclic antidepressants. South Med J. 1980;73:1585–6.
38. Ketterer MW. Cognitive/behavioral therapy of anxiety in the medically ill: cardiac settings. Semin Clin Neuropsychiatry. 1999;4:148–53.
39. McQuay HJ, Moore RA. Antidepressants and chronic pain. Br Med J. 1997;341:763–4.
40. Goldberg RJ, Sokol MS, Cullen LO. Acute pain management. In: Soudemire A, Fogel BS, editors. Principles of medical psychiatry. Orlando: Grune & Stratton; 1987.
41. Rull JA, Quibrera R, Gonzalez-Millan H. Symptomatic treatment of peripheral diabetic neuropathy with carbamazepine (Tegretol): double blind crossover trial. Diabetologia. 1969;5:215–8.
42. Houtchens MK, Richert JR, Sami A. Open label gabapentin treatment for pain in multiple sclerosis. Mult Scler. 1997;3:250–3.
43. Sist TC, Filadora VA, Miner M. Experience with gabapentin for neuropathic pain in the head and neck: report of ten cases. Reg Anesth. 1997;22:473–8.
44. Beecher HK. The powerful placebo. J Am Med Assoc. 1955;159:1602–6.
45. Levine JD, Gordon NC, Fields HL. The mechanism of placebo analgesia. Lancet. 1978;2:654–7.
46. Shapiro AK. Attitudes toward the use of placebos in treatment. J Nerv Ment Dis. 1960;130:200–11.
47. DeVaul RA, Zisook S. Chronic pain: the psychiatrist's role. Psychosomatics. 1978;19:417–21.
48. Fordyce WE. In: Sternbach RA, editor. Learning processes in pain. New York: Raven Press; 1978.
49. Keefe FJ, Bradley LA. Behavioral and psychological approaches to the assessment and treatment of chronic pain. Gen Hosp Psychiatry. 1984;6:49–54.
50. Budzynski T. Biofeedback in the treatment of muscle contraction headache. Biofeedback Self Regul. 1978;3:409–35.
51. Blanchard EB, Andrasik F. Psychological assessment and treatment of headache: recent development and emerging issues. J Consult Clin Psychol. 1982;50:859–79.
52. Kabat-Zinn J. Full catastrophe living: using the wisdom of your body and mind to face stress, pain, and illness. New York: Bantam Dell; 2013.
53. Schmid S, Grossman P, Schwarzer B, et al. Treating fibromyalgia with mindfulness-based stress reduction: results from a 3-armed randomized controlled trial. Pain. 2011;52:361–9.
54. Wong SY, Chan FW, Wong RL, et al. Comparing the effectiveness of mindfulness-based stress reduction and multidisciplinary intervention programs for chronic pain: a randomized comparative trial. Clin J Pain. 2011;27:724–34.

55. Fordyce WE, Fowler US, Lehman JR. Operant conditioning in the treatment of chronic pain. Arch Phys Med Rehabil. 1973;54:399–408.
56. Bernardy K, Klose P, Busch AJ, et al. Cognitive behavioral therapies for fibromyalgia. Cochrane Database Syst Rev. 2013;9:CD009796. https://doi.org/10.1002/14651858.CD009796.pub2.
57. Monticone M, Cedraschi C, Ambrosini E, et al. Cognitive-behavioral treatment for subacute and chronic neck pain. Cochrane Database Syst Rev. 2015;5:CD010664. https://doi.org/10.1002/14651858.CD010664.pub2.
58. Jensen KB, Kosek E, Wicksell R, et al. Cognitive behavioral therapy increases pain-evoked activation of the prefrontal cortex in patients with fibromyalgia. Pain. 2012;153:1495–503.

Part III
Specific Physical Disorders

Chapter 15
Approach to Depression in Patients with Brain Diseases: Stroke, Parkinson's Disease, and Dementia

15.1 Introduction

Brain diseases such as stroke, Parkinson's disease, and dementia [1] often result in major changes in a person's life such as loss of health, occupation, social roles, and independence. The physical and/or psychological sequelae caused by these diseases may be devastating for both the patient and family. In particular, depression during the illnesses not only complicates diagnosis and treatment but also hinders therapeutic efforts.

This chapter addresses the management options available for depression related to each of stroke, Parkinson's disease, and dementia. The management of these diseases focuses on psychopharmacotherapy as well as nonpsychopharmacological interventions including cognitive behavioral approach.

15.2 Stroke

Stroke, defined as a sudden loss of blood supply to the brain leading to permanent damage caused by thrombotic, embolic, or hemorrhagic events, ranks as the leading cause of death in patients aged 50 years and older [2].

The prevalence rates of poststroke depression vary from 20% to 65%. Poststroke depression has been considered the most common neuropsychiatric condition after stroke [3–5]. According to a systematic review by Hackett and Anderson [6], several factors, such as stroke severity, physical disability, and cognitive impairment, have been consistently and positively associated with depression following stroke. In particular, the severity of disability is one of the strongest and most consistent risk factors of poststroke depression [7]. A prospective, longitudinal epidemiological study has also revealed that the risk of developing poststroke depression is

K. B. Koh, *Stress and Somatic Symptoms*,
https://doi.org/10.1007/978-3-030-02783-4_15

increased in patients with more functional and cognitive impairment, greater dependency with regard to activities of daily living, speech and language dysfunctions, and apraxia [8].

Grief and demoralization would be expected as normal, but withdrawal associated with hopelessness and refusal to participate in potentially effective rehabilitation efforts would be considered maladaptive [9]. Stoke can also damage the patient's self-esteem [10]. Other consequences of poststroke depression include increased disability [11], increased cognitive impairment [12, 13], poor rehabilitation outcome [14, 15], higher health costs, diminished social abilities, increased risk of vascular-related events, and increased suicidality and mortality [16–18].

A key problem is that both the patient and physician often do not accept this condition as a treatable illness [19]. A more worrying problem is that when evaluating an older patient, the physician concentrates on other aspects of the patient and dismisses depressive symptoms. Unfortunately, it has been estimated that 80% of poststroke depression patients may not be diagnosed by nonpsychiatric clinicians [20].

15.2.1 Assessment of Poststroke Depression

Clinically, there are differences between depressed younger and older people. Among depressed younger adults, symptoms of fatigue, sleep disturbance, psychomotor retardation, and hopelessness about the future are more commonly reported, whereas subjective complaints of poor memory and lack of concentration are more commonly reported among depressed older adults [21].

There are a number of possible instruments that may help in screening for poststroke depression including the Center of Epidemiological Studies-Depression Scale (CESD), Hamilton Depression Rating Scale (HDRS), and Patient Health Questionnaire (PHQ)-9. They seem to be the optimal measures for screening of poststroke depression. However, not all tools are satisfactory for case finding. Therefore, such scales should be used in conjunction with a more detailed clinical assessment, rather than in isolation [22]. In particular, the Geriatric Depression Scale (GDS) has been considered reliable for use in elderly stroke patients [23]. The GDS is most useful in the diagnosis of depression among patients with higher levels of function and only mild cognitive impairment [24].

In addition, the following factors contribute to the difficulty in diagnosing poststroke depression: (1) lack of proper training of mental health care professionals for recognizing which symptoms are more related to stroke than depression and (2) medical care providers usually have limited knowledge about the differences between depression and typical signs of aging and stroke [25]. Therefore, clinicians should define a set of valid criteria for diagnosing poststroke depression [26].

15.2.2 *Management of Poststroke Depression*

Early and aggressive treatment of poststroke depression is required to minimize the cognitive and performance deficits that depression inflicts on the patient during the recovery period [10]. The biopsychosocial approach to depression is highly recommended because poststroke depression may result from a combination of biological, psychological, and social factors [1].

All treatments must be modified according to the patient's needs, including the cost, accessibility, and availability. Effective treatment will generally include the participation of the family and other support networks. Under all circumstances, the treating clinician should monitor a patient presenting with depression at least weekly for the first 6 weeks to evaluate mood changes, suicidal thinking, physical safety, social life, and adverse effects of any drugs that have been prescribed [6].

Major goals of such a treatment regimen are to improve mood and quality of life, use health care resources appropriately, and reduce the risks of medical complications [27]. The management of poststroke depression includes pharmacotherapy, psychotherapy, and physical exercise.

15.2.2.1 Psychopharmacotherapy

Overall, studies demonstrate that antidepressants are well tolerated in stroke patients and that over 60% of patients with poststroke depression respond to medication [1]. However, psychopharmacotherapy may be particularly complicated in elderly poststroke depression patients, who often have high rates of medical comorbidity and polypharmacy and are more vulnerable to the adverse effects of antidepressants [28]. First of all, the antidepressants used should be effective in controlling mood disorders. It is also important that the antidepressants lack adverse effects on cognitive function since patients who have had strokes often experience cognitive impairment [29]. There are many variables involved in the psychopharmacotherapy of elderly patients, including pharmacokinetic changes associated with aging and their increased vulnerability to drug interactions with other medications, preexisting illnesses, and adverse effects of the drugs [28].

Antidepressants

Antidepressants can be effective in treating most moderate and severe depressive disorders such as major depressive disorder, but antidepressants are generally not indicated for mild forms because the balance of benefit and risk is not satisfactory for elderly stroke patients [28]. Evidence suggests that about 65% of patients with poststroke depression improve with psychoactive drugs as compared to 44% of patients treated with placebo [30]. Selective serotonin receptor inhibitors (SSRIs) and venlafaxine are better tolerated than tricyclics due to less anticholinergic effects, and significant antidepressant efficacy has been demonstrated for sertraline and citalopram [31, 32]. In particular, sertraline, paroxetine, and venlafaxine are preferred because their half-life is relatively short [32]. Furthermore, SSRIs have their lower potential for drug interactions [28]. Therefore, it is advisable to treat post-stroke depression with SSRIs of proven efficacy and switch to nortriptyline if there is no significant improvement after an adequate trial and there are no contraindications for the use of tricyclics [31].

An important finding in a meta-analysis [30] is that the benefit of psychoactive agents in reducing depressive symptoms is significant after 3 or 4 weeks of treatment and increases with continued treatment. Maintenance treatment may also be recommended in order to achieve optimal outcomes and prevent relapse [31]. Thus, antidepressants should be continued at least for 4 months after initial recovery and should be changed if no response is seen after 6 weeks [33]. Antidepressant treatment can then be slowly withdrawn, or in case of relapse, it can be continued for a longer duration [34, 35].

15.2.2.2 Nonpsychopharmacological Interventions

Psychological interventions are the preferred method of treatment for patients with mild mood disorders [6] and are reserved for those in whom antidepressants are either inappropriate or not tolerated [36]. Psychological treatments include behavioral therapy, cognitive behavioral therapy (CBT), problem-solving therapy, and life review therapy [37]. Additionally, Watkins et al. [38] recently showed that motivational interviewing may be effective in improving patients' mood 3 months after stroke.

Treatment of adjustment disorder after a stroke is primarily psychosocial. The focus should be on nonspecific support, education, and psychotherapeutic clarification of the individual's conflicts in the context of the physical illness [9]. In particular, emphasis should be placed on maintaining the person's self-esteem in psychotherapy [10]. Support from family and friends is also essential in treatment.

Cognitive Behavioral Therapy (CBT)

CBT has a very strong and positive effect on poststroke depression because it not only builds confidence but also improves daily lifestyle through a range of activities. CBT is designed to challenge dysfunctional thoughts or beliefs that are associated with low mood and to collaboratively establish more functional thoughts or beliefs [26]. CBT is based on providing insight using psychoeducation, collaborative empiricism, and active problem-solving, assessing the nature and quality of support, and improving the patient's adaptation to a new lifestyle after a stroke [39]. Patients examine how their thoughts may contribute to feelings and how they can transform their feelings [40]. However, patients with cognitive impairment and/or aphasia are not suited to this treatment form [28].

In general, approximately six to eight regular sessions should be provided to patients over a period of 10–12 weeks, with most people experiencing improvements in mood and/or a reduction in symptoms after 2 months of therapy. Responses to therapy should be reviewed after eight sessions. A therapy extension period of 6 months is considered necessary for a person who has multiple issues or severe comorbidity [6].

However, in a randomized controlled trial, Lincoln et al. [41] demonstrated that CBT was not effective in the treatment of poststroke depression. Additionally, a Cochrane review of depression interventions after stroke found that psychotherapeutic intervention for poststroke depression including CBT failed to provide evidence of effectiveness [42].

Given these contradictory results, psychotherapy should be combined with antidepressants to reduce residual symptoms and the risk of relapse in patients with severe depression and in those with moderate or severe depression who refuse antidepressants [43].

Physical Exercise, Activity, Physical and Speech Therapy

Physical exercise during the subacute recovery phase of stroke has a beneficial effect on depressive symptoms [44]. In most psychological treatments, a behavioral activation component is often involved, which addresses the problem of limitations in activity. Some of these approaches primarily focus on the meaningfulness of the activity during the treatment, which may help intensify and maintain cognition and target depression [45]. Additionally, physical therapy and speech therapy may also be helpful for poststroke depression patients in regaining a sense of sound body and self-esteem.

15.2.2.3 Integrated Care

The integrated care pathway (ICP) may be a suitable model for a systematic approach to poststroke depression [34, 46]. This system includes screening for depression and assessing the severity of depression using psychological instruments, such as the Hamilton Depression Rating Scale, Beck Depression Inventory-II (BDI-II) [47], and a clinical interview. This ICP model also suggests selecting a treatment such as the use of a formal psychiatric consultation and psychopharmacotherapy. Sometimes other instruments such as the Structured Assessment for Depression in Brain Damaged (SADBD) [48] individuals and the Stroke Aphasic Depression Questionnaire (SAD) [49] may be required to assess depression in those with severe language or communication deficits.

However, a multidisciplinary approach needs to be included in this program to facilitate more effective management of these patients. Thus, treatment of depression after stroke should include psychiatrists or psychologists, neurologists or neurosurgeons, rehabilitation medicine specialists, nurses, physical therapists, and speech therapists.

The following two cases [50] demonstrate multidisciplinary and integrative approaches in patients with poststroke depression.

Case 1

A 49-year-old female patient was admitted to the department of neurosurgery via the emergency room with a sudden onset of headache and loss of consciousness. She underwent surgery with the diagnosis of aneurysmal rupture at the middle cerebral artery. However, she suffered from its sequelae, including right hemiparesis, aphasia, impaired orientation to time, memory disturbance, and diminished intellectual functioning. She was then transferred to the department of rehabilitation medicine, where she underwent physical therapy and speech therapy. She was referred to the department of psychiatry after being discharged from the hospital.

On her first visit to the outpatient psychiatry department, a mental status examination revealed signs of an organic mental disorder and of an adjustment disorder with depression: weeping spells, loss of self-esteem caused by loss of bodily functions, impaired memory, and slurred speech. She received supportive psychotherapy and medication including haloperidol and fluoxetine biweekly for 3 months and then monthly for 2 years. Additionally, she underwent physical therapy and speech therapy at the department of rehabilitation medicine. Despite her many disabilities, she continued to practice writing and speaking briefly.

Physical therapy helped her lift her right hand to some degree, but not completely. It was possible for the patient to communicate with her family members and friends with the help of the speech therapist, but it was still difficult for her to form sentences. She was sometimes frustrated by her limited ability to speak and lift her arm, but she looked joyful as her slurred speech improved. She continued to exercise outside her house and to receive physical therapy at home everyday.

About 5 months later, she reported feeling thankful for her husband's warm and encouraging attitude. Her speech had drastically improved, and she was able to talk with her friends on the phone, albeit fast. She was surprised that she was again able to say numbers in German as she had forgotten how to immediately after her illness. Her memory also improved. However, she still exhibited bouts of sudden tearfulness, particularly when recalling her survival from her near-death experience. She began to write letters to her friends and her two sons who had been studying abroad. She was able to recall the names of her friends completely. Her stuttering also notably improved. Her friends encouraged her by saying, "Now you can talk better than one month ago" and "You do not stutter at all," although she did not notice those changes.

She continued to exercise at the fitness center. She was able to go outside without being accompanied by her husband. She began to understand the Chinese characters she had forgotten after her illness. Additionally, her vocabulary use and understanding increased. She was also able to speak in a low tone and was surprised that she was still able to completely lift her right arm.

Case 2
A 70-year-old male patient with stroke was admitted to the department of neurology. His brain lesion was found to have multiple diffuse embolisms, the prognosis of which was judged to be irreversible and hopeless by the neurologist. The patient was transferred to the department of rehabilitation medicine for supportive care of the stroke sequelae, including hemiparesis and aphasia. He required physical therapy and speech therapy but declined treatment and refused to eat.

He was referred to the department of psychiatry for consultation. He was severely depressed because he could no longer live as an independent person and instead had to be absolutely dependent on his wife. He was diagnosed with major depressive disorder, and an antidepressant, sertraline (Zoloft), was administered. His wife, who had devoted most of her time to taking care of him, was also tearful and appeared tired because of her husband's pessimistic and uncooperative attitude. After 4 weeks of treatment with the antidepressant, his depression was greatly improved. Thereafter, he began to participate in physical therapy and speech therapy. Even after being discharged from the hospital, he continued to exercise and to receive physical therapy and speech therapy. They moved to Canada where their daughter was living. After 7 years, he returned to Korea with his wife and was assessed at the hospital. He was observed to be able to put on his shoes, stand up and walk with the help of his wife, and even talk, which was very surprising given his status at the last visit.

These two cases show the impact that stroke sequelae have on patients' and their partners' emotions and self-esteem. This suggests that a multidisciplinary approach could be effective in assessing and treating poststroke depression. In particular, treatment of poststroke depression should be integrative, including biological treatment such as antidepressants, psychotherapy, physical exercise, and physical and speech therapy.

15.3 Parkinson's Disease

Parkinson's disease has been regarded as idiopathic degeneration of dopaminergic neurons in the substantia nigra of the midbrain, resulting in loss of transmission of motor impulse to the corpus striatum. This disease is characterized by slow movement with akinesia, rigidity and abulia, coupled with masked face and unblinking stare. On the other hand, the patients may have tremor at rest and with movement, explosive weeping and laughing, pressured speech, festination, and akathisia. Initial symptoms may include resting tremor of one hand, usually progressing to generalized symptoms of tremor, bradykinesia, and rigidity. Later, gait disturbance and dysphagia may occur. Dementia has consistently been reported to be a concomitant of Parkinson's disease [51].

Depression is highly prevalent in patients with Parkinson's disease and may exacerbate the disease [51]. There are many hypotheses about the mechanisms of depression in Parkinson's disease. Among them, it is the most well-known that deficiency of dopamine, norepinephrine, or serotonin related to subcortical nuclei can affect mood regulation. In these patients, alteration in serotonin metabolism was found [52, 53]; depression was correlated with low CSF 5-hydroxyindoleacetic acid (HIAA), suggesting a reduction in central serotonin [53].

Most of neuroimaging studies generally suggest increased neural activity in the prefrontal regions and decreased functional connectivity between the prefrontal-limbic networks in depressed patients with Parkinson's disease. Both nigrostriatal and extra-nigrostriatal pathways (particularly the frontal regions and its connecting areas) may be affected in mood disorders of patients with Parkinson's disease [54].

15.3.1 Assessment of Depression

There are several valid tools for detecting depression in patients with Parkinson's disease: the 15-item Geriatric Depression Scale (GDS-15), Beck Depression Inventory, Montgomery-Åsberg Depression Rating Scale, and Unified Parkinson's Disease Rating Scale. Among these tools, practitioners should choose one that fits their clinical practice [55]. In addition, the Hamilton Depression Rating Scale (HAMD-17) and the GDS scales are recommended for screening and measuring the severity of depression in Parkinson's disease. The GDS-15 may be a preferred choice due to its brevity and ease-to-use design for older adults [56].

15.3.2 Psychopharmacotherapy of Depression

The treatment of psychiatric illness in patients with Parkinson's disease should focus on improving mood and function, while avoiding exacerbation of motor symptoms and delirium [51].

Tricyclic antidepressants such as imipramine and nortriptyline were reported to be effective in depressed patients with Parkinson's disease [57]. Tricyclics should be started at a low dose and increased gradually [51]. However, it should be avoided to use MAO inhibitors because its combination with L-dopa may cause side effects such as hypertension or orthostatic hypotension [32].

Bupropion, dopamine-related antidepressant, was found to be effective in about half of patients with Parkinson's disease with respect to depression and movement

[58]. SSRIs are supposed to help improve depression in patients with Parkinson's disease. However, some SSRIs including fluoxetine should be used with caution because they may cause extrapyramidal syndrome, leading to the exacerbation of symptoms of Parkinson's disease [59, 60].

15.3.3 Psychosocial Treatment of Depression

Pharmacologic treatments of depression can have negative side effects in patients with Parkinson's disease, including the exacerbation of symptoms of Parkinson's disease (e.g., extrapyramidal syndrome). There is a critical need for alternative treatment approaches that address depression among patients with Parkinson's disease. In general, psychosocial or behavioral approaches are known to be effective for depression, but there have been few studies on psychosocial treatments that specifically assess changes in depression among patients with Parkinson's disease [61]. CBT is potentially not only a useful treatment for patients with Parkinson's disease and comorbid depression [62] but also can help people overcome some of the challenges in living with Parkinson's disease by maximizing well-being and quality of life [63].

Results for CBT and other modes of therapy are promising for acute management of depression, but the longer term effects of treatment have been variable. Therefore, there is a need for additional studies on the long-term effects of psychosocial interventions in patients with Parkinson's disease [61].

Overall, therapeutic approaches to Parkinson's disease and its associated psychiatric symptoms including depression must be individualized and may involve a combination of antiparkinson drugs, psychopharmacological treatment, and/or psychotherapeutic intervention [64].

15.4 Dementia

Dementia is a chronic impairment of cognitive ability secondary to cerebral cortical or subcortical cellular dysfunction [65]. Dementia is not a diagnosis per se and is not always irreversible. At least 20% of cases diagnosed as dementia are at least partially reversible [66]. Early signs of dementia include lack of initiative, increased irritability, loss of interest in life activities, and difficulties learning new information or carrying out activities that require original thinking. In the chronically medically ill, an early sign of dementia may be an impaired coping with the tasks of daily living that is due to a decline in cognitive capacity rather than solely to a decline in physical status [65].

Early dementing processes are best detected through the systematic performance of serial mental status examinations supplemented by regular inquiries about activities of daily living such as the handling of personal finances, arrangement of transportation and driving, cooking, shopping, housework and chores, and communication with friends and relatives. Such inquiry enables the physicians to detect changes that may be denied by patients themselves, and family interviews are critical to an assessment of the patient as well [65].

Depression is one of the most common neuropsychiatric disturbances in Alzheimer disease [67–69]. Patients with dementia can become depressed, and aged patients with chronic depression can develop dementia during the course of illness. It was estimated that the prevalence of depression in patients with dementia was about 20–30% [70–73]. The prevalence of depression in patients with Alzheimer disease is known to be inversely correlated with the severity of dementia [74].

In the early stages and even middle stages of dementia, the patient may appear to be depressed [75]. Depression with reversible cognitive impairment may be a prodrome for dementia rather than a separate and distinct disorder [76].

15.4.1 Assessment of Depression

There are many validated tools for the detection of depression in individuals with dementia. Tools that incorporate physicians' interview with patients and collateral histories, the Cornell Scale for Depression in Dementia (CSDD) and Hamilton Depression Rating Scale (HDRS), have higher sensitivities, which would ensure fewer false-negatives [77].

In addition to the CSDD, the Dementia Mood Assessment Scale (DMAS) is recommended for evaluating depressive symptoms, and the Cohen-Mansfield Agitation Inventory (CMAI) is useful for evaluating the full range of agitation symptoms [78].

15.4.2 Treatment of Depression

Treating depression is a key clinical priority to improve the quality of life of people with dementia as well as their caregivers. Nonpharmacological approaches and watchful waiting should be attempted first in patients who present with mild to moderate depression and dementia [79]. Randomized clinical trials have demonstrated that depression in patients with dementia responds to specific psychosocial treatments (e.g., behavioral therapy) [76]. However, in cases of severe depression or depression not able to be managed through nonpharmacological means, antidepressant therapy should be considered [79].

15.4.2.1 Psychopharmacotherapy

Available evidence offers weak support to the contention that antidepressants are effective for patients with depression and dementia [80]. However, randomized clinical trials have demonstrated that depression in dementia patients responds to specific psychopharmacologic treatments [76].

Aged patients with dementia are not only sensitive to anticholinergic effects of tricyclic antidepressants but also their cognitive impairment can be exacerbated by these drugs. Confusion may also occur in patients without dementia receiving the antidepressants. Therefore, the use of these drugs should be avoided in patients with dementia. In addition, MAO inhibitors are not recommended because they can cause orthostatic hypotension [32].

Bupropion, SSRIs, and venlafaxine are preferred drugs for depressed patients with dementia because they cause less cognitive impairment and sedative action than tricyclic antidepressants. In particular, sertraline is known to be superior to placebo for the treatment of major depressive disorder in Alzheimer disease patients. Antidepressants can improve quality of life (e.g., lessened behavior disturbance and improved activities of daily living), although they do not improve cognition [81]. However, bupropion and SSRIs should be cautiously used in patients with dementia because they may cause emotional turmoil [32].

Overall, it is likely that a combined use of behavioral treatment and of antidepressant medication will provide the optimal management of depression in Alzheimer disease [82].

15.5 Conclusions

The physical and/or psychological sequelae caused by stroke, Parkinson's disease, and dementia may be devastating for both the patient and family. Depression during these illnesses not only complicates diagnosis and treatment but also hinders therapeutic efforts. SSRIs and tricyclic antidepressants are known to be effective in poststroke depression. These antidepressants should be continued at least for 4 months after initial recovery and should be changed if no response is seen after 6 weeks. Psychotherapy including cognitive behavioral therapy can be tried for patients with milder depression and those with side effects or contraindications to the use of antidepressants. Multidisciplinary and integrative approaches are recommended for assessing and treating poststroke depression. Tricyclic antidepressants as well as bupropion and SSRIs help improve depression in patients with Parkinson's disease. However, bupropion, SSRIs, and venlafaxine are preferred drugs for depressed patients with dementia because they cause less cognitive impairment and sedative action than tricyclic antidepressants. Overall, therapeutic approaches to Parkinson's disease or dementia comorbid with depression may involve a combination of psychopharmacological treatment and psychotherapeutic interventions including behavioral treatment.

References

1. Whyte EM, Mulsant BH. Post-stroke depression: epidemiology, pathophysiology, and biological treatment. Biol Psychiatry. 2002;52:253–64.
2. Robinson RG, Spalletta G. Poststroke depression: a review. Can J Psychiatr. 2010;55:341–9.
3. Robinson RG. Neuropsychiatric consequences of stroke. Annu Rev Med. 1997;48:217–29.
4. Wolfe CDA. The impact of stroke. Br Med Bull. 2000;56:275–86.
5. Williams LS, Ghose SS, Swindle RW. Depression and other mental health diagnoses increase mortality risk after ischemic stroke. Am J Psychiatry. 2004;161:1090–5.
6. Hackett M, Anderson C. Treatment options for post-stroke depression in the elderly. Aging Health. 2005;1:95–105.
7. Murphy E. Social origins of depression in old age. Br J Psychiatry. 1982;141:134–42.
8. De Ryck A, Brouns R, Fransen E, et al. A prospective study on the prevalence and risk factors of poststroke depression. Cerebrovasc Dis Extra. 2013;3:1–13.
9. Cohen-Cole SA, Harpe C. Assessment of depression in the medically ill. In: Stoudemire A, Fogel BS, editors. Principles of medical psychiatry. Orlando: Grune & Stratton; 1987.
10. Cassem NH. Depression. In: Cassem NH, editor. MGH handbook of general hospital psychiatry. St. Louis: Mosby-Year Book; 1991.
11. Lenze E, Rogers J, Martire L, et al. The association of late-life depression and anxiety with physical disability: a review of the literature and prospectus for future research. Am J Geriatr Psychiatry. 2001;9:113–35.
12. Austin M, Mitchell P, Goodwin G. Cognitive deficits in depression: possible implications for functional neuropathology. Br J Psychiatry. 2001;178:200–6.
13. Butters M, Becker J, Nebes R, et al. Changes in cognitive functioning following treatment of late-life depression. Am J Psychiatry. 2000;157:1949–54.
14. Gillen RTH, McKee TE, Gernert-Dott P, et al. Depressive symptoms and history of depression predict rehabilitation efficiency in stroke patients. Arch Phys Med Rehabil. 2001;82:1645–9.
15. Paolucci S, Antonucci G, Grasso M, et al. Poststroke depression, antidepressant treatment and rehabilitation results: a case-controlled study. Cerebrovasc Dis. 2001;12:264–71.
16. Schulz R, Beach S, Ives D, et al. Association between depression and mortality in older adults: The Cardiovascular Health Study. Arch Intern Med. 2000;160:1761–8.
17. Ensinck K, Schuurman A, van den Akker M, et al. Is there an increased risk of dying after depression? Am J Epidemiol. 2002;156:1043–8.
18. Glassman A, Shapiro P. Depression and the course of coronary artery disease. Am J Psychiatry. 1998;155:4–11.
19. Rabins P. Barriers to diagnosis and treatment of depression in elderly patients. Am J Geriatr Psychiatry. 1996;4:79–83.
20. Schubert D, Taylor C, Lee S, et al. Detection of depression in the stroke patient. Psychosomatics. 1992;33:290–4.
21. Christensen H, Jorm A, Mackinnon A, et al. Age differences in depression and anxiety symptoms: a structural equation modeling analysis of data from a general population sample. Psychol Med. 1999;29:325–39.
22. Meader N, Moe-Byrne T, Llewellyn A, et al. Screening for poststroke major depression: a meta-analysis of diagnostic validity studies. J Neurol Neurosurg Psychiatry. 2014;85:198–206.
23. Agrell B, Dehlin O. Comparison of six depression rating scales in geriatric stroke patients. Stroke. 1989;20:1190–4.
24. Carod-Artal F, Ferreira Coral L, Trizotto D, et al. Poststroke depression: prevalence and determinants in Brazilian stroke patients. Cerebrovasc Dis. 2009;28:157–65.
25. Strober LB, Arnett PA. Assessment of depression in three medically ill, elderly populations: Alzheimer's disease, Parkinson's disease, and stroke. Clin Neuropsychol. 2009;23:205–30.
26. Laidlaw K. Poststroke depression and CBT with older people. In: Dolores G-T, Ann MS, Lary WT, editors. Handbook of behavioral and cognitive therapies with older adults. New York: Springer; 2007.

27. Alexopoulos G, Buckwalter K, Olin J, et al. Comorbidity of late life depression: an opportunity for research on mechanisms and treatment. Biol Psychiatry. 2002;52:543–58.
28. Lokk J, Delbari A. Management of depression in elderly stroke patients. Neuropsychiatr Dis Treat. 2010;6:539–49.
29. Gusev E, Bogolepova A. Depressive disorders in stroke patients. Neurosci Behav Physiol. 2009;39:639–43.
30. Chen Y, Guo JJ, Zhan S, et al. Treatment effects of antidepressants in patients with post-stroke depression: a meta-analysis. Ann Pharmacother. 2006;40:2115–22.
31. Starkstein SE, Mizrahi R, Power BD. Antidepressant therapy in post-stroke depression. Expert Opin Pharmacother. 2008;9:1291–8.
32. Cunningham LA. Depression in the medically ill: choosing an antidepressant. J Clin Psychiatry. 1994;55(Suppl AJ):90–7.
33. Snow V, Lascher S, Mottur-Pilson C. Pharmacologic treatment of acute major depression and dysthymia: clinical guideline, part 1. Ann Intern Med. 2000;132:738–42.
34. Turner-stokes L, Hassan N. Depression after stroke: a review of the evidence base to inform the development of an integrated pathway. Part 1: diagnosis, frequency and impact. Clin Rehabil. 2002;16:231–47.
35. Williams LS. Depression and stroke: cause or consequence? Semin Neurol. 2005;25:396–409.
36. Paolucci S. Epidemiology and treatment of post-stroke depression. Neuropsychiatr Dis Treat. 2008;4:145–54.
37. Scogin F, Welsh D, Hanson A, et al. Evidence-based psychotherapies for depression in older adults. Clin Psychol Sci Pract. 2006;12:222–37.
38. Watkins C, Auton M, Deans C, et al. Motivational interviewing early after acute stroke: a randomized, controlled trial. Stroke. 2007;38:1004–9.
39. Gallagher-Thompson D, Steffen A, Thompson L, et al. Handbook of behavioral and cognitive therapies with older adults. New York: Springer; 2008.
40. Gebretsadik M, Jayaprabhu S, Grossberg G. Mood disorders in the elderly. Med Clin North Am. 2006;90:789–805.
41. Lincoln N, Flannaghan T. Cognitive behavioral psychotherapy for depression following stroke: a randomized controlled trial. Stroke. 2003;34:111–5.
42. Hackett M, Anderson C, House A. Interventions for treating depression after stroke. Stroke. 2009;40:e487–e8.
43. Australian R. Australian and new Zealand clinical practice guidelines for the treatment of depression. Aust N Z J Psychiatry. 2004;38:389–407.
44. Lai SM, Studenski S, Richards L, et al. Therapeutic exercise and depressive symptoms after stroke. J Am Geriatr Soc. 2006;54:240–7.
45. Fiske A, Wetherell J, Gatz M. Depression in older adults. Ann Rev Clin Psychol. 2009;5:363–89.
46. Turner-Stokes L, Hassan N, et al. Managing depression in brain injury rehabilitation: the use of an integrated care pathway and preliminary report of response to sertraline. Clin Rehabil. 2002;16:261–8.
47. Beck AT, Ward CH, Mendelssohn MJ, et al. An inventory for measuring depression. Arch Gen Psychiatry. 1961;4:561–71.
48. Gordon WA, Hibbard MR, Egelko S, et al. Issues in the diagnosis of post-stroke depression. Rehabil Psychol. 1991;36:71–87.
49. Sutcliffe LM, Lincoln NB. The assessment of depression in aphasic stroke patients: the development of the Stroke Aphasic Depression Questionnaire. Clin Rehabil. 1998;12:506–13.
50. Koh KB. Poststroke depression: mechanisms and management. In: Koh KB, editor. Somatization and psychosomatic symptoms. New York: Springer; 2013.
51. McNamara ME. Neurology. In: Stoudemire A, Fogel BS, editors. Principles of medical psychiatry. Orlando: Grune & Stratton; 1987.
52. Mayeux R, Stern Y, Cote L. Altered serotonin metabolism in depressed patients with Parkinson's disease. Neurology. 1984;34:642–6.

53. Mayeux R, Stern Y, Williams JB. Clinical and biochemical features of depression in Parkinson's disease. Am J Psychiatry. 1986;143:756–9.
54. Wen MC, Chan LL, Tan LC, et al. Depression, anxiety, and apathy in Parkinson's disease: insights from neuroimaging studies. Eur J Neurol. 2016;23:1001–19.
55. Goodarzi Z, Mrklas KJ, Roberts DJ, et al. Detecting depression in Parkinson disease: a systematic review and meta-analysis. Neurology. 2016;87:426–37.
56. Torbey E, Pachana NA, Dissanayaka NN. Depression rating scales in Parkinson's disease: a critical review updating recent literature. J Affect Disord. 2015;184:216–24.
57. Cummings JL. Depression and Parkinson's disease: a review. Am J Psychiatry. 1992;149:443–54.
58. Goetz CG, Tanner CM, Klawans HL. Bupropion in Parkinson's disease. Neurology. 1984;34:1092–4.
59. Bouchard RH, Pourcher E, Vincent P. Fluoxetine and extrapyramidal side effects [letter]. Am J Psychiatry. 1989;146:1352–3.
60. Meltzer HY, Young M, Metz J. Extrapyramidal side effects and increased serum prolactin following fluoxetine, a new antidepressant. J Neural Transm. 1979;45:165–75.
61. Yang S, Sajatovic M, Walter BL. Psychosocial interventions for depression and anxiety in Parkinson's disease. J Geriatr Psychiatry Neurol. 2012;25:113–21.
62. Armento ME, Stanley MA, Marsh L, et al. Cognitive behavioral therapy for depression and anxiety in Parkinson's disease: a critical review. J Parkinsons Dis. 2012;2:135–51.
63. Egan SJ, Laidlaw K, Starkstein S. Cognitive behavioral therapy for depression and anxiety in Parkinson's disease. J Parkinsons Dis. 2015;5:443–51.
64. Quelhas R. Psychiatric care in Parkinson's disease. J Psychiatr Pract. 2013;19:118–41.
65. Slaby AE, Cullem LO. Dementia and delirium. In: Stoudemire A, Fogel BS, editors. Principles of medical psychiatry. Orlando: Grune & Stratton; 1987.
66. McCarthy JR, Palmateer LM. Assessment of cognitive deficit in geriatric patients: a study of physician behavior. J Am Geriatr Soc. 1985;33:467–71.
67. Doody RS, Stevens JC, Beck C, et al. Practice parameter: management of dementia(an evidence based review): report of the Quality Standards Subcommittee of the American Academy of Neurology. Neurology. 2001;56:1154–66.
68. Lyketsos CG, Olin JT. Depression in Alzheimer disease: overview and treatment. Biol Psychiatry. 2002;52:243–52.
69. Olin JT, Schneider LS, Katz IR, et al. National Institute of Mental Health-Provisional Diagnostic Criteria for Depression of Alzheimer Disease: rationale and background. Am J Geriatr Psychiatry. 2002;10:125–8.
70. Reifler BV, Larson E, Teri L. Dementia of the Alzheimer's type and depression. J Am Geriatr Soc. 1986;34:855–9.
71. Lazarus LW, Newton N, Cohler B. Frequency and presentation of depressive symptoms in patients with primary degenerative dementia. Am J Psychiatry. 1987;144:41–5.
72. Burns A, Jacoby R, Levy R. Psychiatric phenomena in Alzheimer disease, III: disorders of mood. Br J Psychiatry. 1990;157:81–6.
73. Lyketsos CG, Steinberg M, Tschantz J, et al. Mental and behavioral disturbances in dementia: findings from the Cache County study on memory in aging. Am J Psychiatry. 2000;157:708–14.
74. Fischer P, Simanyi M, Danielczyk W. Depression in dementia of the Alzheimer type and in multi-infarct dementia. Am J Psychiatry. 1990;147:1484–7.
75. Reding M, Haycox J, Blass J. Depression in patients referred to a dementia clinic: a three year prospective study. Arch Neurol. 1985;42:894–6.
76. Katz IR. Diagnosis and treatment of depression in patients with Alzheimer's disease and other dementia. J Clin Psychiatry. 1998;59(Suppl 9):38–44.
77. Goodarzi ZS, Mele BS, Roberts DJ, et al. Depression case finding in individuals with dementia: a systematic review and meta-analysis. J Am Geriatr Soc. 2017;65:937–48.

78. Conn D, Thorpe L. Assessment of behavioral and psychological symptoms associated with dementia. Can J Neurol Sci. 2007;34(Suppl 1):S67–71.
79. Gutzmann H, Qazi A. Depression associated with dementia. Z Gerontol Geriatr. 2015;48:305–11.
80. Bains J, Birks J, Denning T. Antidepressants for treating depression in dementia. Cochrane Database Syst Rev. 2002;21:CD003944.
81. Lyketsos CG, DelCampo L, Steinberg M, et al. Treating depression in Alzheimer disease: efficacy and safety of sertraline therapy, and the benefits of depression reduction: the DIADS. Arch Gen Psychiatry. 2003;60:737–46.
82. Raskind MA. The clinical interface of depression and dementia. J Clin Psychiatry. 1998;59(Suppl 10):9–12.

Chapter 16
Approach to Depression in the Medically Ill

16.1 Introduction

Fifteen percent to 70% of the medically ill were reported to have depression [1–13]. The most frequent reason for referral to psychiatry is known to be depression [14]. Depressive disorders are the most commonly diagnosed mental disorder in patients referred for psychiatric consultation [15–18].

Patients with physical diseases frequently reveal depression by complaining of physical symptoms such as pain rather than cognitive symptoms or mood. In this case, depression tends to be overlooked because such physical symptoms may be caused by physical diseases [19]. Therefore, they are likely to be misdiagnosed as physical diseases rather than depressive disorders [20]. In particular, Korean depressive patients show somatization tendency [3, 21] and then tend to visit departments other than psychiatry for treatment. In general, however, nonpsychiatric physicians do not consider patients' psychological problems during their evaluation process but only give attention to their physical symptoms. As a result, they tend to overlook depression. In one study based on medical records [22], it was reported that 50% of depressive disorders were missed in the medical setting.

Despite the difficulties in screening for depression in medically ill patients due to the overlap of symptoms between the two disorders, it is important to recognize and treat depression in these patients because of the significant likelihood of improvement in quality of life [23] as well as positive impacts on outcomes of physical diseases [24].

K. B. Koh, *Stress and Somatic Symptoms*,
https://doi.org/10.1007/978-3-030-02783-4_16

16.2 Outcomes of Comorbid Depression in the Medically Ill

Mood disorders such as depression result in impaired physical recovery and more intricate treatment regimen [25]. In addition, comorbid depressive symptoms in medically ill patients are associated with poorer survival, longer hospitalization stay, persistent smoking, increased symptom burden, and poorer physical and social functioning [24]. These may be because depressive symptoms in the medically ill are not recognized well so that they are not treated adequately. About 15% of untreated patients with major depressive disorder commit suicide [26]. On the other hand, depression can lead to exacerbation of physical diseases, resulting in higher mortality than simply expected from the physical diseases [27, 28]. Depression can contribute to increased cost of medical care as well as higher morbidity of physical diseases [29].

16.3 Relationship Between Physical Diseases and Depression

Depression can manifest itself as symptoms related to either physical diseases or medication, responses to physical diseases, and comorbidity of physical diseases and psychiatric disorders. First, biological factors can cause depression. Neurotransmitters such as serotonin and norepinephrine are associated with depression. In addition, other biological factors include hormones, nutritional status, electrolytes, endocrine abnormalities, effects of medication, systemic diseases, and cerebral diseases [30]. Second, severe physical diseases act as stressors and make an influence on body image, self-esteem, a sense of identity, the ability to work, marital life, familial relationship, and the ability to maintain social life, leading to depression [12]. Finally, patients with physical diseases may have preexisting psychiatric disorders such as depressive disorders.

However, clinical reports indicate that the relationship between systemic and psychiatric illnesses is bidirectional, further increasing the complexity of the underlying pathophysiological processes [25].

16.4 Emotional Reaction to the Diagnosis of a Chronic Illness

The emotional reaction to the diagnosis of a chronic illness can be a greater challenge than coping with the physical manifestations of the illness. There are a variety of determinants of the emotional reaction to the diagnosis of a chronic illness: (1) personality before the illness; (2) previously unresolved anger or grief; (3) the suddenness, extent, and duration of lifestyle changes mandated by the illness; (4) familial and individual resources for dealing with stress; (5)

stages of individual and family life cycle; (6) previous experience with illness or crisis; and (7) codependency in the family system [31]. People who receive diagnoses of chronic illness may find their emotional reaction more disabling than the illness itself until they go through the adjustment process to embrace the new persons they have become through the illness [31].

16.5 Psychodynamics of Depression in the Medically Ill

Psychodynamic understanding of depression can help assess and treat depressed patients with physical diseases. Patients with physical diseases are likely to be depressed because individuals' conflicts and vulnerabilities can be fostered by such diseases. In particular, a sense of loss is a universal phenomenon seen in patients with severe physical diseases [32, 33], and decreased self-esteem plays a central role in psychodynamics of depression [34].

Physical experiences and physical integrity are important elements of a sense of self during periods of childhood and adulthood. Kohut regarded depressed mood related to severe physical diseases as a manifestation of an injured sense of self [35]. With respect to psychodynamics of physical diseases, the meaning of a specific disease is likely to depend on physical status and individual characteristics. In addition, clinical significance of depression can greatly be affected by coping strategies [36] and social support [37].

Considering these aspects, as Akiskal and McKinney [38] mentioned, depression can represent the final common psychobiological pathway through which a variety of factors interact.

16.6 Why Physicians Miss Depression in the Medically Ill?

First, depressive symptoms can be regarded as part of symptoms of physical diseases. For example, somatic symptoms such as poor appetite, weight loss, fatigue, and insomnia are noted in physical diseases as well as depressive disorders.

Second, physicians tend to see depression as a normal reaction to physical diseases. For example, naturally a patient with lymphadenoma must be depressed due to his/her illness. However, most patients with physical diseases are not depressed. Thus, it is not desirable for physicians to see depression as a normal reaction to illness. If physicians give up treatment of depression with such false ideas, patients are likely to suffer more distress due to their dual disorders. However, depression can certainly be treated if the patient is willing to receive care.

For differential diagnoses, physicians need to focus more on psychological symptoms such as anhedonia, hopelessness, crying, guilt, reduced self-esteem, unworthiness, and suicidal ideation than physical symptoms [39]. These symptoms are common in patients with major depressive disorder, but rare in patients with mild or moderate severity of physical diseases or their sequelae [40].

16.7 Clinical Evaluation of Depression

Depression is generally underdiagnosed in the medically ill [41], and the syndrome can be long lasting and debilitating [42]. Furthermore, even when depression is recognized by primary physicians, the patients are often treated inadequately [43].

Clinicians need to pay particular attention to the psychological symptoms of depression and anhedonia (loss of pleasure) in the medically ill. If patients do not feel pleasure or interest for at least 2 weeks, the possibility of major depressive disorder should be considered. Sometimes it may help therapists make a diagnosis of major depressive disorder to ask the patients about their ability to concentrate, their sense of self-esteem or guilt, and their thoughts about death [44].

Clark et al. [45] found out seven cognitive and emotional symptoms in the medically ill. They include suicidal ideation, a sense of failure, self-reproach, reduced social interest, crying, irresolution, and dissatisfaction.

Personal and family histories of the patients are important because a prior personal or family history of major depressive disorder can increase the likelihood of a current episode. Previous response to treatment can also provide useful information for diagnosis and treatment of depression, along with high prediction of similar responses with the same treatment [46, 47].

16.8 Evaluation of Major Psychological Symptoms in Depressed Patients with Physical Diseases

16.8.1 Depressed Mood and Anhedonia

It is not easy to evaluate if patients with physical diseases have interest or pleasure. In particular, elderly patients may deny depressed mood or anhedonia but show a sense of hopelessness and helplessness. These feelings are regarded as identical to depression. When they avoid people and have no interest in their self-care and other activities, these symptoms can be considered anhedonia [48].

16.8.2 Unworthiness and Excessive Guilt

Patients with major depressive disorder have bad feelings about themselves rather than situations. For example, they express their unworthiness by saying "I am bad" and "I feel bad about myself," whereas they express their self-reproach by saying "I am bad because I am a burden." They express excessive or inappropriate guilt by saying "It is a punishment that I am ill" [48, 49].

16.8.3 Suicidal Ideation

Patients with major depressive disorder can show repetitive thoughts on suicide. On the other hand, patients with serious physical diseases can say "I would like to die." However, death can not only be considered another rational method for the patient's intolerable pain associated with a physical disease, but also can be seen logical by his/her family and physician. In this case, such expression should not be considered suicidal ideation [50].

16.9 Biopsychosocial Evaluation

Biopsychosocial evaluation should precede treatment of depression in the medically ill [12].

16.9.1 General Psychiatric Evaluation

Diagnosis of depression, evaluation of suicidal risk, presence and absence of other mental disorders, and past psychiatric history should be checked [12].

16.9.2 Use of Psychological Instruments

Psychological instruments were developed to evaluate depression in the medically ill. These instruments help differentiate somatic symptoms related to depression from those related to physical diseases, because they are not dependent on somatic symptoms [51]. The Beck Depression Inventory is useful for screening of depression, whereas the Hamilton Rating Scale for Depression is useful for both screening and evaluation of the degree of depression [52]. In addition, there are the Depression in the Medically Ill-18 (DMI-18) questionnaire, Hospital Anxiety and Depression Scale (HADS), and Patient Health Questionnaire-9 (PHQ-9). In particular, the DMI-18 was reported to stand out for its sensitivity [53].

16.9.3 Find Out Precipitating Factors of Depression

The presence and absence of social support, adaptation to job, the role of family, sexual function, body image, and the meaning of illness should be checked [12].

16.9.4 Identify Physical Diseases and Medications Related to Depression

Endocrine and metabolic system diseases, infectious diseases, central nervous system diseases, cancer, and drug toxicity should be checked. Mood disorders associated with medical conditions (depressive disorder due to another medical condition in DSM-5) are similar to major depressive disorder, although their etiology is organic [54]. The physical diseases and medications which have been most commonly reported to be associated with depression are as follows [23, 55]:

1. Physical diseases: cancer (brain and pancreas cancer), cerebrovascular disease (stroke), collagen-vascular disease (systemic lupus erythematosus), chronic obstructive pulmonary disease (COPD), endocrine diseases (hypothyroidism, Cushing syndrome, hypoglycemia), lymphoma, Parkinson's disease, pernicious anemia (B_{12} deficiency), viral infections (influenza, hepatitis, mononucleosis, Epstein-Barr virus), coronary heart disease, end-stage renal disease, chronic pain, Alzheimer disease, and seizure disorder
2. Medications: antihypertensives (reserpine, propranolol, methyldopa), barbiturates, cimetidine, corticosteroids, guanethidine, indomethacin, levodopa, psychostimulants (amphetamine, cocaine in the post-withdrawal phase), benzodiazepines, diuretics (thiazides, spironolactone), clonidine, and oral contraceptives

Depression associated with medications is termed 'substance/medication-induced depressive disorder' in DSM-5. Mood disorders due to medical conditions (depressive disorder due to another medical condition in DSM-5) do not mean that all physical diseases are etiologically associated with depression. However, it is important for clinicians to always consider physical diseases or medications that might contribute to a patient's depressive symptoms [55].

The treatment of mood disorder due to medical conditions should first focus on the medical treatment of the underlying physical diseases or on the removal of the offending medications. However, in cases in which the physical disease cannot be treated, or the medication cannot be removed, clinicians should cautiously initiate the biopsychosocial approach used in the treatment of major depressive disorder without organic causes [55].

16.9.5 Evaluate the Risks and Advantages of Treatment of Depression

In patients with physical disease whose depressive symptoms are severe and not responsive to treatment of physical diseases or brief psychotherapy, psychopharmacological treatment should be considered. In these patients, tricyclic antidepressants can primarily be tried but should be cautiously used in elderly patients with physical diseases, considering changes in pharmacokinetic and drug-drug interaction and risks of drug toxicity [56]. For example, anticholinergic effects of tricyclic antidepressants, such as dry mouth and constipation, can make patients with gastrointestinal symptoms more distressed. In these patients, antidepressants with less anticholinergic effects need to be chosen.

16.10 Psychosocial Treatment

Psychosocial treatment for depressive patients with physical diseases is different from that for depressive patients without physical diseases.

16.10.1 Patients with Physical Diseases Are Resistant to Psychiatric Approach

Depressive patients with physical diseases often deny being depressed and refuse to see psychiatrists. They often feel angry and humiliated when primary physicians see their problems as psychiatric, rather than physical. In these cases, it is difficult for physicians to perform a diagnostic evaluation or to provide psychotherapy to them. Physicians should start conversation with empathy in regard to the patients' anger and frustration [43], as in somatizing patients [57].

16.10.2 Despondency Consequent to Serious Illness

Despondency in serious illness appears to be a natural response but is regarded as the psychic damage done by the disease to the patients' self-esteem. Depression is also defined as a response to narcissistic injury [58], but the response is here called despondency because it does not meet the criteria for depressive disorders. In any serious illness, the mind sustains an injury of its own, as though the illness, for example, myocardial infarction (MI) produces an ego infarction [59].

16.10.2.1 Management of Acute Despondency

Despondency caused by illnesses can threaten work and interpersonal relationship [60]. It is essential to let patients know that such concern is a normal reaction to the illness and that this concern will probably disappear gradually as health returns. In particular, physicians should focus on maintaining patients' sense of self-esteem. Even patients who have good recovery potential are often vulnerable to self-esteem injury. At this time, physicians encourage the patient to feel not only unique but appreciated by asking personal questions [59].

16.10.2.2 Management of Chronic Despondency

Patients who returned home from the hospital feel weak and experience a home-coming depression [61]. Invariably they attribute their weakness to the injury caused by the disease. However, a large part of this weakness is due to muscular atrophy and the systemic effects of immobilization [59].

Patients may find any unusual sensation a threat. It is helpful to inform the patients in advance that such hypersensitivity to bodily sensations commonly occurs, that it is normal, and that it is time-limited. Sometimes patients may feel afraid to leave the house. Moreover, they are likely to regard routine activities like walking as too dangerous [59]. The best treatment for such psychological constriction is a program that emphasizes early and progressive mobilization in the hospital and exercise after discharge [62–65]. Even when the body has no room for improvement, it should be emphasized that the mind can usually be rehabilitated [59].

16.11 Biological Treatment: Antidepressants in the Medically Ill

16.11.1 General Principle

The biological model in which chemical imbalance is corrected by psychopharmacological agents can help clinicians establish therapeutic alliance with the psychologically resistant patients as insulin is helpful for patients with diabetes. Ultimately, however, the patients should be approached biopsychosocially. In these cases, it should be emphasized that psychosocial problems related to the onset and exacerbation of diabetes or hypertension can cause depression and that psychosocial intervention can help treat depression [43].

In the medically ill with depression, diagnoses of physical diseases, the presence and absence of complications of physical diseases, and medications used for physical diseases should be checked. In addition, assessment of the side effects of antidepressants is important. The side effects can be a double-edged sword. In some cases, sedation is more required, but in other cases, it can lead to intolerable risks. Experienced clinicians can adjust such side effects to patients' symptoms, resulting in optimal outcomes [39].

16.11.2 Drug-Disease and Drug-Drug Interactions

Prior to administration of antidepressants in the medically ill, clinicians should answer the following three questions [39].

First, does the physical disease affect medication?

Patients with liver diseases cannot metabolize antidepressants effectively. Renal diseases reduce clearance of antidepressants. Therefore, in patients with renal and liver diseases, clinicians should start using antidepressants at a low dose.

Second, how does the drug affect the physical disease?

Tricyclic antidepressants can increase post-myocardial infarction mortality [66]. These drugs can cause severe orthostatic hypotension in patients with congestive heart failure. Trazodone can cause arrhythmia in patients with the existing unstable heart [67]. Antidepressants blocking dopamine receptor can exacerbate Parkinson's disease, whereas dopamine agonists can improve the disease. Since Alzheimer disease is linked to choline system abnormality, drugs with anticholinergic effects can exacerbate the disease [39].

Third, is there the possibility of drug-drug interactions?

Tricyclic antidepressants can block antihypertensive effects of clonidine, methyldopa, and guanethidine while potentiating the effect of prazosin [68]. A combined use of MAO inhibitors and meperidine, one of sympathomimetic amine series, can cause hypertensive crisis, leading to fatality [39].

SSRIs are likely to block oxidative metabolism by inhibiting cytochrome P450 IID6 isoenzyme in the liver [68]. Among SSRIs, sertraline is the most preferred drug in terms of drug-drug interactions because it inhibits the enzyme least [69]. Venlafaxine is known to be unrelated to drug-drug interactions through inhibition of P450 IID6 [70].

16.11.3 Psychostimulants as Antidepressants in the Medically Ill

The available evidence suggests possible effectiveness of methylphenidate for depressive symptoms including fatigue and apathy in various medically ill populations, although there have been conflicting results [71]. Ten milligrams to 40 mg per day of methylphenidate is known to have little cardiovascular risk [70].

16.12 Use of Antidepressants in Specific Physical Diseases

The use of antidepressants in patients with stroke, Parkinson's disease, dementia, cancer, cardiovascular diseases, diabetes, gastrointestinal diseases, and chronic pain has already been mentioned in other chapters. Herein, the use of antidepressants in patients with other diseases such as renal diseases, hepatic diseases, respiratory diseases, and insomnia are reviewed.

16.12.1 Renal Diseases

Depression occurs frequently in end-stage renal disease (ESRD) patients because they experience a lot of loss. In addition to a loss of energy and strength, these patients have to be dependent on dialysis treatment, sexual function is lowered, and their previous occupational life following dialyses cannot be sustained. In particular, the evaluation of dialysis patients for depression is complicated by the fact that the symptoms and signs of ESRD and its treatment may be identical to those of depression, such as anorexia, dry mouth, constipation, fatigue, and diminished sexual interest and ability [72].

Renal diseases can affect not only the excretion of drugs but also the absorption, distribution, and metabolism. A large amount of drugs are required to maintain steady-state blood levels of water-soluble lithium and psychotropics including protein-binding drugs such as tricyclic antidepressants in patients with uremia. If these patients require long-term use of antidepressants, it is desirable to start with a low dose and then gradually increase the dosage [73].

In general, drugs with less than 500 Dalton such as lithium are excreted by dialyses. However, most of antidepressants except venlafaxine are not significantly excreted by dialyses due to their protein-binding effects [74–76]. It is desirable to reduce the dose of drugs and increase the intervals of their administration in patients with renal diseases. The dosage of medication is regulated by using the index of renal function such as creatinine clearance [69].

Tricyclic antidepressants are not relatively water-soluble and not well dialyzed, although they have small molecules [77]. Patients with ESRD are likely to show toxic responses to therapeutic doses of tricyclic antidepressants. Their therapeutic effects and clinical signs of toxicity can be more reliable index for regulation of dosage [73].

SSRIs such as fluoxetine are not significantly affected by disturbance of renal function [78, 79]. Half-life of venlafaxine in patients with renal diseases is prolonged 50% longer, and its clearance rate is 24% lower. Therefore, these drugs should be started at a low dose and then gradually increased [80]. Regarding the efficacy of SSRIs in patients with non-dialysis-dependent chronic kidney disease and major depressive disorder, however, one study found that 12 weeks of sertraline treatment did not significantly improve depressive symptoms [81].

16.12.2 Hepatic Diseases

If patients with liver diseases complain of depression, insomnia, and hypersomnia, clinicians should check whether they have hepatic encephalopathy. These patients often show hypersensitivity to sedative effects of psychotropics [82]. Therefore, it is desirable to use antidepressants with low sedative action for insomnia in patients with liver diseases [70].

Cognitive function should be thoroughly examined before the use of antidepressants in patients with liver diseases. It should be periodically re-evaluated in order to confirm if psychotropics exacerbate cognitive function. Restlessness and sleep disturbance such as awakening during nights due to physical distress caused by ascites may be bigger problems when liver disease is progressing. In this case, it is desirable to recommend good sleep habit before the use of hypnotics. However, for patients with both liver diseases and depression, antidepressants should be used. At this time, antidepressants need to be selected, considering their sedative action and the necessity of patients' activities [70]. Generally, the degree of liver damage is reflected by the degree of drugs' binding to plasma protein [67]. In patients with ascites, the serum or plasma levels of tricyclic antidepressants can be lower than expected from the dosage administered. Therefore, the dose of medication should be regulated after evaluating therapeutic effects and side effects of drugs [70].

Liver diseases affect metabolism of most psychotropics. Exceptionally, liver diseases do not affect metabolism of some water-soluble drugs such as lithium and lorazepam [70]. Tricyclic antidepressants with narrower range of therapeutic safety tend to be more affected by protein-binding capacity than SSRIs with wider range of therapeutic safety. If tricyclic antidepressants or SSRIs with high protein-binding capacity are used, it should be kept in mind that these drugs can interfere with protein-binding capacity of nonpsychotropic drugs [73]. Venlafaxine has little possibility of interfering with protein binding of drugs administered for liver diseases due to its weak protein-binding capacity. Sedative action of this drug can be used for depressed patients with insomnia. However, anorexia and nausea related to liver diseases may be exacerbated by this drug [70].

Clearance rate of fluoxetine is lower, and its half-life is two times longer in patients with liver cirrhosis compared with healthy individuals [78]. Half-life of other SSRIs such as paroxetine and fluvoxamine may be prolonged in patients with liver diseases [83–85]. Sertraline with shorter half-life and less inhibition of cytochrome P450-mediated metabolism is better than fluoxetine in the treatment of depression associated with liver diseases [73].

In patients with liver diseases, reducing the doses of trazodone is appropriate because clearance may be prolonged. However, in patients with encephalopathy, its severe sedation should be considered relative contraindication [73].

Based on research suggesting that serotonin promotes the development and growth of hepatocellular carcinoma (HCC), one study tested the hypothesis of whether exposure to SSRIs is associated with an increased risk of HCC in chronic hepatitis C virus (HCV) infection patients. However, analysis of a large cohort of HCV patients did not support the hypothesis [86].

16.12.3 Respiratory Diseases

Some patients with respiratory diseases may experience significant depression as well as loss of self-esteem. The extent of their depression is variable, ranging from an adjustment disorder with depressed mood to a severe major depressive disorder [87]. In particular, medication such as corticosteroids may cause emotional instability and depression and suppress immune function. Depression has also been found to suppress immune response, and thus it may exacerbates upper respiratory infections [88]. Side effects of corticosteroids such as moon face, hirsutism, and acne may also cause depression [89]. Patients with asthma are likely to feel lonely because they have to be educated to avoid allergens so that their activities as well as their interpersonal relationship are limited.

The incidence of suicide and suicidal attempts is significantly higher in patients with bronchial asthma compared with those with hypertension [90]. Suicidal ideation may not be expressed directly, but may be expressed in more passive fashion by poor adherence to medical treatment [89].

Clinicians have a tendency to view a depression related to an emotionally traumatic diagnosis such as bronchial asthma as understandable and not to treat it appropriately. On the other hand, the symptoms of depressive disorders such as hopelessness, helplessness, guilt, and psychomotor retardation may interfere with appropriate medical treatment [89].

The diagnosis of major depressive disorder may be difficult in patients with symptoms of chronic respiratory diseases, since many depressive and pulmonary symptoms overlap, including fatigue, lassitude, weight loss, anorexia, and loss of interest [89].

Tricyclic antidepressants such as imipramine and SSRIs such as citalopram are known to improve the status of asthma as well as depression in patients with bronchial asthma and depression [89, 91]. As with benzodiazepines, the dose of antidepressants may need to be smaller in these patients compared with those with no physical diseases [89]. Doxepin may act as a mild bronchodilator [92]. In one study [93], a remission trend was observed favoring escitalopram, one of the SSRIs over placebo on depression measures in patients with asthma and major depressive disorder.

The less sedating antidepressants should be used in patients with compromised pulmonary status (e.g., COPD, sleep apnea) in order to prevent respiratory depression. However, most antidepressants are known to have little effect on respiratory status as far as they are appropriately used [87, 92]. It remains unclear whether SSRIs should be favored over TCAs in the treatment of depressed COPD patients [94], although SSRIs might have fewer side effects than TCAs [95].

16.12.4 Sleep Disorders

For sleep disorders in depressive patients with physical diseases, the use of antidepressants with sedative action may have the benefit of preventing complications caused by medications rather than the combined use of antidepressants and hypnotics. Sedative action is more potent in tricyclic antidepressants, mirtazapine, and trazodone compared with SSRIs, venlafaxine, bupropion, and nefazodone [96–99]. Sedative effect can be accomplished by modifying the dose of medication, but otherwise it is desirable to choose other series of drugs.

Antidepressants such as MAO inhibitors, SSRIs, venlafaxine, and bupropion can often cause insomnia. This may be due to side effects of the antidepressants, such as akathisia, hypomania or mania, and nocturnal myoclonus. If sleep duration is reduced by antidepressants, clinicians should decrease their dose and consider changing to other antidepressants [96]. The addition of 50–100 mg of trazodone sometimes improves quality of sleep.

16.12.5 Other Symptoms

Tricyclic antidepressants are used in other conditions than depression. For example, such conditions include enuresis, chronic pain, migraine, and peptic ulcer. Tricyclic antidepressants can have dual effects for depressed patients with these physical symptoms. SSRIs are also effectively used for chronic pain and migraine [39].

The use of tricyclic antidepressants should be avoided in patients with the history of eye diseases because their anticholinergic effects can facilitate narrow-angle glaucoma. However, SSRIs can be safely used in patients with glaucoma. SSRIs, bupropion, and venlafaxine are more recommended than tricyclic antidepressants or MAO inhibitors for patients with depression and obesity, because they do not cause weight gain [39].

Case

A 59-year-old female patient was referred from the department of gynecology for psychiatric consultation at the outpatient clinic and then admitted to the department of psychiatry. At that time, she showed severe depression, agitation, suicidal rumination, and social withdrawal and complained of a variety of somatic symptoms such as weakness, anorexia, insomnia, generalized ache, palpitation, and lethargy. Six months earlier, she had undergone surgery for uterus cancer at the department of gynecology, after which she developed thrombosis in the left leg. She was admitted to the department of transplantation surgery for about 2 weeks, where she received medication such as 5 mg of warfarin (Coumadin), 300 mg of triflusal (Disgren), and 1 mg of lorazepam per day. She had been almost unable to walk for 1 month while suffering from the above symptoms.

The patient was diagnosed with major depressive disorder. Her husband took care of her all the time during admission. Amitriptyline 25 mg twice per day and ethyl loflazepate 1 mg before sleep were administered orally. She continued to complain of weakness and generalized ache, showing irritability for the first few days after admission. Around this time, when a psychiatric resident visited her, she showed signs of hopelessness, saying "Are you here to see me dying?" She was also anxious, saying "It looks like my illness won't get better." The next day, however, her sleep improved, and she began to complain less frequently of her somatic symptoms. Eight days after hospitalization, she walked to another room to watch TV. The day after, she began to try to walk a little more, and her mood also improved. Thereafter, she continued to walk, had a better appetite, and started to have hopes for her improved physical condition. She once recalled with a bright facial expression, "I have enjoyed playing golf for a long time, but because I thought I could never play golf anymore when I was unable to walk, I lost my joy and meaning of life."

The patient was discharged 18 days after hospitalization, at which time she was able to walk by herself, felt better, and began to regain her physical strength. After eating out with her family, she said "I am considering traveling abroad in the near future."

This patient experienced damage to her self-esteem while she was weak and unable to walk due to thrombosis in the leg as a sequelae of her cancer treatment. Thereafter, she was psychologically constricted and extremely limited in her own activities, showing hypersensitivity to minimal physical changes. Her frequently used cognitive coping mechanisms were extremism, catastrophism, and pessimism. However, increased physical activity as recommended by her therapist as well as improvements in sleep and in her depressed mood as a result of treatment with tricyclic antidepressants, along with her family's emotional support, especially her husband's devoted care, helped her gradually regain her self-confidence and self-respect.

16.13 Future Directions

Cognitive behavioral therapy (CBT), physical rehabilitation, and antidepressant treatment have positive impacts on the quality of life as well as mood in depressed patients with physical diseases (e.g., COPD) [23, 100–102]. In particular, patients who received mindfulness-based cognitive therapy (MBCT) had a reduced risk of depressive relapse when compared with those who did not receive MBCT [103]. However, mindfulness-based stress reduction (MBSR) therapy was found to have small effects on depression, anxiety, and psychological distress in people with chronic somatic diseases, suggesting that integration of MBSR in behavioral therapy may enhance the efficacy of mindfulness-based interventions in these patients [104].

Collaborative care interventions are known to be effective in medically ill patients with depression because psychosocial quality of life and satisfaction with care are enhanced in patients receiving such interventions compared with usual care, although physical quality of life is not [105]. Complex psychological and/or lifestyle interventions that include an exercise component significantly improve symptoms of depression in patients with COPD [106]. In addition, a variety of treatment modalities including medications, psychotherapy, social support, and spiritual intervention need to be considered for management of depression in the medically ill. Therefore, clinicians' therapeutic approach should be tailored to the specific needs of such patients in terms of biopsychosociospiritual perspectives [107].

16.14 Conclusions

It is desirable to evaluate patients' medical and psychiatric status at the same time and consider multidimensional approaches in order to make a diagnosis of depression in the medically ill. Sometimes psychological instruments can be used to assess depression. For treatment, first, it is important to get rid of organic factors than any other things. Second, therapists should address patients' resistance to psychiatric approaches and despondency response to severe physical diseases. Third, it is important to choose appropriate antidepressants as biological treatment. The selection of antidepressants in the medically ill should be considered after evaluating patients' primary depressive symptoms, drug kinetics and dynamics, and side effects of antidepressants. Therapists also need to pay attention to drug-disease and drug-drug interactions. Antidepressants such as SSRIs, bupropion, and venlafaxine are effective for depression in the medically ill. However, tricyclic antidepressants can still be used effectively for patients with pain. In addition, collaborative care interventions are found to be effective in medically ill patients with depression. Therefore, clinicians' therapeutic approach should be tailored to the specific needs of such patients in terms of biopsychosociospiritual perspectives.

References

1. Ban KH, Yum TH, Han HM. Report on depression assessed by Beck Depression Inventory in medical patients. J Korean Neuropsychiatr Assoc. 1987;26:464–73.
2. Oh BH, Cho DY, Kim NK. A study on anxiety and depression in cancer and non-cancer patients. J Korean Neuropsychiatr Assoc. 1986;25:121–31.
3. Lee SD, Cho SH, Kwak DI. The extent of depression and anxiety in medical inpatients. J Korean Neuropsychiatr Assoc. 1990;29:353–67.
4. Lee HS, Hong CH, Byun WT. A study on anxiety and depression in patients admitted at a general hospital. J Korean Neuropsychiatr Assoc. 1989;28:258–67.
5. Ha HK. A study on anxiety and depression in cancer patients. J Korean Neuropsychiatr Assoc. 1982;21:665–74.
6. Yang CK, Han HM. A study on patterns of depression symptoms in medical inpatients. J Korean Neuropsychiatr Assoc. 1995;34:379–90.
7. Yun SJ, Yang CK, Han HM. A study on depression, anxiety and sleep disturbance in patients on hemodialysis. J Korean Neuropsychiatr Assoc. 1999;38:997–1005.
8. Bukberg J, Penman D, Holland JC. Depression in hospitalized cancer patients. Psychosom Med. 1984;46:199–212.
9. Grassi L, Rosti G, Albieri G, et al. Depression and abnormal illness behavior in cancer patients. Gen Hosp Psychiatry. 1989;11:404–11.
10. Hinrichen GA, Lieberman JA, Pollack S, et al. Depression in hemodialysis patients. Psychosom Med. 1989;30:284–9.
11. Popkin MK, Callies AL, Mackenzie TB. The outcome of antidepressant use in the medically ill. Arch Gen Psychiatry. 1985;42:1160–3.
12. Rodin G, Voshart K. Depression in the medically ill: an overview. Am J Psychiatry. 1986;143:696–705.
13. Yang L, Zuo C, Su L, Eaton MT. Depression in Chinese medical inpatients. Am J Psychiatry. 1987;144:226–8.
14. Rodin GM. Renal dialysis and the liaison psychiatrist. Can J Psychiatr. 1980;25:473–7.
15. Koh KB, Min SH, Min SK. The changing patterns of psychiatric consultations in a ten-year period. J Korean Neuropsychiatr Assoc. 1988;27:23–30.
16. Shevitz SA, Silberfarb PM, Lipowski ZJ. Psychiatric consultations in a general hospital—a report on 1,000 referrals. Dis Nerv Syst. 1976;37:295–300.
17. Lipowski ZJ, Wolston EJ. Liaison psychiatry: referral patterns and their stability over time. Am J Psychiatry. 1981;138:1608–11.

18. Bustamente JP, Ford CV. Characteristics of general hospital patients referred for psychiatric consultation. J Clin Psychiatry. 1983;42:338–41.
19. Katon W. Depression: relationship to somatization and chronic medical illness. J Clin Psychiatry. 1984;45:4–11.
20. Katon W, Roy-Byrne PP. Antidepressants in the medically ill: diagnosis & treatment in primary care. Clin Chem. 1988;34:829–36.
21. Kim KI. A symptomatological study on depression: 2. Patterns of depression symptoms in Koreans. J Korean Neuropsychiatr Assoc. 1977;16:46–52.
22. Nielsen AC, Williams TA. Depression in ambulatory medical patients. Arch Gen Psychiatry. 1980;37:999–1004.
23. Wilson I. Depression in the patient with COPD. Int J Chron Obstruct Pulmon Dis. 2006;1:61–4.
24. Ng TP, Niti M, Tan WC, et al. Depressive symptoms and chronic obstructive pulmonary disease: effect on mortality, hospital readmission, symptom burden, functional status, and quality of life. Arch Intern Med. 2007;167:60–7.
25. Duric V, Clayton S, Leong ML, et al. Comorbidity factors and brain mechanisms linking chronic stress and systemic illness. Neural Plast. 2016;5460732. https://doi.org/10.1155/2016/5460732. Epub 8 Feb 2016.
26. Regier DA, Farmer ME, Rae DS. Comorbidity of mental disorders with alcohol and other drug abuse: results from the Epidemiologic Catchment Area (ECA) study. JAMA. 1990;264:2511–8.
27. Katon W, Sullivan MD. Depression and chronic medical illness. J Clin Psychiatry. 1990;51(Suppl 6):3–11.
28. Rovner BW, German PS, Brant LJ. Depression and mortality in nursing homes. JAMA. 1991;265:993–6.
29. Simon GE, Vonkorff M, Barlow W. Health care costs of primary care patients with recognized depression. Arch Gen Psychiatry. 1995;52:850–6.
30. Hall RCW. Depression in psychiatric presentations of medical illness: somatopsychic disorders. New York: SP Medical & Scientific Books; 1980.
31. Lewis KS. Emotional adjustment to a chronic illness. Lippincotts Prim Care Pract. 1998;2:38–51.
32. Freud S. Mourning and melancholia. In: Jones E, editor. Collected papers, vol. 4. 1950. London: Hogarth Press; 1917.
33. Spitz R. Anaclitic depression: an inquiry into the genesis of psychiatric conditions in early childhood. Psychoanal Study Child. 1942;2:313–42.
34. Bibring E. The mechanism of depression. In: Greenacre P, editor. Affective disorders. New York: International Universities Press; 1965.
35. Kohut H. The restoration of the self. New York: International Universities Press; 1977.
36. Cohen F, Lazarus RS. Coping with the stresses of illness. In: Stone GC, Cohen F, Adler NE, editors. Health psychology. San Francisco: Jossey-Bass; 1979.
37. Lin N, Dean A. Social support and depression: a panel study. Soc Psychiatry. 1984;9:83–91.
38. Akiskal HS, McKinney WT. Overview of recent research in depression. Arch Gen Psychiatry. 1975;32:285–305.
39. Cohen-Cole SA, Brown FW, McDaniel JS. Assessment of depression and grief reactions in the medically ill. In: Stoudemire A, Fogel BS, editors. Psychiatric care of the medical patient. New York: Oxford University Press; 1993.
40. Cunningham LA. Depression in the medically ill: choosing an antidepressant. J Clin Psychiatry. 1994;55(Suppl AJ):90–7.
41. Schulberg HC, Saul M, McClelland M. Assessing depression in primary medical and psychiatric practices. Arch Gen Psychiatry. 1985;42:1164–70.
42. Maguire P. The recognition and treatment of affective disorder in cancer patients. Int Rev Appl Psychol. 1984;33:479–91.

43. Keller M, Klerman G, Lavori P. Treatment received by depressed patients. JAMA. 1982;248:1848–55.
44. Spitzer RL, Endicott J, Robins E. Research diagnostic criteria. Arch Gen Psychiatry. 1978;35:773–82.
45. Clark DC, Cavanaugh SV, Gibbons RD. The core symptoms of depression in medical and psychiatric patients. J Nerv Ment Dis. 1983;171:705–13.
46. Hirschfeld RMA, Koslow SH, Kupfer DJ. The clinical utility of the dexamethasone suppression test in psychiatry. J Am Med Ass. 1983;250:2172.
47. Akiskal HS, Djenderedjian AH, Bolinger JM. The joint use of clinical and biological criteria for psychiatric diagnosis. In: Akiskal HS, Webb WL, editors. Psychiatric diagnosis: exploration of biological predictors. New York: Spectrum Publications; 1978.
48. Cavanaugh S. Depression in the medically ill. In: Judd FK, Burrows GD, Lipsitt DR, editors. Handbook of studies on general hospital psychiatry. Amsterdam: Elsevier Science Publishers BV (Biomedical Division); 1991.
49. Cavanaugh S, Clark D, Gibbons R. Diagnosing depression in the hospitalized medically ill. Psychosomatics. 1983;24:809–15.
50. Cavanaugh S. Depression in the medically ill: critical issues in diagnostic assessment. Psychosomatics. 1995;36:48–59.
51. Kathol RG, Mutgi A, Williams J. Diagnosis of major depression in cancer patients according to four sets of criteria. Am J Psychiatry. 1990;147:1021–4.
52. Yang CK, Woo CH, Han HM. A study on depression in medical inpatients. J Korean Neuropsychiatr Assoc. 1992;31:1073–83.
53. Orive M, Padierna JA, Quintana JM, et al. Detecting depression in medically ill patients: comparative accuracy of four screening questionnaires and physicians' diagnoses in Spanish population. J Psychosom Res. 2010;69:399–406.
54. Stoudemire A. Selected organic brain syndromes. In: Hales R, Yudofski, editors. Textbook of neuropsychiatry. Washington, DC: APA Press; 1987.
55. Cohen-Cole SA, Harpe C. Diagnostic assessment of depression in the medically ill. In: Stoudemire A, Fogel BS, editors. Principles of medical psychiatry. Orlando: Grune & Stratton; 1987.
56. Massie MJ, Holland JC. Diagnosis and treatment of depression in the cancer patient. J Clin Psychiatry. 1984;45:25–8.
57. Koh KB. An effective approach to somatization assessment and management. In: Koh KB, editor. Somatization and psychosomatic symptoms. New York: Springer; 2013. p. 99–111.
58. Bibring E. The mechanism of depression. In: Greenacre P, editor. Affective disorders: psychoanalytic contributions to their study. New York: International Universities Press; 1953.
59. Cassem NH. Depression. In: Cassem NH, editor. MGH handbook of general hospital psychiatry. 3d ed. Baltimore: Mosby Year Book; 1991.
60. Cassem NH, Hackett TP. Psychiatric consultation in a coronary care unit. Ann Intern Med. 1971;75:9–14.
61. Wishnie HA, Hackett TP, Cassem NH. Psychologic hazards of convalescence following myocardial infarction. JAMA. 1971;215:1292–6.
62. Unger KM, Moser KM, Hanser P. Selection of an exercise program for patients with chronic obstructive pulmonary disease. Heart Lung. 1980;9:68–76.
63. Pardy RL, Rivington RN, Despas PJ. Inspiratory muscle training compared with physiotherapy in patients with chronic airflow limitation. Am Rev Respir Dis. 1981;123:421–5.
64. Gift AG, Plaut SM, Jacox A. Psychologic and physiologic factors related to dyspnea in subjects with chronic obstructive pulmonary disease. Heart Lung. 1986;15:595–602.
65. Andrews JL Jr. Pulmonary rehabilitation. Pract Cardiol. 1986;12:127–37.
66. Glassman AH, Roose SP, Bigger JT. The safety of tricyclic antidepressants in cardiac patients [letter]. JAMA. 1993;269:2673–5.
67. Janowsky D, Curtis G, Zisook S. Ventricular arrhythmias possibly aggravated by trazodone. Am J Psychiatry. 1983;140:796–7.

68. Crewe HK, Lennard MS, Tucker GT. The effect of paroxetine and other specific serotonin reuptake inhibitors on cytochrome P450IID6 activity in human liver microsomes. Br J Clin Pharmacol. 1991;32:658–9.
69. Preskorn SH. Pharmacokinetics of antidepressants: why and how they are relevant to treatment. J Clin Psychiatry. 1993;54(Suppl 9):14–34.
70. Beliles K, Stoudemire A. Psychopharmacologic treatment of depression in the medically ill. Psychosomatics. 1998;39:S2–S19.
71. Hardy SE. Methylphenidate for the treatment of depressive symptoms, including fatigue and apathy, in medically ill older adults and terminally ill adults. Am J Geriatr Pharmacother. 2009;7:34–59.
72. Levy NB. Chronic renal failure and its treatment: dialysis and transplantation. In: Stoudemire A, Fogel BS, editors. Psychiatric care of the medical patient. New York: Oxford University Press; 1993.
73. Beliles KE, Stoudemire A. Psychopharmacokinetics: clinical applications in medical illnesses. In: Stoudemire A, Fogel BS, editors. Medical psychiatric practice, vol. 3. Washington, DC: American Psychiatric Press Inc; 1995.
74. Clouse RE. Antidepressants for functional gastrointestinal syndromes. Dig Dis Sci. 1994;39:2352–63.
75. Gambertoglio JG. Effects of renal disease-altered pharmacokinetics. In: Benet LZ, Massoud N, Gambertoglio JG, editors. Pharmacokinetic basis for drug treatment. New York: Raven; 1984.
76. Levy NB. Psychopharmacology in patients with renal failure. Int J Psychiatry Med. 1990;20:325–34.
77. Brater DC, Vasko MR. Pharmacokinetics. In: Chernow B, Lake CR, editors. The pharmacologic approach to the critically ill patient. 2nd ed. Baltimore: Williams & Wilkins; 1988.
78. Bergstrom RF, Beasley CM, Levy NB. The effects of renal and hepatic disease on the pharmacokinetics, renal tolerance, and risk-benefit profile of fluoxetine. Int Clin Psychopharmacol. 1993;8:261–6.
79. Aronoff GR, Bergstrom RF, Pottratz ST. Fluoxetine kinetics and protein binding in normal and impaired renal function. Clin Pharmacol Ther. 1984;36:138–44.
80. Stoudemire A, Fogel BS. Psychopharmacology in medical patients: an update. In: Stoudemire A, Fogel BS, editors. Medical-psychiatric practice, vol. 3. Washington, DC: American Psychiatric Press; 1995.
81. Hedayati SS, Gregg LP, Carmody T, et al. Effect of sertraline on depressive symptoms in patients with chronic kidney disease without dialysis dependence: the CAST randomized clinical trial. JAMA. 2017;318:1876–90.
82. Holm E, Uhl W, Stamm S. Safety of fluvoxamine for patients with chronic liver disease: biochemical variables, psychometric performance and EEG. Adv Pharm. 1986;2:151–65.
83. Dalhoff K, Almdal TP, Bjerrum K. Pharmacokinetics of paroxetine in patients with cirrhosis. Eur J Clin Pharmacol. 1991;41:351–4.
84. Dechant KL, Clissold SP. Paroxetine: a review of its pharmacodynamic and pharmacokinetic properties, and therapeutic potential in depressive illness. Drugs. 1991;41:225–3.
85. van Harten J, Duchier J, Devissaguet J. Pharmacokinetics of fluvoxamine maleate in patients with liver cirrhosis after single-dose oral administration. Clin Pharmacokinet. 1993;24:177–82.
86. Pocha C, Knott A, Rector TS, et al. Are selective serotonin reuptake inhibitors associated with hepatocellular carcinoma in patients with hepatitis C? J Clin Psychiatry. 2014;75:e1122–6.
87. Thompson WL, Thompson TL II. Treating depression in asthmatic patients. Psychosomatics. 1984;25:809–12.
88. Reite M, Harbeck R, Hoffman A. Altered cellular immune response following peer separation. Life Sci. 1981;29:1133–6.
89. Thompson WL, Thompson TL II. Pulmonary disease. In: Stoudemire A, Fogel BS, editors. Principles of medical psychiatry. New York: Grune & Stratton; 1987.

90. Levitan H. Suicidal trends in patients with asthma and hypertension: a chart study. Psychother Psychosom. 1983;39:165–70.
91. Brown ES, Vigil L, Khan DA, Liggin JD, et al. A randomized trial of citalopram versus placebo in outpatients with asthma and major depressive disorder: a proof of concept study. Biol Psychiatry. 2005;58:865–70.
92. Thompson WL, Thompson TL II. Use of medications in patients with chronic respiratory disease. Adv Psychosom Med. 1985;14:136–48.
93. Brown ES, Howard C, Khan DA, et al. Escitalopram for severe asthma and major depressive disorder: a randomized, double-blind, placebo-controlled proof-of-concept study. Psychosomatics. 2012;53:75–80.
94. Yohannes AM, Alexopoulos GS. Pharmacological treatment of depression in older patients with chronic obstructive pulmonary disease: impact on the course of the disease and health outcomes. Drugs Aging. 2014;31:483–92.
95. Fritzsche A, Clamor A, von Leupoldt A. Effects of medical and psychological treatment of depression in patients with COPD – a review. Respir Med. 2011;105:1422–33.
96. McElroy SL, Keck PE, Friedman LM. Minimizing and managing antidepressant side-effects. J Clin Psychiatry. 1995;56(Suppl 2):49–55.
97. Nelson JC. Safety and tolerability of the new antidepressants. J Clin Psychiatry. 1997;58(Suppl 6):26–31.
98. Settle EC Jr. Antidepressant side effects: issues and options. J Clin Psychiatry. 1992;10:48–61.
99. Teicher MH, Cohen BM, Baldessarini RJ. Severe daytime somnolence in patients treated with an MAOI. Am J Psychiatry. 1988;145:1552–6.
100. Kunik ME, Veazey C, Cully JA, et al. COPD education and cognitive behavioral therapy group treatment for clinically significant symptoms of depression and anxiety in COPD patients: a randomized controlled trial. Psychol Med. 2008;38:3853–96.
101. Smith SM, Sonego S, Ketcheson L, et al. A review of the effectiveness of psychological interventions used for anxiety and depression in chronic obstructive pulmonary disease. BMJ Open Respir Res. 2014;e000042:1.
102. Sirey JA, Raue PJ, Alexopoulos GS. An intervention to improve depression care in older adults with COPD. Int J Geriatr Psychiatry. 2007;22:154–9.
103. Kuyken W, Warren FC, Taylor RS, et al. Efficacy of mindfulness-based cognitive therapy in prevention of depressive relapse: an individual patient data meta-analysis from randomized trials. JAMA Psychiat. 2016;73:565–74.
104. Bohlmeijer E, Prenger R, Taal E, et al. The effects of mindfulness-based stress reduction therapy on mental health of adults with a chronic medical disease: a meta-analysis. J Psychosom Res. 2010;68:539–44.
105. Baumeister H, Hutter N. Collaborative care for depression in medically ill patients. Curr Opin Psychiatry. 2012;25:405–14.
106. Coventry PA, Bower P, Keyworth C, et al. The effect of complex interventions on depression and anxiety in chronic obstructive pulmonary disease: systematic review and meta-analysis. PLoS One. 2013;e60532:8.
107. Rackley S, Bostwick JM. Depression in medically ill patients. Psychiatr Clin North Am. 2012;35:231–47.

Chapter 17
Approach to Anxiety in the Medically Ill

17.1 Introduction

Anxiety occurs in a wide range of medical conditions [1, 2]. Anxiety symptoms may worsen the outcome of the medical illness and increase health-care utilization [3]. The evaluation of anxiety in the medically ill requires a biopsychosocial approach [4].

Herein, this chapter focuses on approach to medical disorders presenting as anxiety, concurrent psychiatric disorders, and psychosocial anxiety in medical patients.

17.2 Sources of Anxiety in Medical Patients

Effective approach for these patients needs to address three sequential dimensions: (1) the clinician should look for the possibility of an underlying medical basis for the anxiety, (2) a complete past personal and psychiatric history should be obtained to determine if the patient's anxiety is part of some underlying psychiatric disorders, and (3) it should be assessed whether the anxiety represents a psychologic adjustment response [5].

17.2.1 Physical Diseases and Substances Presenting as Anxiety

Physical diseases that can present with anxiety as a prominent symptom (anxiety disorder due to another medical condition in DSM-5) include neurological (e.g., complex partial seizures, postconcussion syndrome, acute neurological injury), cardiovascular (e.g., angina pectoris, cardiac arrhythmias), respiratory (e.g.,

K. B. Koh, *Stress and Somatic Symptoms*,
https://doi.org/10.1007/978-3-030-02783-4_17

hyperventilation syndrome, bronchial asthma, chronic obstructive pulmonary disease (COPD), recurrent pulmonary embolism), endocrine (e.g., hyperthyroidism, hypoparathyroidism/hyperparathyroidism) and metabolic diseases (e.g., hypoglycemia) [1, 5]. In addition, pheochromocytoma, Cushing syndrome, hypomagnesemia, hyponatremia, renal failure, and other electrolyte imbalance may be associated with anxiety [6–10].

Substance-induced anxiety disorders (substance/medication-induced anxiety disorder in DSM-5) include intoxication with caffeine, cocaine, amphetamine, and neuroleptics and withdrawal from alcohol, nicotine, sedative-hypnotics, and narcotics [1]. In addition, α-adrenergic stimulants (e.g., phenylpropanolamine, ephedrine), bronchodilators (e.g., isoproterenol, epinephrine, theophylline), calcium channel blockers (e.g., verapamil, nifedipine, diltiazem), and antihistamines all have been reported to produce anxiety [11–16].

17.2.2 Psychosocial Anxiety in Medical Patients

No evaluation of the anxious medical patient is complete without an inquiry into the psychosocial dimensions of the patient's experience. Potential psychologic sources of anxiety include isolation, loss of independence, loss of bodily integrity, and dying. For example, a sense of panic may occur in the chronic dialysis patient who cannot tolerate the dependence on the machine [5]. As long as patients with life-threatening illness function adaptively, denial plays an important role in continued function [17]. However, recurrence of disease often erodes initial optimism and creates a situation in which the patient for the first time deals with issues of dying [5].

17.2.2.1 Misinterpretations of Physical Sensations

According to the cognitive model, panic attacks occur when catastrophic misinterpretations of ambiguous physical sensations (e.g., shortness of breath, increased heart rate) increase arousal, creating a positive feedback loop that results in panic. In this regard, dyspnea in COPD patients is open to catastrophic misinterpretation [18]. In another study, more catastrophic interpretations of shortness of breath, higher anxiety sensitivity, higher magnitude of recent stressful life events, and worse disease severity were each found to be significant predictors of panic-spectrum psychopathology in COPD [19]. In addition, noncardiac chest pain (e.g., gastroesophageal reflux) can be misinterpreted as a serious cardiac disease, causing anxiety. However, because anxiety-like symptoms overlap with symptoms of ischemic heart disease (e.g., chest pain, dyspnea, dizziness, palpitations) and can be caused by organic factors, the diagnosis and treatment of anxiety in patients with noncardiac chest pain require special considerations [20].

17.2.3 *Anxiety in the Intensive Care Setting*

There are many psychosocial factors contributing to the experience of anxiety in patients with myocardial infarction often seen in the intensive care setting: misconceptions about the meaning of myocardial infarction and its course, misunderstanding of information provided by staff, and misinterpretation of the displays and alarms from the cardiac monitors in their rooms. As mentioned earlier, they may also have fears of death or disability and anxiety related to restriction on ability to perform usual activities, which may be associated with feelings of helplessness and loss of control [21–23]. In these patients, transfer from the cardiac care unit (CCU) to a general medical ward is often accompanied by a marked increase in anxiety, attributed by many to the loss of constant supervision and intensive monitoring [24]. The life problems that they were confronting prior to admission and the effects that the illness and hospitalization might have on their ability to handle these problems can cause anxiety [25, 26]. In particular, patients who witness a cardiac arrest may be likely to develop anxiety [23].

17.2.4 *Concurrent Psychiatric Disorders in Medical Patients*

The second step in evaluating the presentation of anxiety in a medical patient is to evaluate the possibility of underlying psychiatric disorder, such as generalized anxiety disorder, panic disorder, or somatoform disorder (or somatic symptom and related disorder in DSM-5), mood disorder, and borderline personality disorder [5].

17.3 Evaluation for Differential Diagnosis

When anxiety symptoms occur in medically ill patients, the psychiatrist's ability to rapidly identify anxiety and perform a proper differential diagnosis is important because it can be lifesaving. For example, a patient with deteriorating cardiac or pulmonary function may be misidentified as primarily "anxious" and referred to the psychiatrist. The change in the patient's medical status is missed until the situation becomes critical [27]. In this regard, a proper search for the underlying cause of the anxiety is essential if the clinician is to make a correct diagnosis and initiate appropriate treatment.

Two aspects of the patient's history are particularly important during assessment: the duration and severity of medical illness (and treatments) and the duration and severity of anxiety symptoms [28]. When acute anxiety is encountered, the clinician must rule out a rapidly worsening medical condition, substance-induced anxiety (toxicity or withdrawal), and a psychological reaction to stressors or fear associated with the medical illness [27, 28]. Because medication side effects can cause anxiety symptoms in medically ill patients, it is important for the psychiatrist to have knowledge of medications commonly associated with such side effects [27].

During evaluation of medically ill individuals with chronic anxiety, the clinician must rule out medical disorders that can mimic anxiety disorders, psychiatric disorders associated with anxiety symptoms, and poor adjustment to the medical illness. It is also worth remembering that anxiety disorders occur with increased frequency in individuals who have chronic medical illness [28].

For a clinician to conclude that a patient has anxiety disorder due to a general medical condition (anxiety disorder due to another medical condition in DSM-5), the patient should have anxiety as the predominant symptom and should have a specific causative nonpsychiatric medical disease. To ascertain the degree to which a general medical condition is causative for the anxiety, the clinician should know whether the medical condition and the anxiety symptoms have been closely related in the literature [1].

In a patient with a known medical illness, the condition and its associated complications and treatment should be suspected. For example, in the asthmatic patient, hypoxia, respiratory distress, and sympathomimetic bronchodilators may all contribute to the experience of anxiety [29, 30].

The lack of a significant emotional trauma (stressor) or the occurrence of anxiety only coincidental with particular physical events (e.g., a run of ventricular tachycardia on a cardiac monitoring) may suggest the presence of an organic anxiety syndrome [31]. In addition, a lack of personal or family history of anxiety disorders and a poor response to standard antianxiety agents may suggest the presence of an organically based anxiety syndrome [29].

Even for the apparently healthy patients, particular scrutiny should be directed at more common conditions associated with anxiety: arrhythmias, thyroid abnormalities, excessive caffeine intake, and other drug use. In addition to intoxication, withdrawal from medication or substances of abuse should be suspected. Anxiety-like symptoms may be the first clue to a withdrawal syndrome in a patient with unreported regular sedative-hypnotic (e.g., benzodiazepine) or alcohol use [32].

The clinical presentation of anxiety in the medical setting takes many forms [33]. The relative contribution of situational, psychiatric, and physiological factors to the presentation of anxiety-like symptoms in a medical patient is often murky [34].

17.4 Management

Management of the physical disease-induced anxiety should be preceded by treatment of the physical diseases [35]. The primary treatment of substance-induced anxiety disorder is the removal of the causally involved substance. Treatment then must focus on finding an alternative treatment if the substance was a medically indicated drug and on limiting the patient's exposure if the substance was introduced through environmental exposure. When anxiety disorder symptoms are present for a significant period after the physical disease has been treated or the substance use has stopped, treatment of the anxiety disorder symptoms with psychopharmacotherapeutic or psychotherapeutic modalities or both may be appropriate. In addition, behavioral therapy can be tried [1]. There is some experimental and clinical evidence for the utility of cognitive behavior therapy (CBT), based on the cognitive model of panic, for panic attacks in medically ill patients, especially COPD patients. Therefore, mental health professionals need to collaborate with multidisciplinary medical teams in order to prevent and treat panic attacks and panic disorder in these patients [18].

17.4.1 Psychopharmacological Management

Psychopharmacotherapy such as the use of benzodiazepines and antidepressants (e.g., selective serotonin reuptake inhibitors; SSRIs) may be helpful in decreasing anxiety symptoms in the medically ill [1, 3]. However, nonbenzodiazepine anxiolytics such as buspirone may be preferable to benzodiazepines in some cases.

17.4.1.1 Benzodiazepines

The benzodiazepines are well absorbed orally, and each peak blood level after a single dose varies from 2 to 6 h. These drugs fall into long-acting (e.g., diazepam) and short-acting (e.g., lorazepam) classes. Repeated use of long-acting benzodiazepines may lead to accumulation, with potential impairment of cognitive and motor performance. Such drug accumulation is a special risk to be kept in mind with the long-acting benzodiazepines, especially for older patients and those with liver impairment [36, 37]. Lorazepam is promptly absorbed intramuscularly [38], whereas diazepam is poorly absorbed from IM sites [39].

The most common adverse effects of the benzodiazepines involve CNS depression: muscle weakness, ataxia, dysarthria, vertigo, somnolence, and confusion [5]. The benzodiazepines may be associated with the development of amnesia [40].

Withdrawal symptoms of the benzodiazepines may include anxiety, insomnia, dizziness, headache, anorexia, hypotension, hyperthermia, neuromuscular irritability, tinnitus, blurred vision, shakiness, and psychosis. In particular, the short-acting benzodiazepines are associated with a greater prevalence and severity of withdrawal reactions. Withdrawal symptoms can be minimized by tapering the drugs. During withdrawal, autonomic symptoms can be relieved by a β-adrenergic blocker [40].

Clinically, the benzodiazepines are not used only for anxiety. For example, alprazolam is mainly used as an antianxiety agent, but triazolam as a hypnotic, and clonazepam as an anticonvulsant. Clonazepam is also helpful in relieving anxiety of obsessive-compulsive disorder [41]. The dosage and half-life of the benzodiazepine anxiolytics are described in Table 17.1.

Table 17.1 Dosage and half-life of benzodiazepine anxiolytics

	Daily dosage (mg)	Half-life (h)
Chlordiazepoxide (Librium)	5–100	12–48
Diazepam (Valium)	2–40	20–90
Ethyl loflazepate (Victan)	1–4	77 (average)
Lorazepam (Ativan)	1–4	10–20
Clonazepam (Klonopin)	0.5–5.0	18–28
Alprazolam (Xanax)	0.25–5.0	12–19
Triazolam (Halcion)	0.125–0.25	2.5–3.5

17.4.1.2 Buspirone

Buspirone is a nonbenzodiazepine anxiolytic agent. Unlike the benzodiazepines, buspirone lacks muscle relaxant, anticonvulsant, and hypnotic activity. This drug is notably less sedative than benzodiazepines [42, 43]. The major side effects include dizziness, headache, and nervousness. No withdrawal syndrome has been reported. However, it is important to be aware that the anxiolytic effects of buspirone may take several weeks to occur [5]. Therefore, this drug is useful for the chronic treatment of anxiety.

17.4.1.3 Propranolol

Propranolol, β-adrenergic blocker, can antagonize peripheral autonomic symptoms of anxiety such as tachycardia and tremor. In addition, this drug is helpful in relieving nervousness, restlessness, and tension [44]. The most common side effects of the agent are depression and weakness. Contraindications to the use of β-blockers include bradycardia, atrioventricular block, congestive heart failure, and COPD [5].

17.4.1.4 Antidepressants

Antidepressants have been noted to be of value in the treatment of anxiety. Tricyclics such as amitriptyline have been recommended for the treatment of panic attacks [45, 46] and may be effective in the treatment of chronic anxiety [47]. These drugs are also effective in patients with mixed anxiety and depression [48]. In addition, selective serotonin reuptake inhibitors (SSRIs) are known to be effective for anxiety associated with phobia, panic reaction, and obsessive-compulsive symptoms [41].

17.4.2 *Psychosocial Treatment*

Psychosocial treatment includes psychotherapy, behavioral therapy, and family interventions. These methods help provide accurate medical information (e.g., diagnosis and prognosis), explain the role and meaning of the monitoring equipment, provide emotional support and reassurance, and reinforce the appropriate use of denial [26, 49–51]. Providing patients with information about their illness may shorten hospital stays [52].

17.4.2.1 Psychotherapy

Psychotherapy, particularly cognitive behavioral therapy (CBT), is helpful in reducing anxiety in medically ill patients [53]. The attitude of the interviewer must convey a sense of interest in understanding what is concerning the person [5]. In addition to separation and loss, real and symbolic physical threats will be the usual themes to explore in an initial interview [34].

Sharing information about illness and diagnosis should be considered an important means of allowing the patient to resume control and may reduce anxiety in patients. Maintenance of regular contact and communication of concern are valuable positive interventions [5].

With a cognitive approach, the patient with severe anxiety or panic attacks can be helped to systematically assess the reality of his worries and to view panic as catastrophic misinterpretation of otherwise benign bodily sensations [34]. Brief cognitive psychotherapy may help reduce anxiety, shorten hospital stays, reduce medical complications, and lessen functional disabilities at follow-up [54].

17.4.2.2 Behavioral Therapy

Behavioral therapy will usually be limited to relaxation training for anxious patients, but treatment for a phobic patient can be initiated in the hospital with desensitization and exposure techniques, depending on the phobic stimulus [34]. Teaching patients relaxation techniques that they may use as needed may also be an effective strategy to reduce anxiety and enhance self-control and self-efficiency [24].

Most patients with anxiety not caused by organic factors can be taught techniques that include relaxation. Learning to specifically sense and control muscle tension is an effective method for anxiety reduction. The Jacobson method of progressive relaxation depends on systematically tensing and relaxing muscle groups starting with the feet and eventually involving the entire body [55]. This method was devised to induce relaxation by heightening awareness of muscle tension. Meditation has been shown to produce a physiologic state of restful alertness [56].

17.4.2.3 Family Interventions

Family interventions may prove therapeutically expedient, because disrupted relations with family members may be provocative [34].

17.4.3 Comparison of Outcomes of Therapeutic Modalities

In the study which compared CBT group therapy with education for COPD patients with moderate-to-severe anxiety symptoms, both treatments significantly improved quality of life and anxiety over 8 weeks, but the rate of change did not differ between the two groups [57]. In addition to CBT, psychopharmacotherapy (e.g., nortriptyline, buspirone, sertraline) and pulmonary rehabilitation programs have been found to reduce symptoms of anxiety in COPD patients [58].

In one study, among psychoeducation, cognitive, and behavioral programs, the psychoeducation program obtained the best results in reducing anxiety levels in medically ill patients. However, the combination of different psychological techniques, such as providing information to the patient, relaxation training, and cognitive strategies, is desirable in reducing levels of anxiety related with their illness [59].

17.5 Course and Prognosis

The outcome presumably depends on the specific cause; thus, anxiety due to hyperthyroidism may well remit with treatment of the hyperthyroid state, whereas anxiety due to cardiomyopathy with a low-output state may run a more chronic course. On the other hand, the course and prognosis in patients with substance-induced anxiety disorder generally depend on the removal of the causally involved substance. The anxiogenic effects of most drugs are reversible. When the anxiety does not reverse with cessation of the drug, clinicians should consider the possibility that the substance caused irreversible brain damage [1].

17.6 Conclusions

To ascertain the degree to which a general medical condition or substance is a causative factor of a patient's anxiety, the clinician should know whether the medical condition or substance has been closely associated with the anxiety symptoms in the literature. Assessment of anxiety in the medically ill requires examining biologic as well as psychosocial factors. In particular, clinicians should address the major psychologic issues, such as isolation, dependency, loss of bodily integrity, and dying that are known to be commonly associated with anxiety in the medically ill. Management of the physical disease-induced anxiety should be preceded by treatment of the physical diseases. The primary treatment of substance-induced anxiety disorder is the removal of the causally involved substance. However, any successful intervention for these patients should be a biopsychosocial approach that includes psychopharmacological and psychosocial treatment. Benzodiazepine or nonbenzodiazepine anxiolytics and antidepressants may be helpful in decreasing anxiety symptoms in the medically ill. Psychosocial treatment includes providing accurate medical information (e.g., diagnosis and prognosis), explaining the role and meaning of the monitoring equipment, providing emotional support and reassurance, and reinforcing the appropriate use of denial. For patients with persistent anxiety symptoms, cognitive and behavioral strategies can be used.

References

1. Sadock BJ, Sadock VA. Synopsis of psychiatry – behavioral sciences/clinical psychiatry. Philadelphia: Lippincott Williams & Wilkins; 2003. p. 636–42.
2. Fava GA, Porcelli P, Rafanelli C, et al. The spectrum of anxiety disorders in the medically ill. J Clin Psychiatry. 2010;71:910–4.
3. Mago R, Gomez JP, Gupta N, et al. Anxiety in medically ill patients. Curr Psychiatry Rep. 2006;8:228–33.
4. Goldberg RJ. Anxiety: a guide to biobehavioral diagnosis therapy for physicians and mental health clinicians. New York: Free Press; 1982.
5. Goldberg RJ. Anxiety in the medically ill. In: Stoudemire A, Fogel BS, editors. Principles of medical psychiatry. Orlando: Grune & Stratton; 1987.
6. Lishman WA. Organic psychiatry (endocrine disorders and metabolic disorders). London: Blackwell; 1978.
7. Hall RCW, Joffe JR. Hypomagnesemia: physical and psychiatric symptoms. JAMA. 1973;224:1749–51.
8. Gehi MM, Rosenthal RH, Fizette NB, et al. Psychiatric manifestations of hyponatremia. Psychosomatics. 1981;22:739–43.
9. Marshall JR. Neuropsychiatric aspects of renal failure. J Clin Psychiatry. 1979;40:81–5.
10. Webb WL, Gehi M. Electrolyte and fluid imbalance: neuropsychiatric manifestations. Psychosomatics. 1981;22:199–203.
11. Jacobs MA, Senior RM, Kessler G. Clinical experience with theophylline: relationship between dosage, serum concentration, and toxicity. JAMA. 1976;235:1983–6.
12. Bela SV, Raftery EV. The role of verapamil in chronic stable angina: a controlled study with computerized multistage treadmill exercise. Lancet. 1980;1:841–4.
13. Mueller HS, Chahine RA. Interim report of multicenter double-blind placebo-controlled studies of nifedipine in chronic stable angina. Am J Med. 1981;71:645–57.
14. Rickenberger RL, Psytowsky EN, Heger JJ, et al. Effects of intravenous and chronic oral verapamil administration in patients with supraventricular arrhythmias. Circulation. 1980;62:996–1010.
15. Singh BN, Elklrodt G, Peter CT. Verapamil: a review of its pharmacological properties and therapeutic use. Drugs. 1978;15:169–97.
16. Abramowicz M. Drugs that cause psychiatric symptoms. Med Lett. 1984;26:75–8.

17. Dimsdale JE, Hackett TP. Effect of denial on cardiac health and psychological assessment. Am J Psychiatry. 1982;139:1477–80.
18. Livermore N, Sharpe L, McKenzie D. Panic attacks and panic disorder in chronic obstructive pulmonary disease: a cognitive behavioral perspective. Respir Med. 2010;104:1246–53.
19. Livermore N, Sharpe L, McKenzie D. Catastrophic interpretations and anxiety sensitivity as predictors of panic-spectrum psychopathology in chronic obstructive pulmonary disease. J Psychosom Res. 2012;72:388–92.
20. Ketterer MW. Cognitive/behavioral therapy of anxiety in the medically ill: cardiac settings. Semin Clin Neuropsychiatry. 1999;4:148–53.
21. Cassem NH, Hackett TP. Psychiatric consultation in a coronary care unit. Ann Intern Med. 1971;75:9–14.
22. Krantz DS. Cognitive process and recovery from heart attack: a review and theoretical analysis. J Hum Stress. 1980;6:27–38.
23. Stern TA. The management of depression and anxiety following myocardial infarction. Mt Sinai J Med. 1985;52:623–33.
24. Goldstein MG. Intensive care unit syndromes. In: Stoudemire A, Fogel BS, editors. Principles of medical psychiatry. Orlando: Grune & Stratton; 1987. p. 403–21.
25. Cay EL, Vetter N, Philip AE. Psychological status during recovery from an acute heart attack. J Psychosom Res. 1972;16:425–35.
26. Thomas SA, Sappington E, Gross HS. Denial in coronary care patients—an objective reassessment. Heart Lung. 1983;12:74–80.
27. Wise MG, Rieck SO. Diagnostic considerations and treatment approaches to underlying anxiety in the medically ill. J Clin Psychiatry. 1993;54(Suppl):22–6.
28. Wise MG, Griffies WS. A combined treatment approach to anxiety in the medically ill. J Clin Psychiatry. 1995;56(Suppl 2):14–9.
29. Hall RCW. Psychiatric presentations of medical illness. Somatopsychic disorders. New York: SP Medical and Scientific Books; 1980.
30. Rosenbaum JF. The drug treatment of anxiety. N Engl J Med. 1982;306:401–4.
31. Harper M, Roth M. Temporal lobe epilepsy and the phobic anxiety depersonalization syndrome. Compr Psychiatry. 1962;3:120–51.
32. Avant RF. Diagnosis and management of depression in the office setting. Fam Pract Res. 1983;5(Suppl 1):41.
33. MacKenzie TB, Popkin MK. Organic anxiety syndrome. Am J Psychiatry. 1983;140:342–4.
34. Rosenbaum JF, Pollack MH. Anxiety. In: Cassem NH, editor. MGH handbook of general hospital psychiatry. 3rd ed. Baltimore: Mosby Year Book; 1991.
35. Bernstein JG. Handbook of drug therapy in psychiatry. Baltimore: Mosby; 1995.
36. Greenblatt DJ, Allen MD, Harmatz MJ, et al. Diazepam disposition determinants. Clin Pharamcol Ther. 1980;27:301–12.
37. Hoyumpa AM. Disposition and elimination of minor tranquilizers in the aged and in patients with liver disease. South Med J. 1978;71:23–8.
38. Greenblatt DJ, Divoll M, Harmatz JS, et al. Pharmacokinetic comparison of sublingual lorazepam with intravenous, intramuscular and oral lorazepam. J Pharm Sci. 1982;71:248–52.
39. Greenblatt DJ, Koch-Weser J. Adverse reactions to propranolol in hospitalized medical patients: a report from the Boston Collaborative drug surveillance program. Am Heart. 1976;86:478–84.
40. Abernethy DR, Greenblatt DJ, Shader RI. Treatment of diazepam withdrawal syndrome with propranolol. Ann Intern Med. 1981;94:354–5.
41. Jimerson DC, Docherty JP. Psychopharmacology consultation. Washington, DC: Am Psychiatric Press; 1986.
42. Cohn JB, Wilcox CS. Low-sedation potential of buspirone compared with alprazolam and lorazepam in the treatment of anxious patients: a double-blind study. J Clin Psychiatry. 1986;47:409–12.

43. Newton RE, Marunycz JD, Alderdice MT, et al. Review of the side-effect profile of buspirone. Am J Med. 1986;80(Suppl 3B):17–21.
44. Kathol RG, Noyes R Jr, Slymen DJ, et al. Propranolol in chronic anxiety disorders: a controlled study. Arch Gen Psychiatry. 1980;37:1361–5.
45. Klein DF. Medication in the treatment of panic attacks and phobic states. Psychopharmacol Bull. 1982;18:85–90.
46. Pohl R, Berchou R, Rainey JM. Tricyclic antidepressants and monoamine oxidase inhibitors in the treatment of agoraphobia. J Clin Psychopharmacol. 1982;2:399–407.
47. Lipman RS, Covi L, Downing RW, et al. Pharmacotherapy of anxiety and depression. Psychopharmacol Bull. 1981;17:91–103.
48. Paykel ES, Rowman PR, Parker RR, et al. Response to phenelzine and amitriptyline in subtypes of outpatient depression. Arch Gen Psychiatry. 1982;39:1041–9.
49. Cohen-Cole SA. Interviewing the cardiac patient: I. A practical guide assessing quality of life. Qual Life Cardiovasc Care. 1985;2:7–12.
50. Cohen-Cole SA, Bird J. Interviewing the cardiac patient: II. A practical guide for helping patients cope with their emotions. Qual Life Cardiovasc Care. 1986;2:53–65.
51. Munford E, Schlessinger HJ, Glass GV. The effects of psychological intervention on recovery from surgery and heart attacks: an analysis of the literature. Am J Public Health. 1982;72:141–52.
52. Cromwell RL, Butterfield EC, Brayfield FM. Acute myocardial infarction: reaction and recovery. St. Louis: Mosby; 1977.
53. Shaffer KM, Jacobs JM, Coleman JN, et al. Anxiety and depressive symptoms among two seriously medically ill populations and their family caregivers: a comparison and clinical implications. Neurocrit Care. 2017;27:180–6.
54. Gruen W. Effects of brief psychotherapy during the hospitalization period on the recovery process in heart attacks. J Clin Consult Psychol. 1975;43:232–3.
55. Jacobson E. Progressive relaxation. 2nd ed. Chicago: University Press; 1938.
56. Walace RK. Physiological effects of transcendental meditation. Science. 1970;e167:1751–4.
57. Kunik ME, Veazey C, Cully JA, et al. COPD education and cognitive behavioral therapy group treatment for clinically significant symptoms of depression and anxiety in COPD patients: a randomized controlled trial. Psychol Med. 2008;38:385–96.
58. Brenes GA. Anxiety and chronic obstructive pulmonary disease: prevalence, impact, and treatment. Psychosom Med. 2003;65:963–70.
59. Sánchez-Román S, Velasco-Furlong L, Rodríguez-Carvajal R, et al. Effectiveness of a cognitive-behavioral program to reduce anxiety in medically ill patients. Rev Investig Clin. 2006;58:540–6.

Chapter 18
Cognitive Behavioral Therapy for Patients with Chronic Headache

18.1 Introduction

Headaches are one of the most common medical complaints. Headaches are also a major cause of absenteeism from work. Most headaches are not associated with significant organic disease; many persons are susceptible to headaches at times of emotional stress. Psychological stress usually exacerbates headaches, whether their primary underlying cause is physical or psychological [1].

Migraine and tension headache are common and can be disabling [2, 3]. Numerous studies have demonstrated migraine and/or tension headache comorbid with depression and/or anxiety [4, 5]. In addition, patients suffering from chronic tension headache or migraine comorbid with tension headache present a significant impairment of anger control [6].

18.2 Migraine and Tension Headache

In general, chronically stress-related headaches can be subgrouped into migraine and tension headache. Migraine headache is a disorder characterized by paroxysmal and recurrent unilateral headaches, with or without visual aura (e.g., photophobia), and gastrointestinal disturbances (e.g., nausea, vomiting). In contrast to classic migraine as mentioned above, common migraine is without aura such as transient visual, and other sensory or motor disturbances [7]. Cluster headaches are related to migraines. They are unilateral, occur up to eight times a day, and are associated with miosis, ptosis, and diaphoresis [1].

Tension headache is often associated with emotional stress resulting in prolonged contraction of head and neck muscles. A dull, aching pain, sometimes feeling like a tightening band, often begins suboccipitally and may spread over the head. In contrast to migraine, tension headache is usually bilateral and not associated with aura,

K. B. Koh, *Stress and Somatic Symptoms*,
https://doi.org/10.1007/978-3-030-02783-4_18

nausea, or vomiting. The headache may be episodic or chronic and needs to be differentiated from migraine headache, especially with and without aura [1]. Symptom overlap occurs between tension and migraine headache [7].

These chronic headache patients tend to avoid expressing their problems, although they look as if they know the problems well. Such their attitudes are likely to exacerbate and prolong their symptoms by making their stressful situations or conflicts more difficult to resolve [8].

18.3 Pathogenesis of Headache

Migraine headache is seen to be primarily of vascular origin, with vasoconstriction in both the intra- and extracranial arteries occurring during the prodromal phase and vasodilation occurring during the pain associated with a migraine attack [9, 10]. The release and subsequent depletion of vasoactive substances (e.g., serotonin) and reduced pain threshold seem to play an important role in migraine [11]. Over half of migraine attacks were associated with stressful events [12]. However, there is a tendency for migraine symptoms to appear not at the peak of stress but during a period of relaxation immediately following stress [13]. Migraines can be precipitated by cycling estrogen, which may account for their high prevalence in women. Many patients with migraine are overly controlling, perfectionistic, and unable to suppress anger [7].

In contrast, the major pathogenesis of tension headache attributes pain to the sustained contraction of skeletal muscles usually occurring as part of the individual's reaction during life stress [7]. Such pain is thought to result from (1) the stimulation of pain receptors in the contracted muscles and (2) ischemia resulting from the compression of intramuscular arterioles [9, 14]. Tension headache usually occurs during periods of life stress. However, for the most part, headache does not appear to be triggered by dramatic life events but rather by everyday but personally meaningful stressors [15]. Competitive personalities are especially prone to the disorder [1].

18.4 Treatment Modalities in Chronic Headache Patients

To date, pharmacotherapy (antianxiety agents and antidepressants) and nonpharmacotherapy such as exercise, muscular relaxation, and biofeedback treatment are known to be effective for migraine and tension headache patients [16]. However, biofeedback has been found to be not only a costly and time-consuming treatment modality but also provide no additional benefit when compared to simple relaxation techniques alone, in the treatment of migraine and tension headaches in adults [17, 18].

Psychotherapy is an effective treatment for patients chronically afflicted by tension headache. In particular, cognitive behavioral treatment (CBT) such as learning to avoid or cope better with tension is the most effective long-term management approach [1]. Moreover, a combination of exercise, muscular relaxation, self-hypnosis, meditation, and CBT was recommended for treatment of tension headache [19]. In addition, persons with migraine and coexisting tension headache may require more individually tailored interventions to increase the level of physical activity and to improve psychological well-being and perceived stress [3].

18.4.1 Rationale for Use of Cognitive Behavioral Treatment

In addition to depressive and anxiety disorders [20], CBT is likely to be effective in patients with psychological factors affecting other medical conditions (PFAOMC, previously called psychosomatic disorders) whose stress perception levels are lower than those of patients with emotional disorders [13, 21].

CBT has been found to be an efficacious treatment for migraine and tension headache [2, 22]. In particular, cognitive behavioral problem-solving therapy or training might not only reduce levels of stress and depression but also increase life satisfaction in patients with primary headache [23]. The goal of CBT for patients with headache is to alter symptom-related physiological activity indirectly by changing the way clients cope with headache-eliciting stressors [13].

18.4.2 Process of Cognitive Behavioral Treatment

CBT can be divided into education, self-monitoring, and problem-solving or coping skills training. Before treatment is initiated, clients are instructed to record the occurrence of headache and rate the severity of headache along with efforts to record stressors associated with headache and management of headache (e.g., psychological coping strategies) throughout the day [13]. Sometimes psychological tools such as sentence completion test (SCT) can be used as a method to discover cognitive distortions [24].

Holroyd and his colleagues [13] summarized each of the three phases of CBT for patients with headache: (1) the therapist's task is to present an alternative framework emphasizing headache precipitants that are potentially under the client's control. The therapist explains both the ways stress can precipitate headache and the ways cognitive processes shape stress responses; (2) clients are taught to monitor their responses to stressors in their lives. The therapist encourages clients to record their feelings, thoughts, and behavior prior to, during, and following stressful events; (3) the therapist helps the client practice problem-solving and coping skills. However, it may be less crucial to provide clients with specific coping skills than to ensure that they monitor symptoms and can devise methods for interrupting the chain of events that precipitate and aggravate symptoms. In the latter cases, the aim of the therapist's intervention is to increase the client's self-confidence and self-esteem and to provide plausible interpretations of material generated during self-monitoring in terms of historical events in the client's life [25].

18.4.3 *Effects of Cognitive Behavioral Treatment*

CBT group improved significantly more than routine care control group on measures of headaches, depression, anxiety, and quality of life [26]. Cognitive therapy group was more effective than biofeedback treatment group in reducing headaches, and these therapeutic gains were maintained at the 15-week follow-up evaluation [27]. A 2-year follow-up of these participants also found that cognitive therapy might be more effective in maintaining long-term treatment effect than biofeedback treatment [13].

In other studies [28, 29], migraine patients who received self-instruction and were taught coping skills such as thought stopping and assertion training showed more improvement than those with relaxation training. In addition, CBT was found to be effective in each of tension headache, migraine, and mixed groups [30]. Even if CBT proves no more effective than relaxation training in producing the immediate reduction of headache symptoms, it may help promote the long-term maintenance of treatment gains [31].

In addition, stress management (e.g., cognitive coping, relaxation) therapy and tricyclic antidepressant medication each was found to produce larger reductions in headache activity in patients with chronic tension headache than placebo, but antidepressant medication yielded more rapid improvements in headache activity. Moreover, a combined therapy which includes stress management therapy and antidepressant medication is more likely to produce clinically significant reductions in headache index scores than each of stress management therapy and antidepressant medication [32].

18.5 Future Directions

Further studies are needed to determine to what extent CBT increases the effectiveness of relaxation training or if it is effective in patients who do not respond to relaxation training [13]. In addition, the effects of a variety of emerging behavioral therapies, such as acceptance and commitment therapy (ACT) and mindfulness interventions, on headache-related disability and affective distress as well as headache should be investigated in patients with chronic headache. There will have to be more trials, longer follow-up periods, and a need for comparison or integration with established pharmacologic and behavioral migraine treatments in future studies [4].

Case 1

A 32-year-old male patient visited the department of neurology as an outpatient with symptoms of pressing and paralyzing sensations in the left side of the head. Laboratory findings including liver and thyroid function tests revealed no abnormalities. A neurological examination and a brain CT did not show abnormalities either. Psychotropics such as amitriptyline, alprazolam, and propranolol were prescribed by the neurologist for nearly 1 year, but no significant improvement was noted. He was therefore referred to the department of psychiatry.

The patient was usually taciturn, meticulous, and shy. He had been working on a joint project with a university professor for 1 year, but the professor gave up midway. At that time, his superior demanded him to complete the unresolved project quickly. He struggled to complete the project and eventually failed. After that, he started to experience intolerable headaches.

During the first interview, a mental examination revealed that the patient was somewhat talkative, anxious, and very tense, complaining of a pressing sensation in the left side of his head. He also showed suppressed anger and hostility toward his superior. His somatic symptoms such as the paralyzing sensation in the left side of his head and the headache were aggravated by stressors at work. However, these somatic symptoms were relieved at home or while he experienced less stress and felt self-confident.

A combined diagnosis of migraine and tension headache was made. The main stressors exacerbating his somatic symptoms were found to be associated with his work overload and his relationship with his superior. In a series of interviews, his cognitive distortions in relation to these stressors were observed repetitively.

His depressive mood and headache became more severe after he was blamed for his poor job performance, and his demand for going abroad was rejected. In a self-assessment statement, he described, "I was severely scolded for having ordered another staff to do my job. I felt very bad when the superior shouted at me over trivial things. At that time, I got a severe headache and felt like a fool when I didn't say anything while being scolded. I wondered if the superior looked down on me or if I was incompetent." He said, "to other staff, he would not do the same. In spite of my effort, he doesn't seem to trust me at all." As mentioned above, the patient tended to show cognitive distortions such as magnification and selective abstraction. In addition, he showed arbitrary inference, saying "I don't have any prospects in the future at all." In the relationship with his subordinates, he also showed such cognitive distortions. He was very angry when a subordinate was absent from work without asking for a leave. At that time, he experienced a pressing and stiffening sensation of the head, thought that he was really incompetent, and wondered if he was looked down on. In addition, he showed mislabeling ("I am stupid") and "should" statements ("My subordinates should always wait for me; I should command them as their head.").

Maladaptive assumptions seen in this patient were personal ("I must be perfect to be successful and happy") and related to his family and work ("I [or subordinates] should be obedient to seniors [or superiors]"). His statements showed no midway between 100% right and 100% wrong. The therapist tried to make him perceive different degrees of severity in these thoughts as well as in his mood and his headache, by using self-assessment techniques.

As an example, the patient got promoted to section head through fierce competition. The therapist thus pointed out to the patient that this event did not prove his dichotomous thinking, such as "my superior does not trust me at all," but posed a direct challenge to his cognitive distortions. He was also recommended to practice self-assertion when being treated unfairly by his superior.

The patient thought that his superior did not trust him at all when he was scolded, but the next day the superior felt sorry for his behavior, and the patient realized that the superior did not always hate him. During the therapeutic sessions, he was allowed to self-assert and to find alternatives for coping with stress. For example, he was recommended to do pleasurable activities outside of work. He thus started to play tennis after work and to learn how to swim. On weekends, he went hiking or bowling with his wife.

Thereafter, even though the patient still complained of his dissatisfaction toward his superior, the frequency of his thoughts of always being scolded and unfairly treated was markedly reduced. Even when he talked about the superior, he was no longer serious or depressed, and the severity and frequency of his headache were also diminished. In addition, he showed significant changes in his behavior; he went to his superior and complained to him about his transfer to another section.

The following are extracts from the patient's self-assessments during the therapeutic sessions.

*The severity of emotion and symptoms ranges from 1 to 100, and the degree of belief in his/her thoughts ranges from 1% to 100%.

Date: August 28

Situation (event): My request for going abroad was rejected by the director.

Feeling: Depressed (50), pressing sensation of the head and headache (70)

Thought: I probably made a bad impression on the superior (80%)

Reaction or Coping: Busy schedule along with the company's education program, so gave up going abroad and decided to focus on the education program.

Outcome: Depressed (30), pressing sensation of the head and headache (30), initial thought (40%)

Date: September 7

Situation (event): My subordinates were supposed to play tennis with me but left before I got there.

Feeling: A feeling of betrayal (70)

Thought: They seem to ignore me (70%), I am personally inadequate (60%)

Reaction or Coping: Am I reacting too sensitively? I can play tennis with others instead.

Outcome: A sense of betrayal (40), initial thought (50%)

Date: September 17

Situation (event): One of my subordinates was absent from work without notice.

Feeling: Angry (70–80), pressing and stiff sensation of the head (70–80)

Thought: Am I incompetent? (70%)

Reaction or Coping: I won't forgive him if he behaves like this one more time. I will ask him to submit a reason for his absence.

Outcome: Angry (30), pressing and stiff sensation of the head (50), initial thought (30%)

Case 2

A 33-year-old male patient was referred to the department of psychiatry via the department of neurology, where he complained of headache in the left occipital and medial areas, followed by bifrontal headache, poor appetite, and abdominal discomfort. The symptoms had begun to be aggravated 20 days before referral.

The patient had been jovial, self-confident, and hardworking before being transferred to another section of his company. However, he tended to be tense, low-spirited, and lacking in self-confidence after he started working at the new section 5 months before his referral. He had to be at work until late at night and then take his unfinished work home because of the work overload. He could, however, not work at all at home and was extremely worried on Sunday afternoons about things to do during the coming week. Many of his colleagues said "You look sick." He felt so dejected that he often worked with a grimace on the face. He went to church and prayed a lot to seek peace of mind but could not get back to his previous normal state.

During his first interview, his mental status revealed that he was tense, anxious, and fretful and obsessively preoccupied with somatic symptoms. He was sometimes angry and hostile toward his superior but tried to suppress such emotions. He looked lethargic, lacking in drive and self-confidence. He avoided mentioning anything except for his somatic symptoms, but once he began to talk, he expressed his conflicts and difficult situation honestly and in detail.

He was diagnosed with a typical tension headache, primarily related to his work overload and conflict with his superior and secondarily associated with family problems such as serious illnesses of his elder brother and sister-in-law and the resulting economic and psychological burden.

A series of interviews and the results of the sentence completion test (SCT) revealed cognitive distortions. For example, he showed anxiety, saying "my superior used to scold me whenever outcomes were not perfect. It was hard to accept that, and I lost my self-confidence. Moreover, the head interfered in a lot of trivial things and often showed an ambiguous attitude in order to avoid responsibility for important projects. I felt afraid of reporting to the superior and experienced severe headaches whenever I had to meet him."

The therapist and patient discussed whether he could move to another section. However, he said "I am not sure I should move to another section (20%), because it is not easy to adapt to a new environment, and there is little prospect in getting promoted. Now I have no alternatives. I would like to move to another company, but that will take time."

From what he said, the therapist observed cognitive distortions such as negative predictions, for example, arbitrary inferences ("I have no prospect in the future; I have no alternatives"). His maladaptive assumptions seemed to be "I must be perfect in every aspect; I should not be scolded by my seniors."

First of all, the therapist recommended him to do time management because of the work overload. He was instructed to leave work as soon as he finished his job, delegate parts of his job to others, and not to bring any work home if possible. The therapist also proposed him to assess if moving to another section or otherwise to another company might be a solution, considering his ambiguous relationship with his superior and little prospect in the future. Initially, the patient showed skepticism regarding such a possibility, but he later discussed it with his superior, when he realized he had no other alternatives. Eventually, the superior accepted his proposal, and he was moved to another section. After that, his headache disappeared and he regained self-confidence at work. After only six sessions, the patient was able to find effective coping strategies for the stressful relationship with his superior and solve the resulting problems.

In the second case, psychological tools such as sentence completion test (SCT) was used as a method to discover cognitive distortions instead of self-assessments, and a short-term cognitive behavioral therapy was effective, probably because there were only few interpersonal conflicts except for a difficult relationship with the patient's superior. In the first case, however, it took much longer for such a therapy to have an effect on the patient's headache symptoms, because long-term assessments were needed to understand his problems objectively. Moreover, it was not easy to alter the patient's coping methods, because of his rigid and inflexible personality along with various interpersonal conflicts.

18.6 Conclusions

Numerous studies have demonstrated migraine and/or tension headache comorbid with depression and/or anxiety. Cognitive behavioral treatment (CBT) has been found to be an efficacious treatment for migraine and tension headache. The goal of CBT is to alter symptom-related physiological activity indirectly by changing the way clients cope with headache-eliciting stressors. This treatment focuses directly on their cognitive and behavioral changes. CBT can be divided into education, self-monitoring, and problem-solving or coping skills training. The therapeutic processes in two cases with chronic headache were presented, demonstrating their cognitive distortions and maladaptive assumptions. Psychological tools such as sentence completion test (SCT) can be used as a method to discover cognitive distortions instead of self-assessments. The existing literature suggests that cognitive therapy may be more effective in maintaining long-term treatment effect as well as reducing headaches than biofeedback treatment in patients with chronic headache.

References

1. Sadock BJ, Sadock VA. Synopsis of psychiatry – behavioral sciences/clinical psychiatry. 9th ed. Philadelphia: Lippincott Williams & Wilkins; 2003. p. 822–50.
2. Martin PR, Mackenzie S, Bandarian-Balooch S, et al. Enhancing cognitive-behavioural therapy for recurrent headache: design of a randomised controlled trial. BMC Neurol. 2014;14:233.
3. Krøll LS, Hammarlund CS, Westergaard ML, et al. Level of physical activity, well-being, stress and self-rated health in persons with migraine and co-existing tension-type headache and neck pain. Headache Pain. 2017;18:46.
4. Smitherman TA, Wells RE, Ford SG. Emerging behavioral treatments for migraine. Curr Pain Headache Rep. 2015;19:13.
5. Juang KD, Wang SJ, Fuh JL, et al. Comorbidity of depressive and anxiety disorders in chronic daily headache and its subtypes. Headache. 2000;40:818–23.
6. Perozzo P, Savi L, Castelli L, et al. Anger and emotional distress in patients with migraine and tension-type headache. Headache Pain. 2005;6:392–9.
7. Ad Hoc Committee on Classification of Headache. J Am Med Assoc. 1962;179:717–8.
8. Koh KB. Treatment of chronic headache. Drug Inf. 1992;104:34–5.
9. Raskin NH, Appenzeller O. Headache. Philadelphia: Saunders; 1980.
10. Adams HE, Feuerstein M, Fowler JL. Migraine headache: review of parameters, etiology, and interventions. Psychol Bull. 1980;87:217–37.
11. Fanchamps A. The role of humoral mediators in migraine headache. Can J Neurol Sci. 1974;1:189–95.
12. Henryk-Gutt R, Rees WC. Psychological aspects of migraine. J Psychosom Res. 1973;17:141–53.
13. Holroyd KA, Appel MA, Andrasik F. A cognitive-behavioral approach to psycho- physiological disorders. In: Meichenbaum D, Jaremko ME, editors. Stress reduction and prevention. New York: Plenum Press; 1983. p. 219–59.
14. Haynes SN. Muscle-contraction headache: a psychophysiological perspective of etiology and treatment. In: Haynes SN, Gannon LR, editors. Psychosomatic disorders: a psychological approach to etiology and treatment. New York: Holt, Rinehart & Winston; 1981.
15. Howarth E. Headache, personality and stress. Brit J Psychiatry. 1965;111:1193–7.
16. Agras WS. Behavior therapy. In: Kaplan HI, Sadock BJ, editors. Comprehensive textbook of psychiatry. 6th ed. Baltimore: Williams & Wilkins; 1995. p. 1788–806.
17. Mullally WJ, Hall K, Goldstein R. Efficacy of biofeedback in the treatment of migraine and tension type headaches. Pain Physician. 2009;12:1005–11.
18. Holmes DS, Burish TG. Effectiveness of biofeedback for treating migraine and tension headaches: a review of the evidence. J Psychosom Res. 1983;27:515–32.
19. Singer. Neuropsychiatric aspects of headache. In: Kaplan HI, Sadock BJ, editors. Comprehensive textbook of psychiatry. 6th ed. Baltimore: Williams & Wilkins; 1995. p. 251–7.
20. Beck AT, Rush AJ. Cognitive therapy. In: Kaplan HI, Sadock BJ, editors. Comprehensive textbook of psychiatry. Baltimore: Williams & Wilkins; 1989. p. 1541–50.
21. Koh KB. Stress perception of patients with psychosomatic disorders. J Korean Neuropsychiatr Assoc. 1988;27:514–23.
22. Christiansen S, Jürgens TP, Klinger R. Outpatient combined group and individual cognitive-behavioral treatment for patients with migraine and tension-type headache in a routine clinical setting. Headache. 2015;55:1072–91.
23. Eskin M, Akyol A, Çelik EY, et al. Social problem-solving, perceived stress, depression and life-satisfaction in patients suffering from tension type and migraine headaches. Scand J Psychol. 2013;54:337–43.
24. Koh KB. Stress and psychosomatic medicine. 2nd ed. Seoul: Ilchokak; 2011. p. 331–40.
25. Holroyd KA, Andrasik F. Coping and self-control of chronic tension headache. J Consult Clin Psychol. 1978;46:1036–45.

26. Martin PR, Aiello R, Gilson K, et al. Cognitive behavior therapy for comorbid migraine and/ or tension-type headache and major depressive disorder: an exploratory randomized controlled trial. Behav Res Ther. 2015;73:8–18.
27. Holroyd KA, Andrasik F, Westbrook T. Cognitive control of tension headache. Cogn Ther Res. 1977;1:121–33.
28. Mitchell KR, White RG. Control of migraine headache by behavioral self- management: a controlled case study. Headache. 1976;16:178–84.
29. Mitchell KR, White RG. Behavioral self-management: an application to the problem of migraine headaches. Behav Ther. 1977;8:213–21.
30. Bakal DA, Demjen S, Kaganov S. Cognitive behavioral treatment of chronic headache. Headache. 1980;20:163. (Abstract)
31. Lynn SJ, Freedman RR. Transfer and evaluation in biofeedback treatment. In: Goldstein AP, Kanfer F, editors. Maximizing treatment gains: transfer enhancement in psychotherapy. New York: Academic; 1979.
32. Holroyd KA, O'Donnell FJ, Stensland M, et al. Management of chronic tension-type headache with tricyclic antidepressant medication, stress management therapy, and their combination: a randomized controlled trial. JAMA. 2001;285:2208–15.

Chapter 19
Cognitive Behavioral Treatment for Individuals at Risk of Coronary Heart Disease

19.1 Introduction

Behavioral risk factors such as smoking, overeating, physical inactivity, poor compliance with management of diabetes, and type A behavior, hypercholesterolemia, and hypertension are known to be risk factors for coronary heart disease (CHD). These are the main targets for primary preventive interventions, and achieving behavioral change with respect to these risk factors is a major challenge for medicine and psychiatry [1]. In particular, type A behavior and hypertension are not only independent risk factors for CHD [2] but also have been found to be improved by psychological interventions [3, 4]. The recurrence rate of myocardial infarction was reduced following modification of type A behavior [5]. The incidence of CHD was also decreased after psychological interventions for hypertension [6].

Anger is a characteristic feature of individuals with type A behavior and hypertension. In many studies [7–9], hostility and anger were found to play an important role in type A behavior. On the other hand, anger suppression was reported to be consistently associated with hypertension [10–12]. Therefore, anger expression style needs to be modified to effectively manage type A behavior and hypertension.

There is a common physiological pathway for type A behavior and hypertension. In early hypertension, changes in blood pressure were reported to be associated with sympathetic nervous system (SNS) arousal [13]. Pathological responses to type A behavior are in part mediated by excessive hyperactivity of the SNS, aggravating atherosclerosis and then progressing to vascular spasm and arrhythmia. Particularly increased cardiovascular responses to challenges are known to be a characteristic feature of type A behavior [14].

The mechanism of cognitive behavioral therapy (CBT) for type A behavior and hypertension is to remit SNS arousal by using cognitive and relaxation technique [15].

This chapter reviews CBT in individuals with type A behavior and hypertension which are known to be risk factors for CHD.

K. B. Koh, *Stress and Somatic Symptoms*,
https://doi.org/10.1007/978-3-030-02783-4_19

19.2 Cognitive Distortions in Type A Behavior

All-or-nothing thinking, selective attention, personalization, and attribution of causality are often observed in individuals with type A behavior [16]. Type A's express concern that if they say "no" to an opportunity despite too many commitments, they will never get another opportunity [17]. Type A's suppress all stimuli that are peripheral to the main task they are trying to accomplish. Therefore, they are unaware of their early symptoms and signs of CHD [18]. Personalization refers to a tendency to exaggerate one's own importance, beyond normal egocentricity [16]. Beliefs concerning why things happen are called attributions of causality [19]. For example, type A's often attribute their success to effort. Thus, when they fail, they are likely to attribute the cause of their failure to not trying harder [20].

19.3 Cognitive Therapy for Features of Type A Behavior

19.3.1 Time Urgency

Self-defeating time urgency of individuals with type A pattern needs the following intervention: (1) clients should be encouraged to prioritize their daily activities and consider a balance of work and relaxation and productivity and play, (2) clients should be taught methods to cope with job stress more effectively (e.g., relaxation) [21], and (3) clients should be encouraged to change their attitudes to reduce job stress when they try to do something beyond their control. For example, you are stuck in traffic; you will suffer less stress if you can tell yourself that this is just one of those times [16].

19.3.2 Perfectionism

With all-or-nothing thinking tendencies, type A's will automatically equate any mistake or imperfection with total failure [17]. Perfectionism requires the following interventions [16]:

1. The aim of therapeutic intervention is to help clients seek acceptance of imperfection as a goal rather than achievement of perfection.
2. The client should be questioned about perfectionistic rituals and their consequences so that such recognition can set the stage for attitude change.
3. The client should be encouraged to experiment with new behaviors. At this time, it is good to start from minor things if possible.

19.3.3 Achievement Striving

Selective attention greatly works on achievement striving, suppressing awareness of personal limitations. Interventions for these clients help them recognize information that is outside their awareness (i.e., "they are denying"). For example, the therapist provides the client with information on the consequences of type A behavior: positive and negative ones [17].

19.3.4 Excessive Work Involvement

Type A's tend to attribute too much of the outcomes to factors they can control. Therefore, interventions should focus attention on the things within their ability to control and assign external factors to the responsibility for the rest. Occasionally, job demands are so severe that restructuring may not bring about a better adjustment. In this case, it may be worthwhile to consider other job alternatives [16].

19.3.5 Low Self-Esteem

In type A"s, worth equals achievement [16]. One implication of this belief is that one's worth fluctuates with one's accomplishments and approval from others [17]. For treatment of low self-esteem, the therapist questions why being rejected or criticized makes clients so fearful and then can assess realistically the consequences of such an event [16]. The goal of treatment is to help them redress this disproportion of all the sources of self-esteem (e.g., work, relationships with others, and an unconditional sense of self-worth) and then to make them better balanced and develop a sense of adequacy and worth [16].

19.3.6 Hostility

Type A individuals tend to externalize and believe that others should change [22]. Cognitive behavioral approach for hostility is as follows:

1. The therapist needs to help them conceptualize a middle-of-the-road alternative to aggression versus listlessness by giving them an opportunity to discuss some principles of assertiveness [23].
2. The therapist helps the client learn to identify the cognitions that occur when one finds oneself aroused [16].

3. The therapist encourages the client to challenge his/her irrational thoughts along with muscle relaxation [24].
4. The therapist helps the client identify and modify his/her underlying maladaptive assumptions (e.g., the attitudes that "others should do things my way" can be replaced with a more functional alternative such as the attitude that "this is an unfair world." It is also helpful to question the underlying expectation that others should change) [16].

19.3.7 Depression

A large number of type A's have the belief that one has to work for one's worth. Obstacles to accomplishment, such as illness and exhaustion, are likely to cause depression in type A's. The therapist helps the client explore his/her underlying beliefs and expectations. He/she explores them in the context of his present need and situation and gradually begins to exchange the competitive model for one based on cooperation [16].

19.4 Cognitive Behavioral Treatment for Essential Hypertension

Essential hypertension or idiopathic hypertension is the form of hypertension that has no identifiable cause such as kidney disease. Psychological stress is associated with hypertension [25, 26], and hypertensives are known to have higher levels of depression, hostility, and sensitivity in interpersonal relationship as well as higher levels of stress than normal controls [27]. In addition, positive association between perceived stress and serum cholesterol levels was found in individuals with hypertension [27].

Individuals at risk for hypertension are hypothesized to cope with conflicts by suppressing feelings of anger and then expressing anger explosively when such coping mechanism fails. Physiological responses (e.g., increased sympathetic activity) that may be either specific to the arousal of anger or more generally associated with the stress-related emotions are assumed to initiate the hypertensive disease process in genetically susceptible individuals [28].

Indications for cognitive behavioral treatment are hyperreactivity to stress, high levels of occupational stress, and difficulty in tolerating or complying with antihypertensive drugs [29]. In addition, behavioral neurocardiac training with heart rate variability biofeedback modestly lowers ambulatory blood pressure during wakefulness and augments tonic vagal heart rate modulation [30].

19.5 Rationale for Psychological Interventions in Essential Hypertension

Earlier in the disease process, treatments that reduce stress or teach skills for more effective coping with stress may help prevent the hemodynamic cascade toward essential hypertension. Therefore, psychological interventions need to be considered not only for treatment for patients with hypertension but also for prevention for individuals at risk of this disorder. Criteria for screening subjects for preventive intervention might include a family history of essential hypertension, borderline high blood pressure, and cardiovascular reactivity to laboratory stressors [31].

19.6 Process of Cognitive Behavioral Intervention

1. CBT for essential hypertension should begin by explaining the rationale for treatment and the pathogenesis of essential hypertension in nontechnical terms.
2. Patients should be asked to record events that are experienced as stressful and monitor heart rate and blood pressure periodically [28]. This method is known to be effective in patients with mild hypertension [32, 33]. Seeing blood pressure decrease day by day can be a positive feedback to them. However, in some patients so much obsessed with blood pressure, anxiety can arise from taking blood pressure frequently so that it can be recommended to take blood pressure less often.
3. Patients should be encouraged to learn coping skills for stress management. Primarily, self-control relaxation is used as a coping skill for hypertensives. The relaxation treatment begins by teaching them to take a deep breath, to hold it momentarily, and to imagine they are in a peaceful place and then to think the word "relax" as they exhale [28]. Such self-control relaxation training resulted in significantly larger reductions in blood pressure than each of supportive psychotherapy and medical treatment [34].

However, comprehensive treatment altering cognitive and behavioral responses to stress is desirable for these patients. Therefore, in addition to relaxation, treatment needs to include helping the patients recognize and monitor anger-engendering conflict, identify characteristic styles of responding, and experiment with alternative ways of managing anger and conflict [28].

Case

A 58-year-old male patient visited the department of psychiatry as an outpatient with several bouts of chest tightness, dizziness, sensation of impending death, and anxiety. His blood pressure was 180/140 mmHg, and he was diagnosed with panic disorder comorbid with essential hypertension.

Through a series of interviews, it became obvious that his personality was obsessive-compulsive. He always had to put all his clothes and socks in the same places and felt relieved only when the toilet roll was hung in the correct direction. He also felt uncomfortable on days he skipped his exercise, even if it happened only once. His blood pressure was generally high, probably due to his being constantly tense. He used to take his blood pressure several times a day and showed sensitive responses to changes in blood pressure. Atenolol (Tenormin) 50 mg, an antihypertensive drug, was given once a day and ethyl loflazepate 1 mg, an anxiolytic, was given twice a day. He was recommended to do muscle relaxation to relieve tension and anxiety. He was also asked to think and act unlike the way he used to do. He started to challenge his obsessive thinking and compulsive behavior, saying "so what if I take off my socks anywhere?" and "so what if I skip exercise one day?". From that time onward, he felt less anxious and tense.

He did not experience fear of impending death anymore, even though he still felt somewhat anxious. In addition, he was not anxious any more when he did not take his blood pressure and thus decided not to take it anymore. Moreover, he realized that his personality changed markedly, from being rigid and inflexible to being able to listen to others, saying to himself "am I that great?". His anxiety was significantly reduced and his blood pressure remained within the normal range. Eventually, ethyl loflazepate was discontinued, and the patient stayed symptom-free with only Tenormin 25 mg once a day.

19.7 Conclusions

Cognitive behavioral intervention for individuals with risk factors of coronary heart diseases such as type A behavior and hypertension was reviewed. Cognitive strategies misused by patients with type A behavior include all-or-nothing thinking, excessive selective attention, personalization, and attribution of causality. How to apply cognitive behavioral therapy to basic features of the type A pattern such as time urgency, perfectionism, achievement striving, excessive work involvement, low self-esteem, hostility, and depression was described. Cognitive behavioral approach for patients with hypertension helps the clients recognize and monitor anger-engendering conflict, identify characteristic styles of responding, and experiment with alternative ways of managing anger and conflict. The therapist needs to consider therapeutic interventions tailored to each individual's characteristic and problems, because predominant features of type A can vary from person to person.

References

1. Sadock BJ, Sadock VA. Synopsis of psychiatry – behavioral sciences/clinical psychiatry. 9th ed. Philadelphia: Lippincott Williams & Wilkins; 2003.
2. Haynes SG, Matthews KA. The association of Type A behavior with cardiovascular disease: update and critical review. In: Houston BK, Snyder CR, editors. Type A behavior pattern research, theory and intervention. New York: Wiley; 1988.

3. Bennett P, Carroll D. Stress management approaches to the prevention of heart disease. Br J Clin Psychol. 1990;29:1–12.
4. Wadden TA, Luborsky L, Greer S, et al. The behavioral treatment of essential hypertension: an update and comparison with pharmacological treatment. Clin Psychol Rev. 1984;4:403–29.
5. Friedman M, Thorensen CE, Gill JJ, et al. Alteration of type A behavior and its effect on cardiac recurrences in postmyocardial infarction patients: summary of the recurrent coronary prevention project. Am Heart J. 1986;112:653–65.
6. Patel C, Marmot MG, Carruthers M. Trilaxation in reducing coronary risk: four year follow-up. Br Med J. 1985;290:1103–6.
7. Chesney MA, Hecker MA, Black GW. Coronary-prone behavior in the WCGS: a new methodology. In: Houston BK, Snyder CR, editors. Type A behavior pattern: research, theory and intervention. New York: Wiley; 1988.
8. Matthews KA, Glass DC, Rosenman RH, et al. Competitive drive, pattern A, and coronary heart disease: a further analysis of some data from the Western Collaborative Group study. J Chron Dis. 1977;30:489–98.
9. Dembroski TM, Costa PT. Assessment of coronary prone behavior: a current overview. Ann Behav Med. 1988;10:60–70.
10. Spielberger CD, Johnson EH, Russell SF, et al. The experience and expression of anger: construction and validation of an anger expression scale. In: Chesney MA, Rosenman RH, editors. Anger and hostility in cardiovascular and behavioral disorders. Washington, DC: Hemisphere; 1985.
11. Dimsdale JE, Pierce C, Schoenfield D, et al. Suppressed anger and blood pressure: the effect of race, sex, social class, obesity and age. Psychosom Med. 1986;48:430–5.
12. Koh KB, Kim SJ. Comparison of anger between patients with essential hypertension and normal controls. Kor J Psychosom Med. 1995;3:19–27.
13. Obrist PA. Cardiovascular psychophysiology. New York: Plenum Press; 1981.
14. Ward MM, Chesney MA, Swan GE, et al. Cardiovascular responses in type A and type B men to a series of stressors. J Behav Med. 1986;6:39–43.
15. Suinn RM, Bloom LJ. Anxiety management training for pattern A behavior. J Behav Med. 1978;1:25–35.
16. Kinchla J. Cognitive approaches to management of the type A behavior pattern. In: Freeman A, Greenwood V, editors. Cognitive therapy: application in psychiatric and medical settings. New York: Human Sciences Press; 1987. p. 162–82.
17. Price VA. Type A behavior pattern. New York: Academic; 1982.
18. Matthews KA, Brunson BI. Allocation of attention and the type A coronary-prone behavior pattern. J Pers Soc Psychol. 1979;37:2081–90.
19. Kelley HH. Attribution theory in social psychology. In: Levine D, editor. Nebraska symposium on motivation. Lincoln: University of Nebraska Press; 1967. p. 192–238.
20. Margolis LH, McLeroy KR, Runyan CW, et al. Type A behavior: an ecological approach. J Behav Med. 1983;6:245–58.
21. Burman MA, Pennebaker JW, Glass DC. Time consciousness, achievement striving and the type A coronary prone behavior pattern. J Abnorm Psychol. 1975;84:76–9.
22. Powell L. Workshop on the type A behavior pattern. Presented at Society for Behavioral Medicine Convention. 1983.
23. Kiester E. The use of anger. Psychol Today. 1984;18:26.
24. Ellis RA, Harper RA. New guide to rational living. Hollywood: Wilshire Book Co; 1975.
25. Harburg E, Blakelock JL, Roeper J. Resentful and reflective coping with arbitrary authority and blood pressure. Psychosom Med. 1979;41:189–202.
26. Harburg E, Erfurt J, Chape G, et al. Socioecological stressor areas and black-white pressure: Detroit. J Chron Dis. 1973;26:595–611.
27. Kim SJ, Koh KB. The relationship of stress perception with serum cholesterol in patients with essential hypertension. Kor J Psychosom Med. 1993;1:35–44.

28. Holroyd KA, Appel MA, Andrasik F. A cognitive-behavioral approach to psychophysiological disorders. In: Meichenbaum D, Jaremko M, editors. Stress reduction and prevention. New York: Plenum Press; 1983. p. 219–59.
29. Abgrall-Barbry G, Consoli SM. Psychological approaches in hypertension management. Presse Med. 2006;35:1088–94.
30. Nolan RP, Floras JS, Harvey PJ, et al. Behavioral neurocardiac training in hypertension: a randomized, controlled trial. Hypertension. 2010;55:1033–9.
31. Obrist P, Gaebelein C, Teller E, et al. The relationship among heart rate, carotid dp/dt, and blood pressure in humans as a function of the type of stress. Psychophysiology. 1978;15:102–15.
32. Glasgow MS, Gaarder KR, Engel BT. Behavioral treatment of high blood pressure: II. Acute and sustained effects of relaxation and systolic blood pressure biofeedback. Psychosom Med. 1982;44:155–70.
33. Laughlin KD, Fisher L, Sherrard DJ. Blood pressure reduction during self-recording of home blood pressure. Am Heart J. 1979;98:629–34.
34. Taylor CB, Farquhar JW, Nelson E, et al. Relaxation therapy and high blood pressure. Arch Gen Psychiatry. 1977;34:339–42.

Chapter 20
Approaches to Cardiovascular Diseases

20.1 Introduction

Cardiovascular disease is the leading cause of death in most of the industrialized world [1]. Psychosocial factors can not only be considered cofactors in the development of coronary heart disease (CHD) but also play an important role in triggering acute coronary syndrome or acute myocardial infarction (MI) [2]. Autonomic cardiac modulation is profoundly sensitive to acute emotional state such as anxiety, fear, anger, or sadness. Thus, acute emotions, especially anxiety, affect the heart. Instances of sudden cardiac death related to sudden emotional distress have been noted throughout history in all cultures [1].

Psychiatric disorders frequently occur as complications or comorbid conditions in persons with cardiovascular disease [1]. Heart disease itself can result in anxiety, depression, and denial [2–4]. Comorbid depressive disorders worsen the course and prognosis of CHD [2]. Psychosocial treatment for patients with CHD includes behavioral interventions as well as psychotherapy [2].

This chapter reviews psychosocial aspects of cardiac diseases such as CHD, including psychosocial risk factors, psychopathology, and psychiatric disorders. In addition, biopsychosocial interventions such as psychotherapy, psychopharmacotherapy, psychiatric side effects of cardiac drugs, cardiac side effects of psychiatric drugs, and drug interactions are addressed.

20.2 Psychosocial Risk Factors of Coronary Heart Disease

20.2.1 Type A Personality

Type A personality is characterized by aggression, competition, and time urgency and is known to be associated with the prevalence of CHD [5–7]. Prospective studies also found that type A behavior was significantly correlated with the incidence

K. B. Koh, *Stress and Somatic Symptoms*,
https://doi.org/10.1007/978-3-030-02783-4_20

of CHD [8, 9]. Many studies revealed the relationship between type A behavior and the severity of CHD [10–13]. However, other studies reported that type A behavior was not predictive of CHD [14–19].

20.2.2 *Hostility and Anger*

Many studies reported that suppression of anger and hostility was associated with hypertension, a risk factor of CHD [20–25]. Hostility is also associated with increased levels of circulating catecholamines and increased lipid concentrations [1]. In one study, hostility, a feature of type A behavior, was found to be significantly related to the prevalence of myocardial infarction [26]. It was also reported that competitiveness and hostility were associated with CHD [27]. In addition, angina patients are known to have higher levels of anger than patients with MI or healthy controls [28]. The severity of CHD on angiography was reported to be associated with hostility [12–14, 29]. However, other studies did not find the correlation between the hostility scores and the severity of CHD [30, 31].

20.2.3 *Alexithymia*

One study reported that the levels of alexithymia were associated with the severity of stenosis of coronary artery [28]. In contrast, another study found that alexithymia was correlated with previous diagnosis of CHD but related to less severe stenosis group in the patients [32]. On the other hand, MI patients who do not express their emotional problems tend to complain of pain more frequently and to be readmitted [33].

20.2.4 *Type D Personality*

Type D personality is defined as the combination of "negative affectivity" and "social inhibition." Negative affectivity is the tendency to experience negative emotions, and social inhibition is the tendency to inhibit self-expression in social interactions [34]. A series of studies [35–37] have demonstrated that although type D overlaps with depression, it contributes independently to the risk of CHD events.

20.2.5 *Stress*

Stress is known to be associated with cardiovascular diseases such as ischemia, MI, arrhythmias, and hypertension. Stress causes increased blood pressure and heart rate and vasoconstriction by increasing secretion of epinephrine and norepinephrine [33].

One study found that the serum levels of cholesterol were significantly and positively correlated with the levels of perceived stress in patients with essential hypertension [38]. Takotsubo or broken-heart cardiomyopathy is a neurohumorally mediated phenomenon in which sudden emotional shock directly induces cardiomyopathy, although the mechanism is not due to coronary artery atherosclerosis. The mechanism for cardiac injury is still controversial but is thought to be driven by an abrupt increase in sympathetic nervous system activation or circulating catecholamines [39, 40].

It was reported that psychological stress was a risk factor of CHD regardless of age and other risk factors [33]. The levels of perceived stress related to interpersonal changes were also correlated with the degree of coronary artery stenosis, whereas those related to ordinary daily life were correlated with low-density lipid (LDL) cholesterol and total cholesterol levels [41]. In a cross-national study for patients and controls from 52 countries, the number of stressors in the previous year was associated with increased risk of MI [42].

20.2.6 Depression

Depression may significantly affect risk factors such as smoking, hypercholesterolemia, and hypertension. For example, depression is likely to increase the risk of CHD by changing body weight, increasing smoking, and lowering medication compliance [33, 43].

Depression may be more predictive of the development of CHD than type A personality, which indicates that CHD is vulnerable to negative affect rather than time urgency, a feature of workaholics. In particular, major depressive disorder may more greatly affect CHD than a traditional risk factor such as smoking. In addition, depression is known to be associated with sudden death, arrhythmias, and chest pain. Particularly, post-MI depression can be a predictor of 1-year cardiac mortality [44].

Of the proposed mechanisms linking depression and cardiac diseases, abnormal platelet overactivation associated with depression is a biologically plausible mechanism by which depression might exert negative effects on the vascular system and increase cardiac events [45].

20.2.7 Anxiety

The presence of anxiety seems to put one at increased risk of cardiac death [46, 47]. Patients with high anxiety were at significantly increased risk of recurrent myocardial ischemia and infarction, independent of cardiac risk factors for these outcomes [48]. Another study found that higher anxiety scores at 12 months after catheterization in outpatients with CHD were a predictor of angina at a 6-year follow-up [49].

20.2.8 *Denial*

One study found that those with higher denial of emotions in men who had at least minimally positive diagnostic coronary angiograms had a higher likelihood of cardiovascular events [50]. Patients with cardiac diseases who show extreme denial are vulnerable to smoking, overeating, and compulsive working fueled by anxiety or depression [51].

20.2.9 *Lack of Social Support*

Social support can affect the progress of MI [33]. High levels of support predict improvements in depression symptoms over the first post-MI year [44]. In contrast, inadequate support (e.g., low income and the absence of spouse and friends) may increase the mortality of patients with cardiac diseases [32]. Low perceived social support is likely to be associated with mortality and recurrence in patients with MI [32, 52]. Avoidance and distancing were found to be the most ineffective coping strategies in patients with CHD [53]. Therefore, lack of a social support network should be considered a risk factor for subsequent morbidity and mortality after MI [54].

20.3 Cardiac Diseases and Psychiatric Disorders

20.3.1 *Depressive Disorders*

Chronic cardiac diseases evoke depression through narcissistic injury (i.e., limitations in occupational, recreational, and sexual activities related to the loss or threat of loss of functions), object loss, and guilt [51]. However, congestive heart failure may mimic major depressive disorder. Depression may occur in a patient who recovers after a heart attack or cardiac surgery as a result of survivor guilt. This may occur because he/she was able to receive medical or surgical treatment not available to his/her lost loved ones [55].

20.3.2 *Panic Disorder*

The onset of cardiac disease symptoms may play a potent role in provocation of anxiety. Some patients may become fearful of activity, especially work and sex (called "cardiac neurosis"), and emotionally constricted [51]. One study [48] found that anxiety symptoms were elevated roughly twofold above population norms in a cohort of patients hospitalized for acute MI. Angina, arrhythmias, and acute heart failure produce anxiety related to fears of a heart attack, disability, and sudden death.

Panic attacks and cardiac arrhythmias share many symptoms. Psychological stressors can play an important role in the precipitation of each of panic attacks or cardiac arrhythmias [56]. Most often, it is panic disorder that is misdiagnosed as an arrhythmia, usually as paroxysmal atrial tachycardia [33].

20.3.3 Somatoform Disorders (Somatic Symptom and Related Disorders in DSM-5)

Somatoform disorders and cardiac diseases are sometimes mistaken for each other but also frequently coexist [51].

20.3.4 Insomnia

Heart failure produces orthopnea, that is, shortness of breath and inability to sleep in the recumbent position [51].

20.3.5 Delirium

Delirium is much more common after cardiac surgery than after MI. Postoperative delirium is caused by complex factors. Risk factors of delirium include old age, cardiac status, complexity and duration of surgical procedures, preoperative cognitive disturbance, concurrent severe medical diseases, and preoperative psychiatric disorders [33].

20.4 Psychotherapeutic Interventions [51]

Psychotherapeutic interventions for heart disease patients are aimed at reducing anxiety and depression, enhancing compliance, and modifying risk factors. To treat them effectively, the clinician should look beyond the symptoms to their function and meaning:

1. Anxiety: instead of empty reassurance, appropriate psychotherapeutic interventions should be matched to specific fears.

2. Depression: for some, therapy is aimed at improving damaged self-esteem and self-destructive pessimism after MI. For others, unresolved grief over previous losses, sometimes with survivor guilt, must be worked through.
3. Denial: Physicians should avoid directly challenging the patient's claims while showing more concern for the patient and maximizing the patient's sense of control. Since extreme denial usually reflects intense underlying anxiety, trying to scare the patient into cooperating will intensify the denial.

20.5 Effects of Psychosocial Interventions

In one study [57], a part of Recurrent Coronary Prevention Project, a combined intervention of group therapy and behavioral modification was found to reduce type A behavior and halve the recurrence rate compared to each of the interventions in patients with chronic myocardial infarction. At the 1-year follow-up study, the group that changed behavior showed a significant decrease in the recurrence of myocardial infarction compared to the group that did not.

An updated review including randomized controlled trials of psychological interventions compared to usual care found that for people with CHD, there was no evidence that psychological treatments had an effect on total mortality, although the rate of cardiac mortality was reduced and psychological symptoms (depression, anxiety, or stress) were alleviated [58]. Another study also reported that psychosocial intervention group such as cognitive behavior therapy supplemented with a selective serotonin reuptake inhibitor (SSRI) was more effective in reducing depression and social isolation than usual care group but no significant difference was found in event-free survival between the two groups [59].

20.6 Cardiac Rehabilitation

Cardiac rehabilitation (CR) involves early ambulation during hospitalization, prescriptive exercise training, education for patients and family [60], and sexual counseling [61]. Although exercise training may reduce anxiety and depression in cardiac patients [51, 60], severe psychopathology may prevent patients from benefiting from such rehabilitation programs [62]. Compared with no exercise control, exercise-based CR improves health-related quality of life and reduces the risk of cardiovascular mortality and hospitalization [63]. However, no reduction in total mortality was found in people who received education delivered as part of CR, compared to people in control groups [64].

CR for people with CHD should be comprehensive and include educational interventions together with exercise and psychological therapy [64]. For the mentally ill cardiac patients, it is desirable to combine psychiatric treatment with CR [51].

Studies indicate that relaxation training can alter autonomic activation during mental stress, implying a potential therapeutic role of such training in stress-induced ischemia [1]. Therefore, relaxation training can be used as part of CR.

20.7 Countertransference

Physicians old enough to be at risk for CHD could have deep empathy with patients. Otherwise, they may distance themselves from the patients. In contrast, young physicians may become almost messianic in their approach to the patients, enthusiastically attacking risk factors (e.g., smoking and obesity). This usually increases the patient's anxiety, in turn increasing the need to deny the illness [51].

20.8 Psychopharmacotherapy

20.8.1 Antidepressants

Tricyclic antidepressants have a significant cardiovascular side effect profile, particularly pronounced in CHD patients. Adverse cardiac events can include tachycardia, orthostatic hypotension, and cardiac conduction disturbances [43, 65]. For patients with such risk, antidepressants such as SSRI, bupropion, venlafaxine, and nefazodone can be used instead of the tricyclics because they do not produce cardiovascular side effects including orthostatic hypotension [33, 66]. However, mirtazapine also causes orthostatic hypotension [67].

Tricyclics have antiarrhythmic properties (quinidine-like), which have been shown to increase morbidity and mortality in patients with ischemic heart disease [68–70]. SSRIs, bupropion, and venlafaxine are the drugs of first choice for depressed MI patients because they have little quinidine-like property [67].

Patients with serious conduction delays are at risk for complete heart block if treated with traditional antidepressants except trazodone [71–73]. In contrast, fluoxetine and bupropion are known to be safe in patients with bundle branch block. However, atrial fibrillation and bradycardia have been reported in cases who use fluoxetine [33, 74–76]. SSRIs such as sertraline, paroxetine, fluvoxamine, and nefazodone can also cause bradycardia [77, 78]. However, tianeptine, a selective serotonin reuptake enhancer (SSRE), may cause tachycardia [79]. Bupropion [80] and venlafaxine [81] may be occasionally associated with hypertension. Sertraline is known to be a safe drug because it does not significantly interact with digoxin [82].

For patients with depression-related insomnia, trazodone is preferred when anticholinergic and quinidine-like effects of tricyclic antidepressants are likely to exacerbate their heart condition. In this case, however, trazodone should be used with caution because it may contribute to increased ventricular irritability [83, 84].

Fluoxetine does not have a significant effect on anticoagulation activity of warfarin [85], but fluvoxamine and sertraline may increase prothrombin time [86, 87]. Therefore, the use of such drugs should be avoided when bleeding time is supposed to be increased in patients with CHD undergoing surgery [78]. However, venlafaxine is not likely to affect such anticoagulant activity because it has weak bond with serum protein [67].

In general, sertraline and citalopram are recommended as first-line pharmacotherapy for depression, especially for major depressive disorder, in patients with CHD or congestive heart failure. Mirtazapine, bupropion, venlafaxine, and tricyclic antidepressants should be viewed as second- or third-line treatment options [88].

20.8.2 Lithium

Lithium should be used cautiously as it may cause changes in EKG and arrhythmia. Lithium treatment should be initiated at a low dose, then increasing the dosage slowly to avoid side effects [89].

20.8.3 Antipsychotic Agents

Haloperidol can be effectively used in patients with cardiac diseases or following cardiac surgery because it does not produce hypotension as compared to other antipsychotic agents [90]. However, the use of chlorpromazine should be avoided due to risks of changes in the EKG as well as hypotension and arrhythmia [33]. In addition, other antipsychotics should be cautiously used because risperidone may cause tachycardia, whereas olanzapine and quetiapine may cause orthostatic hypotension [79].

20.8.4 Benzodiazepine Antianxiety Agents and Hypnotics

Benzodiazepine antianxiety agents can be used with safety in patients with recent onset of MI because they produce few side effects [90]. However, the therapist must avoid using benzodiazepine antianxiety agents or hypnotics when they are likely to compromise an already impaired respiratory drive [51].

20.8.5 Others

Carbamazepine and β-blockers (e.g., propranolol) may exacerbate congestive heart failure [51].

20.9 Interactions Between Cardiac Drugs and Psychiatric Drugs

Hypotension is the most common side effect observed in interactions between cardiac drugs and psychiatric drugs. Tricyclic antidepressants may prolong the PR, QRS, and QT intervals and then produce AV block synergistically when combined with antiarrhythmic agents (e.g., quinidine, procainamide). Thiazide diuretics and low salt diet are likely to cause lithium toxicity. Trazodone may increase blood levels of digoxin and phenytoin [51].

20.10 Psychiatric Side Effects of Cardiovascular Drugs

Antihypertensive drugs such as reserpine, β-blockers, and methyldopa often cause depression [91, 92]. Among antihypertensive agents, captopril is known to produce less side effects including sexual dysfunction than methyldopa and propranolol [93]. When diuretics cause hypokalemia or hypovolemia, symptoms of organic affective disorder (e.g., anorexia, weakness, depressive mood, delirium) may occur especially in the elderly. Among the antiarrhythmic agents, lidocaine is the most common cause of central nervous system excitement and psychosis. Digitalis toxicity may include visual hallucination, anorexia, depression, and delirium [51].

20.11 Conclusions

Potential psychosocial risk factors of coronary heart disease (CHD) include type A personality, hostility and anger, alexithymia, type D personality, stress, depression, anxiety, denial, and social support. These patients often show psychopathology such as anxiety, depression, and delirium. Psychotherapeutic interventions and psychopharmacotherapy for these psychopathologies were reviewed. Psychotherapeutic interventions with heart disease patient are aimed at reducing anxiety and depression, enhancing compliance, and modifying risk factors. To treat them effectively, the clinician should look beyond the symptoms to their function and meaning. In psychopharmacotherapy, interactions between cardiac drugs and psychiatric drugs need to be examined in addition to cardiac side effects of psychiatric drugs and psychiatric side effects of cardiovascular drugs. For the mentally ill cardiac patients, it is desirable to combine psychiatric treatment with a cardiac rehabilitation. Physicians need to keep in mind that countertransference might influence the progress of a cardiac disease.

References

1. Sadock BJ, Sadock VA. Synopsis of psychiatry – behavioral sciences/clinical psychiatry. Philadelphia: Lippincott Williams & Wilkins; 2003. p. 829–31.
2. Hermann-Lingen C, Meinertz T. Psychosomatic aspects of coronary heart disease. Internist. 2010;51:826–35.
3. Lloyd GG, Cawly RH. Psychiatric morbidity in men one week after first acute myocardial infarction. Br Med J. 1978;2:1453–4.
4. Cassem NH, Hackett TP. Psychological aspects of myocardial infarction. Med Clin N Am. 1977;61:711–21.
5. Friedman M, Rosenman RH. Association of specific overt behavior pattern with blood and cardiovascular findings. J Am Med Assoc. 1959;169:1286–96.
6. Rosenman RH, Friedman M. Association of specific behavior pattern in women with blood and cardiovascular findings. Circulation. 1961;24:1173–84.
7. Kornitzer M, Kittel F, De Backer G. The Belgian Heart Disease Prevention Project: type A behavior pattern and the prevalence of coronary heart disease. Psychosom Med. 1981;43:133–45.
8. De Backer G, Kornitzer M, Kittel F. Behavior, stress and psychological traits as risk factors. Prev Med. 1983;12:32–6.
9. Eaker AD, Abbott RD, Kannel WB. Frequency of uncomplicated angina pectoris in type A compared with type B persons (the Framingham Study). Am J Cardiol. 1989;63:1042–5.
10. Blumenthal JA, Willams RB, Kong Y, et al. Type A behavior and angiographically documented coronary disease. Circulation. 1978;58:634–9.
11. Frank KA, Heller SS, Kornfeld DS, et al. Type A behavior pattern and coronary atherosclerosis. J Am Med Assoc. 1978;240:761–3.
12. Williams RB Jr, Haney TL, Lee KL. Type A behavior, hostility and coronary atherosclerosis. Psychosom Med. 1980;42:539–49.
13. Williams RB Jr, Barefoot JC, Haney TL, et al. Type A behavior and angiographically documented coronary atherosclerosis in a sample of 2,289 patients. Psychosom Med. 1988;50:139–52.
14. Dembroski TM, MacDougall JM, Williams RB, et al. J. Components of type A hostility and anger-in: relationship to angiographic findings. Psychosom Med. 1985;47:219–33.
15. MacDougall JM, Dembroski TM, Dimsdale JE, et al. Components of type A hostility and anger-in: further relationship to angiographic findings. Health Psychol. 1985;4:137–52.
16. Dimsdale JE, Hackett TP, Hutter AM, et al. Type A personality and extent of coronary atherosclerosis. Am J Cardiol. 1978;42:583–6.
17. Dimsdale JE, Hackett TP, Hutter AM, et al. Type A behavior and angiographic findings. J Psychosom Res. 1979;23:273–6.
18. Kornitzer M, Magotteau V, Degre V, et al. Angiographic findings and the type A behavior pattern assessed by means of the Bortner Scale. J Behav Med. 1982;5:313–9.
19. Scherwitz L, McKelvain R, Laman C, et al. Type A behavior, self-involvement and coronary atherosclerosis. Psychosom Med. 1983;45:47–57.
20. Cottington EM, Brock BM, House JS, et al. Psychosocial factors and blood pressure in the Michigan statewide blood pressure survey. Am J Epidemiol. 1985;121:515–29.
21. Diamond EL. The role of anger and hostility in essential hypertension and coronary heart disease. Psychol Bull. 1982;92:410–33.
22. Dimsdale JE, Pierce C, Schoenfield D, et al. Suppressed anger and blood pressure: the effect of race, sex, social class, obesity and age. Psychosom Med. 1986;48:430–5.
23. Hackett TP, Rosenbaum TF, Caddem NH. Cardiovascular disorders. In: Kaplan HI, Sadock BJ, editors. Comprehensive textbook of psychiatry, vol. 2. 5th ed. Baltimore: Williams & Wilkins; 1989.

24. Spielberger CD, Johnson EH, Russell SF, et al. The experience and expression of anger: construction and validation of an anger expression scale. In: Chesney MA, Rosenman RH, editors. Anger and hostility in cardiovascular and behavioral disorders. Washington, DC: Hemisphere; 1985.
25. Koh KB, Kim SJ. Comparison of anger between patients with essential hypertension and normal controls. Kor J Psychosom Med. 1995;3:19–27.
26. Jenkins CD, Rosenman RH, Friedman M. Components of the coronary-prone behavior pattern: their relation to silent myocardial infarction and blood lipids. J Chron Dis. 1966;19:599–606.
27. Hecker MHL, Chesney MA, Black GW, et al. Coronary-prone behaviors in the Western Collaborative Group Study. Psychosom Med. 1988;50:153–64.
28. Koh KB, Cho SY, Kim JW, et al. The relationship of anger expression and alexithymia with coronary artery stenosis in patients with coronary artery diseases. Yonsei Med J. 2004;45:181–6.
29. Siegman AW, Dembroski TM, Ringel N. Components of hostility and severity of coronary artery disease. Psychosom Med. 1987;49:127–35.
30. Helmer OC, Ragland DR, Syme SL. Hostility and coronary artery disease. Am J Epidemiol. 1990;123:112–22.
31. Tennant CC, Langeluddecke PM, Fulcher G, et al. Anger and other psychological factors in coronary atherosclerosis. Psychol Med. 1987;17:425–31.
32. Kauhanen J, Kasplan GA, Cohen RD, et al. Alexithymia may influence the diagnosis of coronary heart disease. Psychosom Med. 1994;56:237–44.
33. Katon W, Sullivan M, Clark M. Cardiovascular disorders. In: Kaplan HI, Sadock BJ, editors. Comprehensive textbook of psychiatry. 6th ed. Baltimore: Williams & Wilkins; 1995.
34. Denollet J. DS14: standard assessment of negative affectivity, social inhibition, and Type D personality. Psychosom Med. 2005;67:89–97.
35. Denollet J, Sys S, Stroobant N, et al. Personality as independent predictor of long-term mortality in patients with coronary heart disease. Lancet. 1996;347:417–21.
36. Denollet J, Pedersen SS, Ong AT, et al. Social inhibition modulates the effect of negative emotions on cardiac prognosis following percutaneous coronary intervention in the drug-eluting stent era. Eur Heart J. 2006;27:171–7.
37. Denollet J, Martens E, Nyklícek I, et al. Clinical events in coronary patients who report low distress: adverse effect of repressive coping. Health Psychol. 2008;27:302–28.
38. Kim SJ, Koh KB. The relationship of stress perception with serum cholesterol in patients with essential hypertension. Kor J Psychosom Med. 1993;1:35–44.
39. Wittstein IS, Thiemann DR, Lima JA, et al. Neurohumoral features of myocardial stunning due to sudden emotional stress. N Engl J Med. 2005;352:539–48.
40. Wittstein IS. The broken heart syndrome. Cleve Clin J Med. 2007;74(Suppl 1):S17–22.
41. Roh KS, Koh KB. The relationship between stress and coronary artery stenosis in patients with coronary artery diseases. Kor J Psychosom Med. 1998;6:126–35.
42. Rosengren A, Hawken S, Ounpuu S, et al. Association of psychosocial risk factors with risk of acute myocardial infarction in 11119 cases and 13648 controls from 52 countries (the INTERHEART study): case-control study. Lancet. 2004;364:953–62.
43. Kent LK, Shapiro PA. Depression and related psychological factors in heart disease. Harv Rev Psychiatry. 2009;17:377–88.
44. Frasure-Smith N, Lespérance F, Gravel G, et al. Social support, depression, and mortality during the first year after myocardial infarction. Circulation. 2000;101:1919–24.
45. Laghrissi-Thode F, Wagner WR, Pollock BG, et al. Elevated platelet factor 4 and betathromboglobulin plasma levels in depressed patients with ischemic heart disease. Biol Psychiatry. 1997;42:290–5.
46. Kawachi I, Colditz G, Ascherio A, et al. Prospective study of phobic anxiety and risk of coronary heart disease in men. Circulation. 1994;89:1992–7.
47. Kawachi I, Sparrow D, Vokonas P, et al. Symptoms of anxiety and risk of coronary heart disease. The Normative Aging Study. Circulation. 1994;90:2225–9.

48. Moser DK, Riegel B, McKinley S, et al. Impact of anxiety and perceived control on in-hospital complications after acute myocardial infarction. Psychosom Med. 2007;69:10–6.
49. Sullivan MD, LaCroix AZ, Spertus JA, et al. Five-year prospective study of the effects of anxiety and depression in patients with coronary artery disease. Am J Cardiol. 2000;86:1135–8. A6, A9
50. Ketterer MW, Huffman J, Lumley MA, et al. Five-year follow-up for adverse outcomes in males with at least minimally positive angiograms: importance of "denial" in assessing psychosocial risk factors. J Psychosom Res. 1998;44:241–50.
51. Levenson JL. Cardiovascular disease. In: Stoudemire A, Fogel BS, editors. Principles of medical psychiatry. New York: Grune & Stratton; 1987.
52. Burg MM, Barefoot J, Berkman L, et al. Low perceived social support and post-myocardial infarction prognosis in the enhancing recovery in coronary heart disease clinical trial: the effects of treatment. Psychosom Med. 2005;67:879–88.
53. Kim JW, Koh KB. The relationship between perceived stress and coping strategies in patients with coronary artery disease. J Korean Neuropsychiatr Assoc. 2000;39:288–96.
54. Mookadam F, Arthur HM. Social support and its relationship to morbidity and mortality after acute myocardial infarction: systematic overview. Arch Intern Med. 2004;164:1514–8.
55. Blacher RS. Paradoxical depression after heart surgery: a form of survivor syndrome. Psychoanal Q. 1978;47:267–83.
56. Lown B, DeSilva RA, Reich P. Psychophysiologic factors in sudden cardiac death. Am J Psychiatry. 1980;137:1325–35.
57. Friedman M, Thoresen CE, Gill JJ, et al. Alteration of type A behavior and reduction in cardiac recurrences in postmyocardial infarction patients. Am Heart J. 1986;108:237–48.
58. Richards SH, Anderson L, Jenkinson CE, et al. Psychological interventions for coronary heart disease. Cochrane Database Syst Rev. 2017;4:CD002902.
59. Berkman LF, Blumenthal J, Burg M, et al. Effects of treating depression and low perceived social support on clinical events after myocardial infarction: the Enhancing Recovery in Coronary Heart Disease Patients (ENRICHD) randomized trial. JAMA. 2003;289:3106–16.
60. Wenger NK, Hellerstein HK. Rehabilitation of the coronary patient. 2nd ed. New York: Wiley; 1984.
61. McLane M, Krop H, Mehta J. Psychosexual adjustment and counseling after myocardial infarction. Ann Int Med. 1980;92:514–9.
62. Cay EL. Psychological aspects of cardiac rehabilitation: unsolved problems. Adv Cardiol. 1982;31:237–41.
63. Anderson L, Thompson DR, Oldridge N, et al. Exercise-based cardiac rehabilitation for coronary heart disease. Cochrane Database Syst Rev. 2016;1:CD001800.
64. Anderson L, Brown JP, Clark AM, et al. Patient education in the management of coronary heart disease. Cochrane Database Syst Rev. 2017;6:CD008895.
65. Glassman AH, Bigger JT. Cardiovascular effects of therapeutic doses of tricyclic antidepressants: a review. Arch Gen Psychiatry. 1981;38:815–20.
66. McElroy SL, Keck PE, Friedman LM. Minimizing and managing antidepressant side-effects. J Clin Psychiatry. 1995;56(Suppl 2):49–55.
67. Beliles K, Stoudemire A. Psychopharmacologic treatment of depression in the medically ill. Psychosomatics. 1998;39:S2–S19.
68. Cohen H, Gibson G, Alderman M. Excess risk of myocardial infarction in patients treated with antidepressant medications: association with use of tricyclic agents. Am J Med. 2000;108:2–8.
69. Tata L, West J, Smith C, et al. General population based study of the impact of tricyclic and selective serotonin reuptake inhibitor antidepressants on the risk of acute myocardial infarction. Heart. 2005;91:465–71.
70. Morganroth J, Goin JE. Quinidine-related mortality in the short-to-medium-term treatment of ventricular arrhythmias. Meta Anal Circ. 1991;84:1977–83.
71. Glassman AH, Walsh BJ, Roose SP. Factors related to orthostatic hypotension associated with tricyclic antidepressants. J Clin Psychiatry. 1982;43:35–8.

72. Roose SP, Glassman AH, Giardina EGV. Tricyclic antidepressants in depressed patients with cardiac conduction disease. Arch Gen Psychiatry. 1987;44:273–5.
73. Vieweg WVR, Yazel J, Ballenger JC. Tricyclic antidepressant use in a patient with bundle branch blocks and ventricular ectopy. J Clin Psychiatry. 1984;45:353–5.
74. Buff DD, Brenner R, Kitane SS. Dysrhythmia associated with fluoxetine treatment in an elderly patient with cardiac disease. J Clin Psychiatry. 1991;52:174–6.
75. Ellison JM, Milofsky JE, Ely E. Fluoxetine-induced bradycardia and syncope in two patients. J Clin Psychiatry. 1990;51:385–6.
76. Feder R. Bradycardia and syncope induced by fluoxetine (letter). J Clin Psychiatry. 1991;52:139.
77. Fisch C. Effects of sertraline on the ECG in nonelderly and elderly patients with major depression (abstract). Biol Psychiatry. 1991;29(suppl):S353–S4.
78. Stoudemire A, Fogel BS. Psychopharmacology in medical patients: an update. In: Stoudemire A, Fogel BS, editors. Medical-psychiatric practice, vol. 3. Washington, DC: American Psychiatric Press; 1995.
79. Koh KB. Stress and psychosomatic medicine. Seoul: Ilchokak; 2011.
80. Roose SP, Dalack GW, Glassman AH, et al. Cardiovascular effects of bupropion in depressed patients with heart disease. Am J Psychiatry. 1991;148:512–6.
81. Johnson EM, Whyte E, Mulsant BH, et al. Cardiovascular changes associated with venlafaxine in the treatment of late-life depression. Am J Geriatr Psychiatry. 2006;14:796–802.
82. Warrington SJ. Clinical implications of the pharmacology of sertraline. Int Clin Psychopharmacol. 1991;6(Suppl 2):11–21.
83. Janowsky D, Gurtis G, Zisook S. Ventricular arrhythmias possibly aggravated by trazodone. Am J Psychiatry. 1983;140:796–7.
84. Lippman S, Bedford P, Manshadi M. Trazodone cardiotoxicity. Am J Psychiatry. 1983;140:1383.
85. Rowe H, Carmichael R, Lemberger L. The effect of fluoxetine on warfarin metabolism in rat and man. Life Sci. 1978;23:807–12.
86. Benfield P, Ward A. Fluvoxamine: a review of its pharmacodynamic and pharmacokinetic properties, and therapeutic efficacy in depressive illness. Drugs. 1986;32:313–34.
87. Wilner KD, Lazar JD, Apseloff G. The effects of sertraline on the pharmacodynamics of warfarin in healthy volunteers (abstract). Biol Psychiatry. 1991;29(Suppl):354S–5S.
88. Shapiro P. Psychopharmacology in cardiac disease. In: Ferrando S, Levenson J, Robinson M, et al., editors. Handbook of psychopharmacology in the medically ill. Washington, DC: American Psychiatric Publishing; 2009.
89. Levenson JL, Mishra A, Bauernfeind RA. Lithium treatment of mania in a patient with recurrent ventricular tachycardia. Psychosomatics. 1986;27:594–6.
90. Risch SC, Groom GP, Janowsky DS. The effects of psychotropic drugs on the cardiovascular system. J Clin Psychiatry. 1982;43:16–31.
91. Avron J, Everitt DE, Weiss S. Increased antidepressant use in patients prescribed B-blockers. JAMA. 1986;255:357–60.
92. DeMuth GW, Ackerman SH. Alphamethyldopa and depression: a clinical study and review of the literature. Am J Psychiatry. 1983;140:534–8.
93. Croog SH, Levine S, Testa MA. The effects of antihypertensive therapy on the quality of life. New Engl J Med. 1986;314:1657–64.

Chapter 21
Approach to Stress and Mental Disorders in Patients with Diabetes

21.1 Introduction

Diabetes mellitus is a disorder of metabolism and the vascular system, manifested by disturbance in the body's control of glucose, lipid, and protein. This disorder results from impaired insulin secretion or action. Heredity and family history are important in the onset of diabetes. However, sudden onset is often associated with emotional stress, which disturbs homeostatic balance in persons who are predisposed to the disorder [1].

Medical treatment and modification of life habits in patients with diabetes mellitus require their consistent and long-term cooperation [2]. The progress of diabetes mellitus largely depends on these patients' compliance with treatment and control of the disease. One of the factors interfering with the control of the disease is stress. In addition, it has been recognized for a period of long time that emotional state of diabetics affects the treatment of the disease [3, 4]. When they are depressed and dejected, they often overeat or overdrink self-destructively and cause their diabetes to get out of control [1].

On the other hand, mental disorders can exacerbate diabetes as well as increase the risk for diabetes. Because coexisting diabetes and mental disorders are so common, one should consider screening patients with diabetes for mental disorders and vice versa [5].

21.2 Relationship Between Stress and Diabetes

It has been reported that in about 78% of diabetic patients, the onset and aggravation of the disorder are associated with psychosocial stressors [6]. Complications of diabetes, long-term diet, and medication which are major stressors of patients with diabetes can cause serious emotional or physical problems. In particular,

K. B. Koh, *Stress and Somatic Symptoms*,
https://doi.org/10.1007/978-3-030-02783-4_21

complications of diabetes such as peripheral neuropathy, retinopathy, hypertension, gangrene, and stroke can cause depression, leading to suicide [7, 8].

A considerable number of type 1 diabetic patients were reported to experience loss of important family members before the diagnosis of diabetes was made [9–11]. Sometimes cumulated ordinary stress can affect the onset of diabetes by reducing defensive functions and inducing emotion-related physiological changes [8]. Recent life events are also known to be associated with poor control of diabetes [12]. In addition, the more frequent the life events, the poorer the index of diabetic control and the more frequent the changes of insulin dosage used [13].

21.3 Mechanism Linking Stress to Diabetes

The effect of stress on glucose metabolism is known to be mediated by counterregulatory hormones (e.g., glucagon, epinephrine, norepinephrine, cortisol, growth hormone, beta-endorphin) which increase blood glucose levels and reduce actions of insulin [14, 15]. These hormones are called stress hormones. They are important in helping healthy people adapt to stressful situations by mobilizing energy. In diabetic patients, however, increased blood glucose induced by stress cannot be metabolized sufficiently due to insulin deficiency. Thus, stress is likely to enhance chronic hyperglycemia [14].

21.4 Psychological Responses and Adaptation

Once the diagnosis of diabetes is made, patients are shocked along with fear [16]. As in patients with other physical diseases, a variety of psychological and behavioral alterations occur in patients with diabetes. They experience anger, hopelessness, and a sense of self-depreciation, which will endanger an important interpersonal relationship [8]. In addition, patients with diabetes are known to have low self-esteem and remarkable depression [17, 18].

Children with diabetes experience isolation and alienation because they should live and behave unlike other healthy children [8]. They often use diet as a means of attracting attention from their parents or expressing their hostility by rejecting or overeating meals [19]. At the onset of diabetes during an adolescent period, their effort to be independent of their parents is threatened so that they may resist treatment of diabetes. At first, adults deny their illness itself and reject treatment. They go through a period of anger, anxiety, depression, and a sense of guilt and then accept the illness and adapt to it by complying with physicians' and nurses' recommendation. This adaptive process depends on the patients' premorbid personality and the degree of their personal maturity [8]. In particular, young adults with type 2 diabetes show more depressive symptoms and are less likely to eat healthily than their older counterparts, suggesting that the former may require more intensive psychological and self-care support than the latter [20].

21.5 Stress Management

Stress management can help control glucose and lipid metabolism. It includes (1) education about diabetes, stress, and the effect of stress on diabetic control, (2) self-regulation training (e.g., relaxation therapy, meditation), (3) cognitive behavioral therapy; this therapy focuses on stress, individuals' psychosocial issues, marital conflicts, familial, occupational, and social problems, and (4) adaptation to changes of lifestyle [15].

The advantage of stress management is not only to reduce unstable metabolic function and the required amount of insulin but also to delay neuropathy and vascular diseases. This can indirectly provide diabetic patients with a sense of achievement through their self-control and can help control diabetes by enhancing active cooperation with their physicians and reducing maladaptive coping strategies. In general, a considerable number of studies on the effects of stress management such as muscle relaxation and biofeedback showed positive results. For example, biofeedback, muscle relaxation, and autogenic training significantly reduced the required amount of insulin and improved the index of diabetic control (the levels of urine sugar and acetone) [21]. A group of patients who received biofeedback and muscle relaxation showed a better effect on glucose tolerance in patients with type 2 diabetes, when compared with the control group [22]. In patients with type 1 diabetes, muscle relaxation also significantly reduced the serum levels of glucose [23, 24]. However, there was a report that muscle relaxation did not improve glucose control in type 1 diabetic patients [25].

21.6 Mental Disorders and Diabetes

Treatment for patients with mental disorders and diabetes should focus first and foremost on improving the mental disorders. As their cognitive functioning improves, it is desirable that focus should be directed toward treating the metabolic parameters (e.g., weight, lipids, blood pressure, glycemic control). Assessment and treatment of both the mental and physical aspects in patients with diabetes will help enhance their long-term survivability and quality of life [5].

21.6.1 Depression and Diabetes

The most common reason for referral to psychiatry in patients with diabetes was depression. Forty-two percent of the patients were diagnosed with depressive disorders which included adjustment disorder with depressed mood, major depressive disorder, and dysthymic disorder [26]. In particular, patients with type 1 diabetes often show severe depression [18]. Young adults with type 1 diabetes who are more depressed are likely to have higher HbA (1c) levels [27].

21.6.2 Prevalence of Depression

The prevalence of depression in diabetics was reported to be between 9% and 27% [28, 29]. Compared with nondiabetic people, the prevalence rate of depression is more than three times higher in patients with type 1 diabetes and nearly twice as high in patients with type 2 diabetes [30].

21.6.3 Depression and Complications of Diabetes

The likelihood of developing depression tends to increase as patients get older and develop more diabetes-related complications; they become more disabled by their disease and face the realization that reversal of their symptoms is unlikely [31]. Diabetic neuropathy is a risk factor for depression predicting both the severity and increments of depression over time [32]. In addition, patients with depression and anxiety are known to be at high risk for coma due to ketoacidosis by neglecting their diet. Such tendency is more prominent in patients with diabetes whose illness has its onset during adolescence [33, 34].

Compared with patients with diabetes alone, those with depression and diabetes demonstrate poorer self-management skills (e.g., following diet and exercise regimens) and more often fail to refill their prescribed medications [35]. Depressed patients frequently adopt a lifestyle that promotes cardiovascular diseases. For example, patients with depression tend to be overweight, are physically inactive, and abuse nicotine more than do age-matched controls [36, 37]. Major depressive disorder has been shown to be associated with a 2.3-fold increase in the risk of mortality for patients with type 2 diabetes [31].

21.7 Psychosocial Approach to Depression

Depression is not always a permanently curable disorder; therefore, the goal of therapy must be directed initially at inducing remission and, over the long term, reducing the likelihood of recurrence. Partial remissions tend to increase the chance of recurrence, implying that patients should be treated until they are free of depressive symptoms and maintained at this level for a minimum of 1 year [36]. In particular, addressing diabetes-specific emotional problems as part of depression treatment in diabetes patients may help improve glycemic outcomes [38].

It is desirable for therapeutic team members including physicians to show friendly attitude as a consultant rather than coercive attitude as an authoritative figure [8]. Physicians' empathetic listening to patients, especially uncooperative ones, can help them ventilate their emotions so that they can manage their emotional reactions to illness, such as anxiety, depression, anger, and guilt. For diabetes education, especially regarding diet, it is desirable to help patients change faulty habits, rather than to use coercion [39].

In addition, it has been reported that confrontation is an effective coping strategy, and social support helps control diabetes by preventing a sense of isolation [12]. Group therapy for adolescents with diabetes is also known to be effective [2].

Diabetes can be exacerbated by stressors so that it is important to identify stressors and to seek psychiatric consultations if necessary. In particular, psychiatric consultation is recommended when severe depression is noted [39]. In patients with complications of diabetes such as diabetic neuropathy comorbid with depression, integrative approaches that target depression while concurrently optimizing treatment and self-management may be most powerful [32]. Moreover, for depressed patients with hopelessness and helplessness, physicians need to minimize the patients' self-esteem injury rather than manage diabetes itself (e.g., diet) [7], as shown in the following case.

Case
A 40-year-old woman with diabetes hospitalized in the department of endocrinology was referred to the department of psychiatry for management of uncontrolled eating. She had suffered from diabetes for a period of 10 years and had difficulty walking due to complications such as peripheral neuropathy. After realizing that diabetes could not be cured completely while reading a pamphlet on the illness, she began to live in a state of self-abandonment, feeling a sense of hopelessness and helplessness. Thereafter, she gave up her diet and ate sweet foods such as cakes and doughnuts carelessly. The internist reproached her for not complying with his diet requests when her blood sugar levels rose above 400 mg/dl even after insulin had been injected several times during her admission. She cried out, saying, "any patient who can control their eating is not a real diabetic patient." After venting her emotions such as anger and resentment toward the physician, the psychiatrist said, "please eat as many doughnuts as you can now, but start trying to cut down on the number one by one." The patient calmed down after that. Later, she followed the internist's diet advice and did not buy any more sweet foods at the cafeteria of the hospital. She also looked peaceful and emotionally stable, reading the Bible in her room.

21.7.1 Cognitive Behavioral Therapy (CBT)

CBT may be effective when diabetic patients show negative thoughts about their physical condition. It is important to explain to patients that most diabetes-related complications may be prevented, delayed, or even reversed if treated intensively [5].

Formation of an optimistic partnership between psychiatrists, primary physicians, and family members is an integral aspect of CBT. CBT has been shown to be effective in achieving remission in 85% of patients with type 2 diabetes mellitus over a 10-week course, and 70% of these patients remained free of depression at the 6-month follow-up visit [40, 41]. One study has found that both individual mindfulness-based cognitive therapy (MBCT) and CBT are effective in improving depression in individuals with type 1 and type 2 diabetes [42]. In another study, it has been reported that CBT is an effective intervention for adherence and glycemic control as well as depression in adults with type 2 diabetes and depression [43]. In addition, group CBT can effectively help type 1 diabetic patients with comorbid depression achieve and maintain better glycemic outcomes [44]. However, in an analysis of randomized controlled trials (RCTs), the evidence for glycemic control is inconclusive for psychological interventions [45].

21.7.2 Behavioral Approach to Depression

The behavioral approaches that may be self-motivating for depressed patients with diabetes are as follows [5]: (1) begin a regularly scheduled exercise program for more than 30 min each day, (2) the physician should encourage patients to develop a positive attitude toward diabetes self-management, (3) it should be explained that depression can be improved once normal neurotransmission is reestablished, because major depressive disorder is neurochemically related disorder, (4) remind patients that the good news is that most individuals will live their life without any major disrupting event (e.g., limb amputation, eye and kidney diseases) secondary to the disease with more advanced management of diabetes.

21.8 Psychopharmacotherapy for Depression

Successful treatment of depression was associated with significant improvement of glycemic control in studies using fluoxetine and sertraline [46, 47]. Selective serotonin reuptake inhibitors (SSRIs) and serotonin norepinephrine reuptake inhibitors (SNRI) such as duloxetine and venlafaxine are the most appropriate antidepressants for managing depression in diabetic patients because of their more favorable side effects [48]. However, some antidepressants should be used with caution. For example, SSRIs such as fluoxetine, sertraline, and paroxetine may cause hypoglycemia [28]. Tricyclic antidepressants such as imipramine may cause hypoglycemia when used for a brief period but hyperglycemia when used for a long-term period [49]. Overall, to maximize response of both depression and diabetic disorder, one should consider SSRIs in preference over tricyclic antidepressants [28]. In general, it is safe to start one-third of the usual adult dosage of antidepressants in elderly patients [48]. The dosage and main side effects of antidepressants used in adult and elderly patients are described in Table 21.1.

To prevent side effects such as anxiety and restlessness as well as recurrence of depression, antidepressant medications should not be abruptly discontinued under any circumstances. Medications should be tapered slowly over a 1- to 2-week period [5, 50].

Sexual dysfunction and weight gain may become apparent within 1 month of starting SSRI. However, it should be noted that more than 50% of patients with major depressive disorder may have sexual dysfunction as a symptom of their depression [51]. Among antidepressants, the SSRI and venlafaxine are more likely to cause sexual dysfunction than are bupropion, nefazodone, and duloxetine [52].

Table 21.1 Dosage and side effects of antidepressants

	Daily doses of adults (elderly) (mg)	Main side effects
TCAs		
Amitriptyline (Elavil)	50–200 (25–75)	Drowsiness, dry mouth, constipation, difficulty in urination, edema, blurred vision, increased appetite, weight gain, orthostatic hypotension, mania, seizure
Imipramine (Tofranil)	50–200 (25–75)	Same as above
SARIs		
Trazodone (Trittico)	50–250 (25–75)	Drowsiness, orthostatic hypotension, dizziness, headache, nausea, priapism
Nefazodone (Serzone)	100–300 (50–200)	Orthostatic hypotension
SSRIs		
Fluoxetine (Prozac)	5–20 (5–10)	Nausea, vomiting, diarrhea, abdominal pain, decreased appetite (early), headache, insomnia, anxiety, tremor, hidrosis, decreased sexual desire
Sertraline (Zoloft)	25–100 (25–50)	Same as above
Fluvoxamine (Luvox)	25–150 (25–50)	Same as above
Paroxetine (Seroxat, Paxil)	10–30 (10–20)	Myoclonus, dry mouth in addition to the above
SNRIs		
Venlafaxine (Effexor)	25–225 (25–75)	Drowsiness, dizziness, nausea, dry mouth, constipation, decreased appetite, listlessness, anxiety, impotence
Duloxetine (Cymbalta)	60–120 (30–60)	Nausea, dry mouth, insomnia, increased blood pressure
NaSSAs		
Mirtazapine (Remeron)	15–45 (15–30)	Drowsiness, dizziness, dry mouth, constipation, edema, increased appetite, weight gain
NDRIs		
Bupropion (Wellbutrin)	150–300 (75–100)	Headache, insomnia, nausea, restlessness, seizure
SSREs		
Tianeptine (Stablon)	25–37.5 (25)	Drowsiness, headache, dizziness, dry mouth, nausea, constipation, decreased appetite, tachycardia, listlessness, tremor

TCA tricyclic antidepressants, *SARIs* serotonin antagonist and reuptake inhibitors, *SSRIs* selective serotonin reuptake inhibitors, *SNRIs* serotonin-norepinephrine reuptake inhibitors, *NaSSAs* noradrenergic and specific serotonergic antidepressants, *NDRI* norepinephrine-dopamine reuptake inhibitors, *SSREs* selective serotonin reuptake enhancers

The following treatment options are available for patients whose depression has improved while taking an antidepressant but in whom sexual dysfunction developed during their course of therapy [5]: (1) reduce the dose of the antidepressant, (2) take a drug holiday, and (3) switch medications (e.g., duloxetine or bupropion).

In addition, weight gain may occur with the use of antidepressants in patients with diabetes [5]. In particular, tricyclic antidepressants such as amitriptyline and SSRIs such as paroxetine can cause weight gain. Fluoxetine may cause weight loss when used for less than 6 months but weight gain when used for more than 6 months [53]. In order to manage weight gain associated with antidepressant treatment, patients are recommended to improve diet and initiate exercise program, and medication should be changed to weight-neutral medications (e.g., duloxetine and bupropion).

21.9 Anxiety Disorder and Diabetes

Results from a meta-analysis study suggest that diabetes is associated with an increased likelihood of having anxiety disorders [54]. Diabetes patients with anxiety symptoms are less likely to adhere to self-care recommendations in relation to eating habits and smoking [55]. However, most diabetic patients with anxiety disorder or anxiety symptoms seem to respond well to supportive psychotherapy and antianxiety agents (e.g., alprazolam)/antidepressants (e.g., SSRIs) for a short period of time unlike diabetic patients with depression.

21.10 Schizophrenic Disorder and Diabetes

The link between schizophrenic disorder and diabetes is known to be high [56]. It is critical that psychotic symptoms should be first stabilized for management of diabetic patients with schizophrenic disorder in order to enhance adherence to medical recommendations [57].

Atypical antipsychotics such as clozapine, olanzapine, risperidone, and quetiapine have been known to induce weight gain. Among them, clozapine and olanzapine are particularly likely to be associated with a high rate of diabetes than are risperidone and quetiapine [58]. Drugs that have the highest affinity toward histamine-receptor blockade, such as olanzapine, are associated with the most weight gain, whereas ziprasidone and aripiprazole with limited histamine receptor activity are associated with the least weight gain [59].

21.11 Bipolar Disorder and Diabetes

A considerable number of patients with bipolar disorder are estimated to be overweight or obese at the time of their initial diagnosis [60]. Medications used for the treatment of bipolar disorder tend to further increase one's weight. Patients who gain 5% or more of their initial weight at any time during therapy may need to be switched to a different therapeutic agent after tapering off the original drug [5].

21.12 Sleep Disorders and Diabetes

Diabetic patients with insomnia demonstrated higher levels of fasting blood glucose and insulin resistance than subjects with normal sleep pattern [61]. Subjects averaging less than 5–6 h per night of sleep have a 28% chance of developing type 2 diabetes, whereas those with difficulty maintaining sleep have an 84% likelihood of developing the disorder [62].

21.12.1 Management of Sleep Disorders

Insomnia needs to be etiologically treated after physical and psychological assessment. For example, for insomnia due to pain, primary treatment should focus on pain, whereas for insomnia due to mental disorders such as depressive or anxiety disorders, psychotherapy or psychopharmacotherapy should be tried [63].

Hypnotics should be used for insomnia of unknown etiology for a short-term period. Their long-term use should be avoided because of potentially high risks for drug abuse and dependence [39]. Hypnotics such as triazolam (Halcion, Zolmin) and zolpidem (Stilnox) can be used for patients who have difficulty in falling asleep. Triazolam has an advantage of less hangover due to its short half-life. Its common side effects include headache, dizziness, dry mouth, restlessness, impaired orientation and memory, hallucination, and aggression. Zolpidem is a nonbenzodiazepine hypnotic and has an advantage of less effect on cognitive function such as memory and less hangover. This drug is recommended for those who work in the daytime because it does not affect cognition and job performance. Unlike triazolam, it has no rebound insomnia after 24 h. Its common side effects include drowsiness, diminished attention, fatigue, headache, dizziness, diplopia, memory impairment, and difficulty in walking. Tremor, seizure, sweating, vomiting, anxiety, and excitement can also occur as withdrawal symptoms so that it should be gradually discontinued [64]. In addition, lorazepam (Ativan) can be considered a sleep-inducing drug because its half-life is short. In elderly patients, half of adult dosage of these drugs is recommended. However, it should be kept in mind that long-term use of these hypnotics and antianxiety agents can lead to drug abuse or dependence [39].

Early awakening or middle insomnia is often associated with depression [63, 65]. Such insomnia can be the only symptom or initial symptom of depressive disorders in some patients. Later they can show their personal conflicts or maladaptation to life. For these insomniac patients, tricyclic antidepressants such as amitriptyline (Elavil) can be effective. However, it has anticholinergic effects such as drowsiness, dry mouth, difficulty in urination, and constipation. Trazodone can be tried for patients with such serious side effects [39].

21.13 Conclusions

The relationship between stress and diabetes, mechanism linking stress to diabetes, psychological response and adaptation, stress management, and approach to mental disorders in patients with diabetes were reviewed. Mental disorders such as depressive disorders, schizophrenic disorder, bipolar disorder (depressive type), and sleep disorders may increase the risk of diabetes. Management for patients with both psychiatric disorders and diabetes should focus first and foremost on improving the psychiatric disorders. Psychosocial approach for diabetic patients with depression should be supportive by allowing the patients to ventilate their emotions, minimizing self-esteem injury, and maintaining hope. In particular, cognitive behavioral therapy is recommended, and appropriate antidepressants need to be used for these patients. It should be noted that antipsychotics can alter metabolic status in patients with schizophrenic disorder and bipolar disorder. Hypnotics should be used for a short-term period. If possible, diabetic patients with potential psychiatric disorders should be referred to psychiatrists for assessment.

References

1. Sadock BJ, Sadock VA. Synopsis of psychiatry – behavioral sciences/clinical psychiatry. 9th ed. Philadelphia: Lippincott Williams & Wilkins; 2003.
2. Rubin RT, King BH. Endocrine and metabolic disorders. In: Kaplan HI, Sadock BJ, editors. Comprehensive textbook of psychiatry, vol. 2. 6th ed. Baltimore: Williams & Wilkins; 1995.
3. Kravitz AR, Isenberg PH, Shore MF, et al. Emotional factors in diabetes mellitus. In: Marble AL, et al., editors. Joslin's diabetes mellitus. 11th ed. Philadelphia: Lea and Ferbiger; 1971.
4. Koch MF, Milnar GD. Psychiatric aspects of patients with unstable diabetes mellitus. Psychosom Med. 1974;36:57–62.
5. Unger J, Schwartz Z. Diabetes management in primary care. 2nd ed. Philadelphia: Lippincott Williams & Wilkins; 2013.
6. Koh KB, Lee HC. Stress perception of patients with non-insulin-dependent diabetes mellitus. J Korean Neuropsychiatr Assoc. 1992;31:1084–91.
7. Koh KB, Bae JH. Coping strategy of patients with diabetes mellitus. J Korean Neuropsychiatr Assoc. 1988;27:685–92.
8. Kimball CP. The biopsychosocial approach to the patient. Baltimore: Williams & Wilkins; 1981.
9. Robinson N, Fuller JH. Role of life events and difficulties in the onset of diabetes mellitus. J Psychosom Res. 1985;29:583–91.
10. Slawson PF, Flynn WR, Kollar EJ. Psychological factors associated with the onset of diabetes mellitus. JAMA. 1963;185:166–70.
11. Stein SP, Charles E. Emotional factors in juvenile diabetes mellitus: a study of early life experience of adolescent diabetics. Am J Psychiatry. 1971;128:700–4.
12. Schwartz LS, Springer J, Flaherty JA. The role of recent life events and social support in the control of diabetes mellitus: a pilot study. Gen Hosp Psychiatry. 1986;8:212–6.
13. Bradley C. Life events and the control of diabetes mellitus. J Psychosom Res. 1979;23:159–62.
14. Surwit RS, Schneider MS. Role of stress in the etiology and treatment of diabetes mellitus. Psychosom Med. 1993;55:380–93.
15. Evans MB. Emotional stress and diabetic control: a postulated model for the effect of emotional distress upon intermediary metabolism in the diabetic. Biofeedback Self Regul. 1985;10:241–54.

16. Koh KB. Psychiatric aspects of diabetes mellitus. New Med J. 1987;30:25–8.
17. Ford CV. The somatizing disorders: illness as a way of life. New York: Elsevier Biomedical; 1984.
18. Surridge DHC, Williams EDL, Lawson JS, et al. Psychiatric aspects of diabetes mellitus. Br J Psychiatry. 1984;145:269–76.
19. Kolb LC, Brodie HK. Modern clinical psychiatry. 10th ed. Philadelphia: WB Sunders Co; 1982.
20. Browne JL, Nefs G, Pouwer F, et al. Depression, anxiety and self-care behaviors of young adults with type 2 diabetes: results from the International Diabetes Management and Impact for Long-term Empowerment and Success (MILES) study. Diabet Med. 2015;32:133–40.
21. Fowler JE, Budzynski TH, Vandenbergh RL. Effects of an EMG biofeedback relaxation program on the control of diabetes. Biofeedback Self Regul. 1976;1:105–12.
22. Surwit RS, Feinglos MN. The effects of relaxation on glucose tolerance in non-insulin dependent diabetes. Proceedings of the 14th Meeting of the Biofeedback Society of America, Denver; 1983.
23. Lammers CA, Naliboff BD, Straatneyer AJ. The effects of progressive relaxation on stress and diabetic control. Behav Res Ther. 1984;22:641–50.
24. Landis B, Jovonovic L, Landis E. Effect of stress reduction on daily glucose range in previously stabilized insulin-dependent diabetic patients. Diabetes Care. 1985;8:624–6.
25. Felinglos MN, Hastedt P, Surwit RS. Effects of relaxation therapy on patients with type I diabetes mellitus. Diabetes Care. 1987;10:72–5.
26. Koh KB. Clinical characteristics of patients with diabetes mellitus referred for psychiatric consultation. J Korean Neuropsychiatr Assoc. 1990;29:1022–8.
27. Johnson B, Eiser C, Young V, et al. Prevalence of depression among young people with type 1 diabetes: a systematic review. Diabet Med. 2013;30:199–208.
28. Goodnick PJ, Henry JH, Buki VMV. Treatment of depression in patients with diabetes mellitus. J Clin Psychiatry. 1995;56:128–36.
29. Anderson RJ, Freedland KE, Clouse RE, et al. The prevalence of comorbid depression in adults with diabetes: a meta-analysis. Diabetes Care. 2001;24:1069–78.
30. Roy T, Lloyd CE. Epidemiology of depression and diabetes: a systematic review. J Affect Disord. 2012;142(Suppl):S8–S21.
31. Katon WJ, Rutter C, Simon G, et al. The association of comorbid depression with mortality in patients with type 2 diabetes. Diabetes Care. 2005;28:2668–72.
32. Vileikyte L, Gonzalez JS. Recognition and management of psychosocial issues in diabetic neuropathy. Handb Clin Neurol. 2014;126:195–209.
33. Hood KK, Huestis S, Maher A, et al. Depressive symptoms in children and adolescents with type 1 diabetes: association with diabetes specific characteristics. Diabetes Care. 2006;29:1389–91.
34. Anderson BJ, Edelstein S, Abramson NW, et al. Depressive symptoms and quality of life in adolescents with type 2 diabetes. Diabetes Care. 2011;34:2205–7.
35. Lustman PJ, Griffith LS, Clouse RE. Depression in adults with diabetes: results of 5-yr follow-up study. Diabetes Care. 1988;11:605–12.
36. Lustman PJ, Clouse RE. Practical considerations in the management of depression in diabetes. Diabetes Spectr. 2004;17:160–6.
37. Katon WJ, Lin EH, Russo J, et al. Cardiac risk factors in patients with diabetes mellitus and major depression. J Gen Intern Med. 2004;19:1192–9.
38. van Bastelaar KM, Pouwer F, Geelhoed-Duijvestijn PH, et al. Diabetes-specific emotional distress mediates the association between depressive symptoms and glycaemic control in type 1 and type 2 diabetes. Diabet Med. 2010;27:798–803.
39. Koh KB. Stress and psychosomatic medicine. 2nd ed. Seoul: Ilchokak; 2011.
40. Williams MM, Clouse RE, Lustman PJ. Treating depression to prevent diabetes and its complications: understanding depression as a medical risk factor. Clin Diabetes. 2006;24:79–86.
41. Lustman PJ, Griffith LS, Freeland KE, et al. Cognitive behavior therapy for depression in type 2 diabetes: a randomized controlled trial. Ann Intern Med. 1998;129:613–21.

42. Tovote KA, Fleer J, Snippe E, et al. Individual mindfulness-based cognitive therapy and cognitive behavior therapy for treating depressive symptoms in patients with diabetes: results of a randomized controlled trial. Diabetes Care. 2014;37:2427–34.
43. Safren SA, Gonzalez JS, Wexler DJ, et al. A randomized controlled trial of cognitive behavioral therapy for adherence and depression (CBT-AD) in patients with uncontrolled type 2 diabetes. Diabetes Care. 2014;37:625–33.
44. Snoek FJ, van der Ven NC, Twisk JW, et al. Cognitive behavioural therapy (CBT) compared with blood glucose awareness training (BGAT) in poorly controlled type 1 diabetic patients: long-term effects on HbA moderated by depression. A randomized controlled trial. Diabet Med. 2008;25:1337–42.
45. Baumeister H, Hutter N, Bengel J. Psychological and pharmacological interventions for depression in patients with diabetes mellitus and depression. Cochrane Database Syst Rev. 2012;12:CD008381. https://doi.org/10.1002/14651858.CD008381.pub2.
46. Williams MM, Clouse RE, Rubin EH, et al. Evaluating late-life depression in patients with diabetes. Psychol Ann. 2004;34:305–12.
47. Daubresse J-C, Kolanowski J, Krzentowski G, et al. Usefulness of fluoxetine in obese non-insulin-dependent diabetics: a multicenter study. Obes Res. 1996;4:391–6.
48. Min SK. New psychiatry. Seoul: Ilchokak; 2006.
49. Kaplan SM, Mass JW, Pixley JM. Use of imipramine in diabetics. JAMA. 1960;174:511–7.
50. Lustman PJ, Clouse RE. Depression in diabetic patients: the relationship between mood and glycemic control. J Diabetes Complicat. 2005;19:113–22.
51. Hirschfield RMA. Management of sexual side effects of antidepressant therapy. J Clin Psychiatry. 1999;60(Suppl 14):27–30.
52. Clayton AH, Pradko JF, Croft HA, et al. Prevalence of sexual dysfunction among newer antidepressants. J Clin Psychiatry. 2002;63:357–66.
53. Deshmukh R, Franco K. Managing weight gain as a side effect of antidepressant therapy. Cleve Clin J Med. 2003;70:614–23.
54. Smith KJ, Béland M, Clyde M, et al. Association of diabetes with anxiety: a systematic review and meta-analysis. J Psychosom Res. 2013;74:89–99.
55. Smith KJ, Pedneault M, Schmitz N. Investigation of anxiety and depression symptom co-morbidity in a community sample with type 2 diabetes: associations with indicators of self-care. Can J Public Health. 2016;106:e496–501.
56. Cassidy F, Ahearn E, Carroll BJ. Elevated frequency of diabetes mellitus in hospitalized manic-depressive patients. Am J Psychiatry. 1999;156:1417–20.
57. Yu BP, Ortiz T, Chong YS, et al. Use of novel antipsychotic medications in diabetes: a retrospective review. Drug Benefit Trends. 2002;14:42–5.
58. Koro CE, Fedder DO, L'Italien GJ, et al. Assessment of independent effect of olanzapine and risperidone on risk of diabetes among patients with schizophrenia: population-based case-control study. Br Med J. 2002;325:243–7.
59. Wirshing DA, Wirshing WC, Kysar L, et al. Novel antipsychotics: comparison of weight gain liabilities. J Clin Psychiatry. 1999;100:3–16.
60. Fagiolini A, Frank E, Houck PR, et al. Prevalence of obesity and weight change during treatment in patients with bipolar 1 disorder. J Clin Psychiatry. 2002;63:528–33.
61. Knutson KL, Cauter EB, Zee P, et al. Cross-sectional associations between measures of sleep and markers of glucose metabolism among subjects with and without diabetes. Diabetes Care. 2011;34:1171–6.
62. Cappuccio FP, D'elia L, Strazzullo P, et al. Quantity and quality of sleep and incidence of type 2 diabetes: a systematic review and meta-analysis. Diabetes Care. 2010;33:414–20.
63. Koh KB. Guidance of drug administration for insomniacs. Drug Inf. 1986;129:86–7.
64. Min SK. Clinical psychopharmacology. Seoul: Jungangmunhwa Co; 2003.
65. Koh KB. Symptoms of depression and differential diagnoses. Drug Inf. 1987;1:48–50.

Chapter 22
Approach to Functional Dyspepsia

22.1 Introduction

Gastrointestinal symptoms are very common in the general population [1, 2]. A considerable number of patients visiting gastrointestinal clinics complain of upper abdominal symptoms without organic abnormalities [3–5]. This means that functional dyspepsia can often be seen in patients with gastrointestinal disorders [6].

The term 'functional dyspepsia (FD)' or 'nonulcer dyspepsia' was used in a number of patients with ulcer-like upper abdominal symptoms without evidence of organic pathology [7]. Patients with FD, defined in the 2016 Rome IV criteria as bothersome clinical dyspepsia symptoms, experience markedly reduced quality of life [8].

About 45% of dyspepsia cases did not have any abnormalities in the upper gastrointestinal tract [9]. In addition, about half of outpatients visiting the department of gastroenterology of general hospitals were found to be functional. Among these patients, 10% had FD [5].

These FD patients were reported to complain of indigestion, cardiac symptoms, musculoskeletal symptoms, and exhaustion more often than patients with duodenal ulcer or healthy controls [10]. This disorder can be comorbid with irritable bowel syndrome (IBS) or gastroesophageal reflux [11]. In particular, IBS-FD overlap is associated with an increased severity of psychopathological features [12].

This chapter reviews the causes and treatment of FD in terms of biopsychosocial perspectives.

K. B. Koh, *Stress and Somatic Symptoms*,
https://doi.org/10.1007/978-3-030-02783-4_22

22.2 Etiology

The causes of FD remain to be established, but several etiologies have been associated with FD. In the Rome IV criteria, the brain-gut axis was acknowledged as an important factor in the etiology of functional gastrointestinal (GI) disorders [8].

22.2.1 Biological Factors

Accumulating data suggest that infections and possibly food may play an important role in subsets of FD. FD does not equate with no pathology; duodenal eosinophilia is now an accepted association, and Helicobacter pylori infection is considered to be causally linked to dyspepsia [13].

In some of these patients, gastritis, smooth muscle disturbance, and gastroesophageal reflux are seen as causes of functional dyspepsia [7]. On the other hand, Colin-Jones [14] regarded FD as a heterogeneous group with multiple causes. In some cases, gastric acid associated with reflux may play a significant role in FD, whereas in others, abnormal motility, infection, and personality may play a more important role.

22.2.2 Psychosocial Factors

Psychosocial factors seem to play an important role in the pathogenesis of FD [15].

22.2.2.1 Mental Disorders

FD was reported to be highly associated with mental disorders, especially anxiety disorders [16–18]. Eighty-six percent of FD patients showed mental disorders, while 25% of patients with other diseases such as gall stone and hiatal hernia did. The most common diagnoses in patients with FD were anxiety disorders, especially generalized anxiety disorder [12].

22.2.2.2 Negative Emotion

FD is associated with a variety of factors such as neuroticism, mood alteration, childhood emotional deprivation, and family history [19, 20]. Anxiety symptoms were found in about two-thirds of patients with FD [17]. They showed higher levels of tension and neurotic traits than the general public [21, 22]. Some studies found that these traits were higher in patients with FD compared with duodenal ulcer patients [16, 19]. Depressive symptoms are also common, ranging from 13% to 41% of FD patients [16, 17, 23, 24]. FD can be comorbid with mental disorders such as anxiety and depressive disorders and personality traits. Therefore, a considerable number of patients with FD can be affected by such mental disorders [25].

Anxiety and depression may occur as secondary responses to chronic diseases such as FD and duodenal ulcer. However, patient with gall stone showed normal personality patterns [26]. Thus, organic diseases with pain do not necessarily cause anxiety or neurosis.

22.2.2.3 Stress

Major psychological factor associated with FD is life stress. Severe life stressors, especially the breaking up of a close relationship, precede the onset of functional abdominal pain significantly more often than the onset of organic abdominal illness [27]. Patients with FD were also found to experience more severe life stressors than healthy controls [28, 29]. Therefore, perceived major life stressors are likely to be more important than perceived minor life stressors in the pathogenesis of FD [30].

It was interesting to find that there were no significant differences between patients with gastritis and those with gastric cancer in the levels of perceived stress as measured by the Global Assessment of Recent Stress (GARS) scale and depression levels as assessed by the Beck Depression Inventory [31]. In addition, one study found that patients with chronic superficial gastritis had lower levels of perceived stress related to work/job and changes in relationship but had higher levels of perceived stress related to somatic symptoms, when compared with patients with gastric ulcer [32]. These results suggest that the levels of perceived stress in patients with gastric diseases may be associated with other factors than the severity of organic pathology. Moreover, there were other studies in which no significant differences were found in the frequency of life events between patients with FD and healthy controls [33, 34].

Case 1
A 60-year-old female patient visited the department of psychiatry, due to continued abdominal discomfort and pain, despite no abnormalities found on gastroendoscopic examination. Accompanied by her elder sister, she looked exhausted but denied any psychological stressor. Her symptoms were considerably improved after a 4-week-long administration of sertraline, an antidepressant, and ethyl loflazepate, an antianxiety agent. Thereafter, she began to complain of her symptoms again with a grimacing face. At that time, she expressed her conflict with her daughter-in-law, saying "She did not visit me during the period of Chuseok (Korean Thanksgiving Day). She also avoided seeing me even when she visited my neighbor. I do not know how to deal with this."

Case 2
A 50-year-old female patient was admitted to the department of internal medicine, due to abdominal pain, nausea, and vomiting, but laboratory findings showed no

abnormalities. She was thus referred and then transferred to the department of psychiatry. Her symptoms were exacerbated whenever she visited her sister-in-law and got back home. Later, she said, "she bought a lot of land with the money we had lent her, and later the price of the land jumped and she got rich. However, she did not thank me at all." She felt very disappointed at her sister-in-law's cold attitude.

As seen in these cases, patients with functional dyspepsia often show resistance to expressing their own conflicts or stressful situations at first. Over time, however, or by using a therapeutic technique such as cognitive behavioral therapy, their stressful situations can be elicited from them.

22.2.2.4 Personality

Dependent personality was reported to be more prominent in patients with FD compared with normal controls [21]. However, conflict associated with dependence was also a unique pattern of personality observed in patients with duodenal ulcer [35]. On the MMPI, patients with FD showed patterns of personality similar to patients with IBS or organic gastrointestinal diseases, whereas the dyspepsia patients showed higher levels of psychopathologies in a variety of subscales than normal controls [36].

22.2.2.5 Alexithymia

Patients with psychological factors affecting other medical condition (PFAOMC; previously called psychosomatic disorders) tend to show alexithymia, that is, difficulties in expressing their emotion verbally [37]. Alexithymia may overexcite the autonomic nervous system. Thus, alexithymia is considered an etiological factor of FD or duodenal ulcer [38]. However, patients with FD do not suppress their emotions consciously [39].

22.2.2.6 Somatothymia

Patients with FD tend to show somatothymia, that is, a tendency to communicate their psychological distresses in somatic symptoms. In particular, this tendency is prominent in patients with low levels of socioeconomic condition [40].

22.2.2.7 Poor Perception

Patients with FD are known to have poorer perception of their own psychological status, physical status, and medical treatment than patients with peptic ulcer or healthy controls [11, 41].

22.2.2.8 Anger

As seen in the above two cases, anger suppression seems to play a role in the pathogenesis of FD. However, no significant differences were found in anger suppression between patients with FD and those with duodenal ulcer [16]. It was also reported that high levels of emotional control were not characteristic of patients with FD [38].

22.2.2.9 Coping Strategies

Patients with FD are likely to use coping strategies which produce anxiety [15]. Examinations by a questionnaire revealed that patients with abdominal pain were closely associated with psychiatric symptoms and that patients with such association had weaker coping abilities than those with no such association [42].

Patients with FD perceive their stressors as more uncontrollable. Compared with patients with rheumatism or healthy controls, FD patients use more action-oriented coping styles but use distraction, acceptance, social support, and muscular relaxation less when handling stressful life events [15]. In a Korean study, patients with chronic superficial gastritis were found to use social support and avoidance-escape less than patients with gastric ulcer [32].

22.2.2.10 Lifestyle

There were differences in lifestyles between patients with FD and those with duodenal ulcer, although both of them have similar symptoms. That is, patients with FD smoke and drink alcohol less, eat more irregularly, and have higher frequency of dyspepsia symptoms than patients with duodenal ulcer [11].

22.2.2.11 Illness Behavior

Illness behavior refers to perceiving and evaluating symptoms and then behaving. It depends on individuals [43]. Patients with FD who sought consultation from general practitioners tended to perceive their symptoms more seriously than those who did not. However, there were no significant differences in the frequency of symptom complaints, the severity of symptoms, and the degree of other symptoms between the two [44].

22.2.2.12 Social Class

The prevalence of FD is not associated with social class. However, patients from lower social classes more frequently sought consultation from general practitioners than those from higher social classes [1].

22.2.2.13 Childhood Experiences

Childhood abdominal pain can persist into adulthood in some patients [45]. In one study, however, no significant differences were found in childhood happiness and parental separation between patients with FD and healthy controls [46].

22.2.2.14 Complex Factors

These days the causes of functional somatic symptoms are regarded as complex [47, 48]. For example, physical abnormalities such as esophageal spasm and gastroesophageal reflux can occur in patients with FD, but such abnormalities do not fully explain their symptoms. Individuals' belief in health, stressful life events, learned behavior during childhood, and personality traits can affect illness behavior as well as the severity and chronicity of symptoms. However, it is not clear to what extent physical and psychological factors are related to symptom formation. The theory on the interaction of multiple causal factors can benefit treatment rather than harm it, because patients may be sufficiently understood and effectively treated when multiple factors are considered [7].

On the other hand, organic diagnoses do not exclude the relevance of psychosocial factors. For example, 20% of patients with organic abdominal pain had psychiatric diagnoses [49], and negative life events were more associated with the onset of peptic ulcer than that of FD [28].

22.3 Diagnosis

FD is a clinical syndrome comprising chronic bothersome early satiety, postprandial fullness, epigastric pain, or burning [10]. FD can be subdivided into postprandial distress syndrome (comprising early satiety and/or postprandial fullness) and epigastric pain syndrome [50]. These two syndromes are increasingly accepted as valid clinical entities, based on new insights into the pathophysiology and the results of clinical trials. Diagnosis is based on the clinical history and exclusion of peptic ulcer and cancer by endoscopy. Evidence is accumulating that FD and gastroesophageal reflux disease are part of the same disease spectrum in a major subset [10].

22.4 Treatment

Symptoms of FD are nonspecific, and the pathophysiology is diverse, which explains in part why a universally effective treatment for FD remains elusive [51].

22.4.1 Psychotherapy

It is important for physicians to consider psychological factors whenever evaluating patients with FD [5, 52, 53]. In addition, a diagnosis of psychogenic abdominal pain should be made based on positive results from psychosocial evaluation rather than by simply excluding organic factors [4]. After psychosocial evaluation during an early period of treatment, primary physicians need to provide explanations for their patients' problems to the extent that they could understand the problems in order to prevent unnecessary physical examinations [7].

If physicians are certain that there are no organic diseases, they should avoid examinations and then explain why. Most patients may not require psychiatric treatment, even though they have prominent psychological factors. If the patients' symptoms are related to their belief in health, they can be usually controlled by simple explanation. One study found that the frequency of referral for consultation or of prescription of drugs for gastrointestinal problems was considerably decreased by simply notifying the patients that there are no abnormalities in their endoscopic findings [54]. Such reassurance ("You have no severe diseases at all") itself is not only therapeutically effective but also plays an important role in controlling repetitive medical examinations in patients with chronic symptoms [7]. However, such reassurance has limitations [55]. In addition to reassurance, changes in lifestyles such as avoiding drinking alcohol and coffee and reduction of body weight can be needed for treatment of FD [16]. If necessary, patients should be counseled about risk factors contributing to their symptoms [12].

Hypnosis and behavioral therapy can be considered therapeutic modalities in patients with chronic gastrointestinal symptoms without organic pathology. These methods were reported to be effective in patients with IBS [56, 57]. Cognitive behavioral therapy including cognitive therapy and muscular relaxation can work in patients with FD [58]. Therapists' explanation for symptoms may help patients recognize the situations eliciting pain as well as the outcome of pain. Whenever pain occurs, patients are encouraged to write a diary in which the pain-related place, person, antecedents (thoughts preceding pain), and activities are included. During therapy sessions, therapists help the patients analyze those situations based on the content in their diary and finally propose alternative behaviors. In addition, the patients are recommended to practice problem-solving approach, self-assertiveness, and cognitive restructuring. They are also taught to train muscular relaxation [12].

Assessment of pain is done by checking the frequency and intensity of pain on their self-assessment, total duration of pain for a period of 1 week, and pain index (calculated by the intensity and duration of pain) [12].

Brief counseling and supportive psychotherapy can be done for FD patients but is known to be more effective in patients with other gastrointestinal diseases. In particular, formal psychotherapy is recommended for patients with persistent symptoms [58].

Psychotherapy should be chosen based on individual patient levels. For anxiety disorders and depressive disorders, traditional psychotherapy can be effective. However, cognitive behavioral therapy can be tried in cases whose persistent symptoms are related to patients' abnormal belief in health or preoccupation with somatic symptoms. This kind of treatment can be applied to a variety of somatizers and patients with hypochondriasis [59, 60] as well as children with chronic abdominal pain [61]. In particular, symptoms of uncertain etiology can be more fit for cognitive behavioral therapy, because the self-assessment and behavioral components of the therapy may help find their causes and improve the symptoms [62].

22.4.2 Biological Treatment

In FD patients with mild symptoms, reassurance and lifestyle adjustments are often sufficient. For those with more severe or persistent symptoms, it is desirable to use proton pump inhibitors (PPIs), prokinetics, and psychotropic agents. In those with *Helicobacter pylori* infection, eradication is recommended. PPIs are the initial therapy of choice for epigastric pain syndrome, while prokinetics such as mosapride and acotiamide are preferred in postprandial distress syndrome [50].

22.4.2.1 Psychopharmacotherapy

It is necessary for physicians to consider using antianxiety agents or antidepressants when patients continue to show anxiety and depression despite explanation and reassurance [12]. Antianxiety agents such as lorazepam and diazepam are known to be more effective than placebo in patients with functional gastrointestinal disorders including FD [63]. However, about 60% of such patients respond to placebo [64]. Therefore, it is desirable to avoid the use of antianxiety agents in the patients unless their quality of life is lowered despite their continued symptoms [11]. In particular, these agents should be used for a short period of time if necessary [65].

About 38% of patients with gastritis are likely to have high levels of depression (scores of greater than 18 on the Beck Depression Inventory) [31]. Tricyclic antidepressants such as amitriptyline can be used for these patients because they do not seem to stimulate the gastrointestinal system. However, anticholinergic effects of these drugs can delay gastrointestinal motility. In such cases, it is desirable to gradually increase the dose of tricyclic antidepressants and assess their plasma levels. This may help prevent complications associated with doses [66]. In particular, the use of these antidepressants is considered for refractory symptoms of FD or epigastric pain syndrome [50]. Mirtazapine is recommended for FD patents with weight loss. However, selective serotonin reuptake inhibitors (SSRIs) are not preferred in these patients [10, 50].

22.4.2.2 Drug-Drug Interaction

Antacids and histamine (H_2) blockers can affect the absorption of tricyclic antidepressants because most of psychotropics are absorbed in the alkaline environment of the small intestine. However, it is not known yet whether the effects of diseases or drugs on changes of gastrointestinal acidity can affect the dose of tricyclic antidepressants [67].

Trazodone is more sedative and less stimulative of the gastrointestinal system than nefazodone. Nefazodone is associated with indigestion and abdominal pain, which occur in patients with the past history of peptic ulcer. In addition, this drug can cause side effects such as dry mouth, nausea, and constipation [66].

Cimetidine inhibits CyP450 isoenzyme in the liver and gastrointestinal tissues. This enzyme is related to the metabolism of nefazodone and tricyclic antidepressants. The combined use of cimetidine and nefazodone/tricyclic antidepressants is at risk for cumulative drug toxicity (e.g., gastrointestinal motility increased by nefazodone, decreased gastrointestinal motility related to anticholinergic effects of tricyclic antidepressants). Cimetidine also inhibits the metabolism of venlafaxine [66]. However, ranitidine does not affect the dynamics of tricyclic antidepressants.

22.5 Prognosis

Prognosis of patients with FD varies depending on the criteria of selection, duration of symptoms, and follow-up period. In general, the prognosis of FD in most patients is good. For example, a 6-year follow-up study found that 76% of 102 patients with FD did not show dyspepsia any longer and only 3% developed peptic ulcer [68]. However, the prevalence of peptic ulcer was found to be much higher in another follow-up study compared with the previous one [69].

FD tends to be chronic. In a follow-up study, among FD patients with negative X-ray findings for a period of 13 years, 34% showed poor prognosis [70]. In another 6-year follow-up study for patients with FD, there were no changes in symptoms [68]. In addition, patients with FD were reported to experience significant levels of physical symptoms and psychological distress after 1-year follow-up [7].

Predictive factors for chronicity of symptoms were known to be psychosocial factors and low pain tolerance [71]. These chronic patients often visit surgical clinics and hospitals and are likely to cause severe social impairment [7].

22.6 Conclusions

It is important for physicians to consider psychological factors whenever evaluating patients with functional dyspepsia (FD). Psychosocial factors associated with either the onset or aggravation of FD include negative emotion such as anxiety or depression, stress, personality, coping strategies, and lifestyles. Explanation for symptoms, reassurance, modification of lifestyles, consultation on risk factors, hypnosis, and cognitive behavioral therapy may help treat these patients. A combination of psychotherapy and muscular relaxation helps reduce the onset of pain and relieve symptoms. In FD patients with mild symptoms, reassurance and lifestyle adjustments are often sufficient. For those with more severe or persistent symptoms, it is desirable to use proton pump inhibitors (PPIs), prokinetics, and psychotropic agents. Tricyclic antidepressants can be used for refractory symptoms of FD, especially in epigastric pain syndrome. In addition, mirtazapine is recommended for FD patents with weight loss. Drug-drug interaction needs to be evaluated when considering the combined use of cimetidine and nefazodone/tricyclic antidepressants in FD patients, because of a risk for cumulative drug toxicity.

References

1. Jones RH, Lydeard SE, Hobbs FOR, Kenure JE, et al. Dyspepsia in England and Scotland. Gut. 1990;31:401–5.
2. Thompson WG, Heaton KW. Functional bowel disorders in apparently health people. Gastroenterology. 1980;79:283–8.
3. Camilleri M, Thompson DG, Malagelada JR. Functional dyspepsia. J Clin Gastroenterol. 1986;8:424–9.
4. Colgan S, Creed F, Klass H. Symptom complaints, psychiatric disorder and abnormal illness behaviour in patients with upper abdominal pain. Psychol Med. 1988;18:887–92.
5. Harvey RF, Shah SY, Read AE. Organic and functional disorders in 200 gastroenterology outpatients. Lancet. 1983;1:632–4.
6. Kane FJ Jr, Strohlein J, Harper RG. Nonulcer dyspepsia associated with psychiatric disorder. South Med J. 1993;86:641–6.
7. Morris C. Invited review: non-ulcer dyspepsia. J Psychosom Res. 1991;35:129–40.
8. Yamawaki H, Futagami S, Wakabayashi M, et al. Management of functional dyspepsia: state of the art and emerging therapies. Ther Adv Chronic Dis. 2018;9:23–32.
9. Thompson WG. Nonulcer dyspepsia. Can Med Assoc J. 1984;130:565–9.
10. Haug TT, Svebak S, Wilhelmsen I, et al. Psychological factors and somatic symptoms in functional dyspepsia: a comparison with duodenal ulcer and healthy controls. J Psychosom Res. 1994;38:281–91.
11. Kellner R. Psychosomatic syndromes and somatic symptoms. Washington, DC: Am Psychiatric Press; 1991. p. 97–110.
12. Piacentino D, Cantarini R, Alfonsi M, et al. Psychopathological features of irritable bowel syndrome patients with and without functional dyspepsia: a cross sectional study. BMC Gastroenterol. 2011;11:94.
13. Talley NJ. Functional dyspepsia: new insights into pathogenesis and therapy. Korean J Intern Med. 2016;31:444–56.
14. Colin-Jones DG. Management of dyspepsia: report of a working party. Lancet. 1988;1:576–9.
15. Cheng C, Hui W, Lam S. Coping style of individuals with functional dyspepsia. Psychosom Med. 1999;61:789–95.
16. Langeluddecke P, Goulston K, Tennant C. Psychological factors in dyspepsia of unknown cause: a comparison with peptic ulcer disease. J Psychosom Res. 1990;34:215–22.
17. Magni G, Di Mario F, Bernasconi G, et al. DSM-III diagnoses associated with dyspepsia of unknown cause. Am J Psychiatry. 1987;144:1222–3.
18. Magni G, Dimario F, Borgherini G. Personality and duodenal ulcer response to antisecretory treatment. Digestion. 1987;38:152–5.

19. Wilson KCM, Whiteoak R, Dewey M, et al. Aspects of personality of soldiers presenting to an endoscopy clinic. J Psychosom Res. 1989;33:85–91.
20. Roberts DM. The psychiatric basis of dyspepsia in the absence of organic disease. J R Army Med Corps. 1978;124:13–8.
21. Talley NJ, Fung LH, Gilligan IJ, et al. Association of anxiety, neuroticism and depression with dyspepsia of unknown cause. Gastroenterology. 1986;90:886–92.
22. Bennett E, Baeurepaire J, Langeluddecke P, et al. Life stress and non-ulcer dyspepsia: a case-control study. J Psychosom Res. 1991;35:579–90.
23. Hill O, Blendis L. Physical and psychological evaluation of non-organic abdominal pain. Gut. 1967;8:221–9.
24. Gomez J, Dally P. Psychologically mediated abdominal pain in surgical and medical outpatient clinics. Br Med J. 1977;1:1451–3.
25. Creed F, Guthrie E. Psychological factors in the irritable bowel syndrome. Gut. 1987;28:1307–18.
26. McIntosh JH, Nasiry RW, Frydmann M, et al. The personality pattern of patients with chronic peptic ulcer. Scand J Gastroenterol. 1983;18:945–50.
27. Creed F, Craig T, Farmer R. Functional abdominal pain, psychiatric illness, and life events. Gut. 1988;29:235–42.
28. Craig TKJ, Brown GW. Goal frustration and life events in the etiology of painful gastrointestinal disorder. J Psychom Res. 1984;28:411–21.
29. Jorgensen LS, Bonlokke L, Christensen NJ. Life strain, life events and autonomic response to a psychological stressor in patients with chronic upper abdominal pain. Scand J Gastroenterol. 1986;21:605–13.
30. Hui WM, Shiu LP, Lan SK. The perception of life events and daily stress in nonulcer dyspepsia. Am J Gastroenterol. 1991;86:292–6.
31. Koh KB, Lee SI, Lee JM. A comparison of stress perception and depression between gastric cancer and gastritis patients. Korean J Psychosom Med. 1994;2:88–97.
32. Oh S, Koh KB. The comparison of perceived stress and coping strategies in patients with gastric ulcer and those with chronic gastritis. Korean J Psychosom Med. 2000;8:11–9.
33. Jonsson BH, Theorell T, Gotthard R. Symptoms and personality in patients with chronic functional dyspepsia. J Psychosom Res. 1995;39:93–102.
34. Talley NJ, Piper DW. A prospective study of social factors and major life event stress in patients with dyspepsia of unknown cause. Scand J Gastroenterol. 1987;22:268–72.
35. Alexander F. Psychosomatic medicine: its principles and applications. New York: WW Norton; 1950.
36. Talley NJ, Phillips SF, Bruce B, et al. Relation among personality and symptoms in nonulcer dyspepsia and the irritable bowel syndrome. Gastroenterology. 1990;99:327–33.
37. Sifneos PE. The prevalence of alexithymic characteristics in psychosomatic patients. Psychother Psychosom. 1973;22:255–62.
38. Talley NJ, Ellard K, Jones M, et al. Suppression of emotions in essential dyspepsia and chronic ulcer: a case-control study. Scand J Gastroenterol. 1988;23:337–40.
39. Adami HO, Bergstrom R, Nyren O, et al. Is duodenal ulcer really a psychosomatic disease? Scand J Gastroenterol. 1987;22:889–96.
40. Yates WR. Gastrointestinal disorders. In: Sadock BJ, Sadock VA, editors. Comprehensive textbook of psychiatry. 7th ed. Philadelphia: Lippincott Williams & Wilkins; 2000.
41. Wilhelmsen I, Haug TT, Ursin H, et al. Discriminant analysis of factors distinguishing patients with functional dyspepsia from patients with duodenal ulcer: significance of somatization. Dig Dis Sci. 1995;40:1105–11.
42. Johnsen R, Jacobsen BK, Forde OH. Associations between symptoms of irritable colon and psychological and social conditions and lifestyle. Br Med J. 1986;292:1633–5.
43. Mechanic D. The concept of illness behaviour. J Chronic Dis. 1961;15:189–94.
44. Lydeard S, Jones R. Factors affecting the decision to consult with dyspepsia: comparison of consulters and nonconsulters. J R Coll Gen Pract. 1989;39:495–8.
45. Christensen MF, Mortensen O. Long-term prognosis in children with recurrent abdominal pain. Arch Dis Child. 1975;50:110–4.

46. Talley NJ, Jones M, Piper DW. Psychosocial and childhood factors in essential dyspepsia: a case-control study. Scand J Gastroenterol. 1988;23:341–6.
47. Barsky AJ, Klerman GL. Overviews: hypochondriasis, bodily complaints and somatic styles. Am J Psychiatry. 1983;140:273–83.
48. Kellner R. Hypochondriasis and somatization. JAMA. 1987;258:2718–22.
49. MacDonald AJ, Bouchier IAD. Non-organic gastrointestinal illness: a medical and psychiatric study. Br J Psychiatry. 1980;136:276–83.
50. Vanheel H, Tack J. Therapeutic options for functional dyspepsia. Dig Dis. 2014;32:230–4.
51. Lacy BE, Talley NJ, Locke GR 3rd, et al. Review article: current treatment options and management of functional dyspepsia. Aliment Pharmacol Ther. 2012;36:3–15.
52. Barbara L, Camilleri M, Corinaldes R, et al. Definition and investigation of dyspepsia. Dig Dis Sci. 1989;34:1272–6.
53. Lennard-Jones JE. Functional gastrointestinal disorders. N Engl J Med. 1983;308:431–5.
54. Jones R. What happens to patients with non-ulcer dyspepsia after endoscopy? Practitioner. 1988;232:75–8.
55. Warwick HMC, Salkovskis PM. Reassurance. Br Med J. 1985;290:1028.
56. Whorwell PJ, Prior A, Colgan SM. Hypnotherapy in severe irritable bowel syndrome: further experience. Gut. 1987;28:423–5.
57. Bennett P, Wilknson S. A comparison of psychological and medical treatment of the irritable bowel syndrome. Br J Clin Psychol. 1985;24:215–6.
58. Bates S, Sjoden PO, Nyren O. Behavioral treatment of non-ulcer dyspepsia. Scand J Behav Ther. 1988;17:155–65.
59. Klimes I, Mayou RA, Pearce MJ, et al. Psychological treatment for atypical noncardiac chest pain: a controlled evaluation. Psychol Med. 1990;20:605–11.
60. Salkovskis PM, Warwick HM. Morbid preoccupations, health anxiety and reassurance: a cognitive-behavioural approach to hypochondriasis. Behav Res Ther. 1986;24:597–602.
61. Sanders MR, Rebgetz M, Morrison M, et al. Cognitive-behavioral treatment of recurrent nonspecific abdominal pain in children. J Consult Clin Psychol. 1989;57:294–300.
62. Koh KB. Stress and psychosomatic symptoms. 2nd ed. Seoul: Ilchokak; 2011. p. 426–38.
63. Baume P, Tracey M, Dawson L. Efficacy of two minor tranquilizers in relieving symptoms of functional gastrointestinal distress. Aust NZ J Med. 1975;5:503–6.
64. Talley NJ, Phillips SF. Non-ulcer dyspepsia: potential causes and pathophysiology. Ann Intern Med. 1988;108:865–79.
65. Holtman G, Talley NJ. Functional dyspepsia: current treatment recommendations. Drugs. 1993;45:918–30.
66. Beliles K, Stoudemire A. Psychopharmacologic treatment of depression in the medically ill. Psychosomatics. 1998;39:S2–S19.
67. Beliles KE, Stoudemire A. Psychopharmacokinetics: clinical applications in medical illnesses. In: Stoudemire A, Fogel BS, editors. Medical psychiatric practice, vol. 3. Washington, DC: American Psychiatric Press, Inc; 1995. p. 1–77.
68. Gregory DW, Davies GT, Evans KT. Natural history of patients with X-ray- negative dyspepsia in general practice. Br Med J. 1972;4:519–20.
69. Spiro HM. Moynihan's disease? the diagnosis of duodenal ulcer. N Engl J Med. 1974;291:567–9.
70. Bonnevie O. Outcome of non-ulcer disease. Scand J Gastroenterol. 1982;17(Suppl 79):135–8.
71. Sloth H, Jorgensen LG. Predictors for the course of chronic non-organic upper abdominal pain. Scand J Gastroenterol. 1989;24:440–4.

Chapter 23
Approach to Irritable Bowel Syndrome

23.1 Introduction

Irritable bowel syndrome (IBS) is a chronic disorder characterized by abdominal pain or discomfort associated with disordered defecation in the absence of identifiable structural or biochemical abnormalities [1]. However, this concept is likely to be outdated. There is epidemiological evidence that, in a major subset of patients, gastrointestinal symptoms arise first and incident mood disorders occur only later. Additionally, possible mechanisms for gut-brain dysfunction have been identified, suggesting primary gut disturbances might be the underlying cause in a subgroup [2].

IBS is known to be second only to the common cold as a cause of absence from work [3]. The prevalence of IBS was 10–20% of the US adult population [4]. About 10% of the total patients visiting general practitioners had symptoms of IBS, whereas 40–50% of the patients visiting gastrointestinal specialists did [5]. The prevalence of this disorder was three times more common in women than in men [3].

IBS is a highly prevalent functional disorder that reduces patients' quality of life [6]. In particular, IBS patients with predominant diarrhea have lower quality of life than those with predominant constipation [1]. Psychological factors as well as the severity of physical symptoms (e.g., diarrhea, abdominal pain, and abdominal distension) are known to be associated with reduced health-related quality of life in patients with functional bowel disorders in primary care [7]. In addition, IBS imposes a significant economic burden on the health-care system, and despite the wide range of medications, to date no completely effective remedy is available [6].

The pathogenesis of IBS is complicated and multifactorial, and the treatment remains clinically challenging [8]. In addition, symptom-based categorization of patients, that is, grouping patients with this disorder into either diarrhea-predominant or constipation-predominant subtypes, promotes heterogeneity. Therefore, an approach based on the underlying pathophysiology is expected to help develop therapies that target causes and ultimately provide a cure for patients with IBS [2, 9].

This chapter reviews clinical features, etiology, treatment, and prognosis of IBS.

K. B. Koh, *Stress and Somatic Symptoms*,
https://doi.org/10.1007/978-3-030-02783-4_23

23.2 Clinical Features

Main symptoms of IBS include altered bowel habit (e.g., diarrhea, constipation, or both), abdominal pain, and abdominal bloating [10]. Symptoms that occur more often in IBS than in organic diseases are characterized by pain relieved by defecation, more frequent stools with pain onset, looser stools with pain onset, abdominal distension, mucus in stool, and feeling of incomplete evacuation after defecation [11]. In addition, there are various noncolonic gastrointestinal symptoms such as nausea, vomiting, dyspepsia, esophageal symptoms, and early satiety [12, 13]. Signs unrelated to the gastrointestinal system and indicative of stress, such as cool and clammy hands and flushing face and neck, are more common in IBS patients than in other patients [14].

About 50% of patients with IBS experience abdominal pain in various sites, but less than 10% complain of diarrhea without pain. Half of the patients also complain of pain in other areas (e.g., headache, backache, myalgia, heartburn, and pelvic pain) [3].

23.3 Etiology

Biological and psychological factors are currently believed to influence the pathogenesis of IBS [15–17]. The onset of the syndrome is likely to be associated with an interaction of biological, psychological, and social factors [3]. To date, the etiological factors of IBS can be subdivided as follows.

23.3.1 Biological Factors

Biological factors known to play an important role in the development of IBS include alteration in gut microbiome, gut motility (e.g., hyperactivity of the large bowel), visceral sensation (e.g., visceral hypersensitivity), intestinal permeability, gut immune function, and brain-gut interactions [15–21]. Other mechanisms that play a role in diarrhea-predominant IBS include altered bile salt metabolism, abnormalities in the serotonin metabolism, and genetic factors [9].

Neural regulation seems to be associated with responses of the large bowel to pain. It was hypothesized that IBS patients have more neural pathways from the intestine to the brain than those from the brain to the intestine. To test this hypothesis clinically, the method of distending many balloons at various sites was used. Pain threshold measured by distending the large bowel in patients with IBS was found to be lower than in healthy individuals. Therefore, these IBS patients are likely to be hypersensitive to pain stimulation and to frequently complain of headache, backache, and menstrual pain [3]. In another study, however, tolerance to pain induced by electrocutaneous stimulation in IBS patients was higher than in healthy subjects [22].

23.3.2 *Psychosocial Factors*

The importance of psychosocial factors and the central nervous system in the pathophysiology of IBS is gradually being recognized. The explanations for these are various, ranging from factors aggravating primary physiological disturbance to psychological factors influencing impairment of normal physiology of the gastrointestinal system [3]. Colonic motility was decreased in patients with a sense of helplessness and self-defeat, whereas the motility was increased in patients with hostility and defensiveness [23].

23.3.2.1 Stressors

More than half of patients with IBS were reported to experience gastrointestinal symptoms caused by environmental stressors. Stressful events were also more common in IBS patients than in other patients [14]. Typically their stressors were associated with work and housework [3]. Most of them experienced uncontrollable marital disharmony and loss such as serious illnesses or death of their relatives [24]. IBS patients may also have a family history of death of parents before the age of 15 and a history of traumatic life events such as sexual and physical abuse [25].

Exposure to stressors results in alterations of the brain-gut interactions ("brain-gut axis") ultimately leading to the development of a broad array of gastrointestinal disorders including IBS and gastroesophageal reflux disease. The major effects of stress on gut physiology include (1) alterations in gastrointestinal motility, (2) increase in visceral perception, (3) changes in gastrointestinal secretion, (4) increase in intestinal permeability, (5) negative effects on regenerative capacity of gastrointestinal mucosa and mucosal blood flow, and (6) negative effects on intestinal microbiota. Mast cells are important effectors of brain-gut axis that translate the stress signals into the release of a wide range of neurotransmitters and proinflammatory cytokines, which may profoundly affect the gastrointestinal physiology [26]. The underlying mechanism of IBS has a close correlation with mucosal immune activation, alterations in the central nervous system, peripheral neurons, and gastrointestinal microbiota. Stress-induced alterations in neuro-endocrine-immune pathways act on the gut-brain axis and microbiota-gut-brain axis and cause symptom flare-ups or exaggeration in IBS [27].

Anger-provoking stimulation increases colonic motility when compared to non-anger-provoking situation [25]. In addition, the levels of epinephrine in urine under stressful conditions are higher in patients with IBS with predominant diarrhea than in other medical patients [28].

Case

A 50-year-old woman continuously suffered from lower abdominal pain and diarrhea. She therefore visited the department of internal medicine of a university hospital, where no laboratory abnormalities were found. She was referred to the department of psychiatry for consultation. Thereafter, she was several times admitted to psychiatry via the emergency room due to repetitive abdominal pain and diarrhea. According to her family, her husband had an extramarital affair with another woman who gave birth to a son. Then the patient took care of the son for a period of 20 years while her husband was living with the woman. Recently her husband got back home. At that time, she began to develop her symptoms. This suggests that her large bowel symptoms are likely to be associated with her suppressed hostility toward her husband.

23.3.2.2 Illness Behavior

Most of patients with IBS do not seek medical help. Patients with IBS who visited hospitals showed more psychopathologies such as hypochondriasis, depression, and hysteria on the MMPI, when compared with those with IBS not seeking medical help and healthy controls [29]. Other studies also found that psychopathologies were more predominant in patients with IBS seeking medical help compared with those not seeking medical help [30, 31]. These results suggest that IBS patients not seeking medical help cope better with life events and somatic symptoms than those seeking medical help.

In addition, IBS patients seeking medical help were poorer in their general health status, suffered from headache more frequently, had parents with more concern about illnesses, and were more absent from school than those not seeking medical help [32]. Patients with IBS complain of symptoms unrelated to gastrointestinal symptoms three times more frequently than controls without dysfunction of the large bowel [3]. Therefore, patients with IBS are likely to seek medical help due to their abnormal illness behavior rather than their symptoms.

23.3.2.3 Social Learning

Mothers who spend most time with their children are known to have experienced more chronic abdominal pain than fathers. In addition, patients with IBS have many siblings [33, 34]. From parents or significant others with IBS, children may learn misconceptions about normal bowel habits. They may also learn that symptoms of IBS are a socially acceptable sign of distress, a way to avoid unpleasant responsibility, and a way to elicit concern and affection from family, friends, and health-care providers. Many of these persons recognize that they have a psychological problem but find it more socially acceptable to be identified as having a medical problem. Therefore, they present themselves to the primary physician as if they do not recognize the psychological problem [35, 36].

23.3.2.4 Psychopathology

A number of studies found that psychopathologies, such as anxiety and depression, were more frequently observed in patients with IBS compared with healthy controls [5, 37]. High levels of hostility were also found in patients with IBS. However, these psychopathologies did not correlate with changes in motility of the large bowel and the severity of symptoms [38]. IBS patients had more psychological problems than those with other diseases [28, 39, 40]. For example, anxiety was more predominant in patients with IBS compared with those with other diseases [38]. IBS patients have a tendency for catastrophizing, and pain catastrophizing is regarded as a significant predictor of gastrointestinal symptoms related to pain. In addition to lower pain thresholds, altered pain perception in IBS may be attributable to affective disturbances, negative emotions in anticipation of or during visceral stimulation, altered pain-related expectations, and learning processes [20]. Somatization is known to be an independent risk factor for IBS. Somatization more than the severity of IBS influences the way the patients perceive their illness, the outcome, and the efficacy of treatment [41].

Patients with IBS were reported to have more mental disorders than patients with other diseases [42, 43]. Forty-three percent of patients with IBS were known to correspond to major depressive disorder [44], but it was noteworthy that patients with IBS who showed depression did not report depression unlike patients with depression visiting the outpatient clinic.

The psychological problems of IBS patients were found to be greater than those found in persons with much more severe and disabling gastrointestinal diseases [28, 39, 40]. This result suggests that their psychological problems are unlikely to be solely a reaction to the gastrointestinal symptoms [28, 45]. Four conclusions based on structured psychiatric interviews are as follows: (1) more than 70% of IBS patients have a psychiatric disorder; (2) a large proportion of these disorders go unrecognized by the attending physicians; (3) from the psychiatric perspective, the patients form a heterogeneous group; (4) psychiatric disorders are more common among IBS patients encountered at teaching hospitals than in private practice [40].

23.3.2.5 Family History

About 32% of patients with IBS and about 2% of controls were reported to have a family history of IBS. However, there were no twin studies that examined the genetic influences in IBS [14]. Loss and separation during childhood was found to be major psychodynamic issues of patients with IBS [46]. In comparison with control patients, married patients with IBS had more conflicts and dependent relationships with their mothers [32].

23.4 Diagnosis

The diagnosis of IBS relies on the identification of characteristic symptoms and the exclusion of other organic diseases. Determining the predominant symptom (IBS with diarrhea, IBS with constipation, or mixed IBS) plays an important role in selection of diagnostic tests [21].

23.5 Differential Diagnosis

Laxatives, β-adrenergic blocker, and abuse of drugs (e.g., tricyclic antidepressants) can cause IBS-like gastrointestinal symptoms [3]. Lactose intolerance characterized by lactase deficiency should be differentiated from IBS. In addition, food allergy needs to be differentiated. IBS patients have higher levels of anxiety and report more severe abdominal pain than patients with inflammatory bowel disease, such as ulcerative colitis, whereas patients with inflammatory bowel disease report more episodes of diarrhea, but they do not rate them as significantly more severe than do the IBS patients [46].

23.6 Treatment

Choosing therapeutic methods depends on the nature and severity of IBS, patients' personality, psychopathology, duration of illness, physicians' expertise, and technique [14]. If main symptoms of IBS are constipation, high-fiber diet or bulking agent can be helpful, whereas anticholinergic agents are effective for diarrhea [3].

23.6.1 Psychopharmacotherapy

Tricyclic antidepressants are effective for IBS patients comorbid with depressive disorders [14]. Anticholinergic effects of tricyclic antidepressants may help improve functional gastrointestinal disorders including IBS, but one study found that there was no significant association between the two [47, 48]. A small amount of tricyclic antidepressants may be effective in patients with generalized anxiety disorder accompanied by gastrointestinal symptoms. However, antianxiety agents and antipsychotics should be avoided because the former may lead to drug dependence and the latter may develop tardive dyskinesia. Antianxiety agents can be cautiously used in patients with anxiety uncontrolled by other methods [14].

23.6.2 *Psychosocial Treatment*

Various dietary, lifestyle, medical, and behavioral interventions have proven effective in randomized clinical trials [21]. When diet and pharmacotherapy do not work, behavioral and psychological treatment such as hypnotherapy and cognitive behavioral therapy (CBT) should be considered. In mild cases, only explanation about the nature of IBS and reassurance may improve symptoms [14]. Sometimes group therapy is helpful for these patients [49].

23.6.2.1 Hypnotherapy

Gut-directed hypnotherapy has beneficial short-term effects in improving gastrointestinal symptoms of patients with IBS [41]. Hypnotherapy may affect IBS partly through changes in colorectal sensitivity and improvement in psychological factors [50]. In particular, hypnotherapy relaxing smooth muscle can be tried when psychotherapy does not work [14]. Hypnotherapy was reported to be more effective than psychotherapy, although both were effective for these IBS patients [51].

23.6.2.2 Behavioral Therapy

A combination of autogenic training and group therapy can be considered in IBS patients, but this treatment takes more time than other forms of treatment. Otherwise, desensitization technique can be tried for patients with IBS whose stressors precede large bowel symptoms [14]. Such behavioral therapy may be appropriate when symptoms are considered resulting from excessive autonomic reaction to certain stimuli. For example, self-assertiveness training, marital therapy, or systematic desensitization technique can be chosen as a treatment modality after situations eliciting symptoms are explored. These stress management methods are aimed at helping the patient either resolve stressful problems or alter their emotional reaction to stressful circumstances that cannot be changed [52]. If anxiety seems to induce IBS symptoms, muscle relaxation can be tried [14].

23.6.2.3 Cognitive Behavioral Therapy (CBT)

CBT focuses on replacing maladaptive coping strategies with more positive cognitions and behaviors. Several studies have shown that CBT is effective in reducing bowel symptoms as well as psychological symptoms in patients with IBS [41, 53]. One study found that CBT had a direct effect on global IBS symptom improvement independently of its effects on psychological distress [54]. It is desirable that gastroenterologists teach these patients about a number of factors such as drugs, diet, and environmental factors. They also should explain the relationship between stressors and large bowel symptoms and focus treatment on symptoms rather than causes. In addition, they can help the patients cope with stressful situations effectively [3]. However, one meta-analysis revealed that for IBS patients, CBT was superior to waiting list, basic support, or medical treatment at the end of treatment but not superior to other psychological treatments [55].

Emotional symptoms often accompany gastrointestinal symptoms. To clarify this, self-reported diary is recommended [56]. This diary includes the severity of specific somatic symptoms (e.g., diarrhea, abdominal pain, and abdominal bloating) and of mood (e.g., anxiety, depression, and anger), precedent factors of somatic symptoms and of mood, thoughts, and behavioral consequences. Through this diary, necessary information can be elicited, and the relevance of psychological phenomenon and physiological information can be clarified. Therapists need to know the physiology of the disease, consider patients' personal characteristics, and be flexible in order to treat them effectively [49].

Overall, the management of IBS should be a multifactorial approach, including pharmacotherapy targeted against the predominant symptom, behavioral and psychological treatment, dietary alterations, education, reassurance, and effective patient-physician relationship [26].

23.7 Prognosis

A large proportion of patients with IBS can improve with placebo alone, but they have a tendency for recurrence [57]. The therapeutic response *to high fiber diets, bulking agents, and explanation* was better in men than in women and in patients with constipation than in those with diarrhea [14]. One study found an association between psychiatric ill health and poor prognosis [58]. Similarly, in another study, prognosis was poorer in IBS patients with psychosocial stressors or emotional disorders compared with those without them [59].

23.8 Conclusions

Irritable bowel syndrome (IBS) is characterized by diarrhea or constipation, abdominal pain, and abdominal bloating. Biological and psychological factors are currently believed to influence the pathogenesis of IBS. Biological factors include alteration in gut microbiome, gut motility, visceral sensation, intestinal permeability, gut immune function, and brain-gut interactions. Some IBS patients are difficult to cope with abdominal symptoms due to their emotional distress. For constipation, high fiber diet or bulking agents can be helpful, whereas for diarrhea, anticholinergic agents are effective. In IBS cases comorbid with anxiety or depressive disorders, tricyclic antidepressants are recommended. However, antianxiety agents and antipsychotics should be avoided because the former may lead to drug dependence and the latter may develop tardive dyskinesia. Explanation, reassurance and supportive psychotherapy can also be helpful for some IBS patients. In addition, hypnosis and cognitive behavioral therapy (CBT) have beneficial effects in improving gastrointestinal symptoms of patients with IBS.

References

1. Singh P, Staller K, Barshop K, et al. Patients with irritable bowel syndrome-diarrhea have lower disease-specific quality of life than irritable bowel syndrome-constipation. World J Gastroenterol. 2015;21:8103–9.
2. Holtmann GJ, Ford AC, Talley NJ. Pathophysiology of irritable bowel syndrome. Lancet Gastroenterol Hepatol. 2016;1:133–46.
3. Garrick TR. Gastrointestinal disorders. In: Kaplan HI, Sadock BJ, editors. Comprehensive textbook of psychiatry, vol. 2. 6th ed. Baltimore: Williams & Wilkins; 1995.
4. Longstreth GF, Wilson A, Knight K, et al. Irritable bowel syndrome, health care use, and costs: a U.S. managed care perspective. Am J Gastroenterol. 2003;98:600–7.
5. Sammons MT, Karoly P. Psychosocial variables in irritable bowel syndrome: a review and proposal. Clin Psychol Rev. 1987;7:187–204.
6. Lazaraki G, Chatzimavroudis G, Katsinelos P. Recent advances in pharmacological treatment of irritable bowel syndrome. World J Gastroenterol. 2014;20:8867–85.
7. Lee V, Guthrie E, Robinson A, et al. Functional bowel disorders in primary care: factors associated with health-related quality of life and doctor consultation. J Psychosom Res. 2008;64:129–38.
8. Deiteren A, de Wit A, van der Linden L, et al. Irritable bowel syndrome and visceral hypersensitivity: risk factors and pathophysiological mechanisms. Acta Gastroenterol Belg. 2016;79:29–38.
9. Holtmann G, Shah A, Morrison M. Pathophysiology of functional gastrointestinal disorders: a holistic overview. Dig Dis. 2017;35(Suppl 1):5–13.
10. Thompson WG. The irritable bowel: one disease, or several, or none? In: Read NW, editor. Irritable bowel syndrome. New York: Grune & Stratton; 1985.
11. Manning AP, Thompson WG, Heaton KW. Towards positive diagnosis of the irritable bowel. Br Med J. 1978;2:653–4.
12. Thompson DG, Laidlow JM, Wingate DL. Abnormal small-bowel motility demonstrated by radiotelemetry in a patient with irritable colon. Lancet. 1979;2:1321–3.
13. Waston WC, Sullivan SN, Corke M. Globus and headache: common symptoms of the irritable bowel syndrome. Can Med Assoc J. 1978;118:387–8.
14. Kellner R. Psychosomatic syndromes and somatic symptoms. Washington, DC: Am Psychiatric Press; 1991. p. 111–44.
15. Crowell MD, Harris L, Jones MP, et al. New insights into the pathophysiology of irritable bowel syndrome: implications for future treatments. Curr Gastroenterol Rep. 2005;7:272–9.
16. Hasler WL. Traditional thoughts on the pathophysiology of irritable bowel syndrome. Gastroenterol Clin N Am. 2011;40:21–43.
17. Pimentel M, Chang C. Inflammation and microflora. Gastroenterol Clin N Am. 2011;40:69–85.
18. Chaudhary NA, Truelove SC. Human colonic motility: a comparative study of normal subjects, patients with ulcerative colitis and patients with irritable colon syndrome. Gastroenterology. 1961;40:1–36.
19. Ritchie J. Pain from distension of the pelvic colon by inflating a balloon in the irritable colon syndrome. Gut. 1973;14:125–32.

20. Elsenbruch S. Abdominal pain in irritable bowel syndrome: a review of putative psychological, neural and neuro-immune mechanisms. Brain Behav Immun. 2011;25:386–94.
21. Chey WD, Kurlander J, Eswaran S. Irritable bowel syndrome: a clinical review. JAMA. 2015;313:949–58.
22. Cook IJ, van Eeden A, Collins SM. Patients with irritable bowel syndrome have greater pain tolerance than normal subjects. Gastroenterology. 1987;93:727–33.
23. Almy TP. Experimental studies on the irritable colon. Am J Med. 1951;10:60–7.
24. Hislop IG. Psychological significance of the irritable colon syndrome. Gut. 1971;12:452–7.
25. Welgan P, Meshkinpour H, Beeler M. Effect of anger on colon motor and myoelectric activity in irritable bowel syndrome. Gastroenterology. 1988;94:1150–6.
26. Konturek PC, Brzozowski T, Konturek SJ. Stress and the gut: pathophysiology, clinical consequences, diagnostic approach and treatment options. J Physiol Pharmacol. 2011;62:591–9.
27. Qin HY, Cheng CW, Tang XD, et al. Impact of psychological stress on irritable bowel syndrome. World J Gastroenterol. 2014;20:14126–31.
28. Esler MD, Goulston KJ. Levels of anxiety in colonic disorders. N Engl J Med. 1973;288:16–20.
29. Drossman DA, McKee DC, Sandler RS. Psychosocial factors in the irritable bowel syndrome: a multivariate study of patients and non-patients with irritable bowel syndrome. Gastroenterology. 1988;95:701–8.
30. Smith RC, Greenbaum DS, Vancouver JB. Psychosocial factors are associated with health care seeking rather than diagnosis in irritable bowel syndrome. Gastroenterology. 1990;98:293–301.
31. Whitehead WE, Bosmajian L, Zonderman AB. Symptoms of psychologic distress associated with irritable bowel syndrome. Gastroenterology. 1988;95:709–14.
32. Lowman BC, Drossman DA, Cramer EM. Recollection of childhood events in adults with irritable bowel syndrome. J Clin Gastroenterol. 1987;9:324–30.
33. Hill OW, Blendis L. Physical and psychological evaluation of non-organic abdominal pain. Gut. 1967;8:221–9.
34. Whitehead WE, Schuster MM. Gastrointestinal disorders: behavioral and physiological basis for treatment. New York: Academic; 1985.
35. Latimer PR. Irritable bowel syndrome: a behavioral model. Behav Res Ther. 1981;19:475–83.
36. Latimer PR, Campbell D. Behavioral medicine and the functional bowel disorders. Int J Ment Health. 1980;9:111–28.
37. Walker EA, Roy-Byrne PP, Katon WJ. Irritable bowel syndrome and psychiatric illness. Am J Psychiatry. 1990;147:365–72.
38. Whitehead WE, Engel BT, Schuster MM. Irritable bowel syndrome: physiological and psychological differences between diarrhea-predominant and constipation-predominant patients. Dig Dis Sci. 1980;25:404–13.
39. Liss JL, Alpers D, Woodruff RA. The irritable colon syndrome and psychiatric illness. Dis Nerv Syst. 1973;34:151–7.
40. Young SJ, Alpers DH, Norland CC, Woodruff RA. Psychiatric illness and the irritable bowel syndrome. Gastroenterology. 1976;70:162–6.
41. Surdea-Blaga T, Baban A, Nedelcu L, et al. Psychological interventions for irritable bowel syndrome. J Gastrointestin Liver Dis. 2016;25:359–66.
42. Fava GA, Pavan L. Large bowel disorders: illness configuration and life events. Psychother Psychosom. 1976/1977;27:93–99.
43. Ford MJ, Miller PM, Eastwood J. Life events, psychiatric illness, and the irritable bowel syndrome. Gut. 1987;28:160–5.
44. Toner BB, Garfinkel PE, Jeejeebhoy KN. Self-schema in irritable bowel syndrome and depression. Psychosom Med. 1990;52:149–55.
45. West KL. MMPI correlates of ulcerative colitis. J Clin Psychol. 1970;26:214–9.
46. Schwarz SP, Blanchard EB, Berreman CF, et al. Psychological aspects of irritable bowel syndrome: comparisons with inflammatory bowel disease and nonpatient controls. Behav Res Ther. 1993;31:297–304.
47. Greenbaum DS, Mayle JE, Vanegeren LE. Effects of desipramine on irritable bowel syndrome compared with atropine and placebo. Dig Dis Sci. 1987;32:257–66.

48. Clouse RE. Antidepressants for functional gastrointestinal syndromes. Dig Dis Sci. 1994;39:2352–63.
49. Wise TN. Gastroenterology. In: Stoudemire A, Fogel BS, editors. Principles of medical psychiatry. New York: Grune & Stratton; 1987.
50. Simrén M. Hypnosis for irritable bowel syndrome: the quest for the mechanism of action. Int J Clin Exp Hypn. 2006;54:65–84.
51. Whorwell PJ, Prior A, Colgan SM. Hypnotherapy in severe irritable bowel syndrome: further experience. Gut. 1987;28:423–5.
52. Latimer PR. Irritable bowel syndromes. In: Dorfman W, Cristofar L, editors. Psychosomatic illness review. New York: Macmillan Publishing Co; 1985.
53. Tang QL, Lin GY, Zhang MQ. Cognitive-behavioral therapy for the management of irritable bowel syndrome. World J Gastroenterol. 2013;19:8605–10.
54. Lackner JM1, Jaccard J, Krasner SS, et al. How does cognitive behavior therapy for irritable bowel syndrome work? A mediational analysis of a randomized clinical trial. Gastroenterology. 2007;133:433–44.
55. Li L, Xiong L, Zhang S, et al. Cognitive-behavioral therapy for irritable bowel syndrome: a meta-analysis. J Psychosom Res. 2014;77:1–12.
56. Kanfer FH, Saslow G. Behavioral analysis. Arch Gen Psychiatry. 1965;12:529–38.
57. Waller SL, Misiewicz JJ. Prognosis in the irritable-bowel syndrome. Lancet. 1969;1:753–6.
58. Lancaster-Smith MJ, Prout BJ, Pinto T, et al. Influence of drug treatment on the irritable bowel syndrome and its interaction with psychoneurotic morbidity. Acta Psychiatr Scand. 1982;66:33–41.
59. Chaudhary NA, Truelove SC. The irritable colon syndrome. Q J Med. 1962;31:307–22.

Chapter 24
Therapeutic Approaches for Cancer Patients

24.1 Introduction

Psychological distress can influence tumor progression via many different pathways (e.g., genetic changes, immune surveillance, and pro-angiogenic processes) [1]. Although some cancers that had a very poor prognosis several decades ago are being cured today, cancer has remained a disease equated with hopelessness, pain, fear, and death. Diagnosis and treatment of cancer often produce severe psychological stress due to the actual symptoms of the disease, as well as to the patient's and family's perceptions of the disease [2]. The universal fears of cancer patients have been termed the six Ds: death, dependence, disfigurement, disability, disruption of interpersonal relationships, and discomfort [3].

The patient's ability to manage these stressors depends on medical, psychological, and social issues. These include the disease itself (i.e., site, symptoms, clinical course, type of treatment), previous level of adjustment to medical illness, and the threat that cancer poses in attaining age-appropriate developmental tasks and goals. In addition, there are issues related to cultural and religious attitudes, the presence or absence of emotionally supportive persons, the patient's potential for physical and psychologic rehabilitation, and the patient's own personality and coping style [4].

Medical development in the diagnosis and treatment of cancer has dramatically improved survival rate. As a result, professional attention has turned from death and dying issues to the physical, psychological, and behavioral consequences of rigorous treatment regimens [2, 5].

To live with cancer is much more than adapting to the treatments and their various side effects. There is a host of psychosocial issues with which to cope other than the threat to mortality. To understand cancer as merely a biologic event is to overlook the innumerable biopsychosocial factors that demand strategic coping from the patient and his family [6]. Therefore, quality of life and delayed treatment effects have become important issues [2].

K. B. Koh, *Stress and Somatic Symptoms*,
https://doi.org/10.1007/978-3-030-02783-4_24

In this chapter are reviewed the most frequently encountered psychosocial issues, psychotherapeutic, pharmacological, and behavioral management of patients with cancer.

24.2 Patients' Reactions to Cancer

Anxiety, depression, anger, and guilt are the most frequent responses to cancer [7, 8]. In general, cancer patients are more anxious and depressed than patients with any other physical diseases. At this time, anger is more associated with anxiety and is usually expressed toward physicians, hospital staff, and family members [7]. Cancer may often be associated not only with guilt occurring when regarded as punishment for being bad (e.g., other people's death and unhappiness, sexual behavior) but also with anger, depression, and overstress. The sense of loss or being rejected constitutes a large part of stress related to having a cancer. Such a sense of loss may be due to the loss of identity, job, role, independence, and a sense of self and changes in body image. Hopelessness and helplessness are also frequent responses to cancer [9].

Denial is the most frequent defense mechanism observed in cancer patients [10, 11]. In one study, about a third of cancer patients receiving radiotherapy denied the diagnosis of cancer, whose psychopathology such as hostility was predominant [12]. Other studies also found that denial was not infrequent in cancer patients and their family members [5, 13–16]. Some view denial as negative, but others view it as positive in terms of maintaining hope [17–19], reducing stress levels related to illness [8], and enhancing autoimmune response [9].

The psychological response stages of denial, depression, anger, bargaining, acceptance, and resolution, as defined by Kubler-Ross [20], do not occur in any patterned progression in cancer patients. Patients rather show daily changes in mood such as optimism and pessimism, related to the medical illness. Intellectual problem-solving and information gathering can provide control over unknown prognosis, side effects of drugs, and feelings of hopelessness. Patients who cope well during terminal illnesses have the ability to blend problem-solving methods with some denial and hope [2].

24.3 Factors Influencing Responses to Cancer

Patients' responses to cancer are influenced by medical, psychological, and interpersonal factors. Medical factors are related to the site of cancer, symptoms, and prognosis [21]. Psychological factors include patients' premorbid personality, previous personal experiences of cancer, life stress, coping ability, strength of ego, process of personality development, past history of psychiatric disorders, and meaning of cancer. Interpersonal factor relates to social support of their family and treatment team. In addition, patients' age may influence their responses to cancer [10, 22]. Therefore, general process of psychological development should be reviewed whenever a diagnosis of cancer is made [22].

24.4 Psychopathology and Psychiatric Disorders in Cancer Patients

Cancer patients often show a sense of hopelessness, helplessness, and disappointment prior to the onset of cancer, which are called preneoplastic feeling [23]. The most frequent symptoms in cancer patients are anxiety, depression, delirium, nausea and vomiting, anorexia, and pain [2]. Breast and pulmonary cancer patients tend to suppress anger [24, 25], whereas pancreatic cancer patients have relatively higher incidence of depression [26]. Cancer patients also tend to suppress emotion than noncancer patients [27], which is known to be a characteristic of cancer patients [15, 28] and to be associated with development and poor prognosis of cancer [29].

Main issues in cancer patients who are supposed to be hospitalized and undergo operation include risks and sequelae of surgery, prognosis, fear of a painful death, and anger. During this period, psychiatric treatment is strongly required because psychological problems often tend to occur [30]. In addition, cancer patients receiving radiotherapy face dual stress; radiotherapy itself can be stressful, and their reaffirmation of cancer can add to emotional distress [12].

Among cancer patients, the spectrum of depressive disorders, encompassing adjustment disorder with depressed mood and major depressive disorder, accounted for the majority of diagnoses, followed by organic mental disorder, personality disorder, and anxiety disorder. In particular, most of these disorders are known to be associated with either reactions to or manifestations of the disease or treatment [31]. The factor most significantly related to severe depression was physical function [32]. Although few cancer patients commit suicide, they may be at a somewhat greater risk for suicide than the general population [33, 34].

24.5 Poor Copers Versus Good Copers in Cancer Patients

Poorly coping patients basically have two main deficits in their coping repertoire. First, they tend to overuse coping strategies that have been less effective in resolving problems (e.g., getting drunk). Second, a hallmark of poorly coping patients is that they are unable to generate a number of alternative coping strategies. In contrast, good copers are able to try a number of problem-solving approaches and to persevere until something effective is found and some degree of resolution is achieved. Also, these patients are able to evaluate and to rank-order their approaches to problem-solving rather than giving each strategy an equal weighting [6].

Active confrontation with a fighting spirit may help patients with breast cancer live longer than surrendering to helplessness and hopelessness [35]. Also, patients who actively confront their illness and the uncertainty that surrounds it have been shown to have better psychological health [36]. Among coping strategies of patients with cancers in general, confrontation was found to have a positive effect and externalization to have a negative effect on the resolution of patients' pending problems [13]. Denial may distort reality but can work as an adaptive means for cancer patients [37]. Cancer patients with the most favorable prognoses were known to express their emotion such as hostilities openly and directly [38].

In one study, the use of active, problem-focused therapy and minimal use of avoidance were associated with fewer physical and psychological symptoms, and patients who coped via problem-solving and emotional regulation had less severe dysfunction [39]. Consistent with this, another study [40] found that avoidance contributed significantly to psychological disturbance following stressful life events in elderly adults. Therefore, counseling and support aimed at promoting engagement, such as actively seeking information about the situation and talking to someone about one's feelings, may reduce anxiety and depression in patients with a potentially life-threatening illness such as breast cancer [36].

24.6 Effective Communication with Cancer Patients

The ability to listen is emphasized over the ability to say something. Therefore, the real question to ask is not "what do you tell your patients?" but rather "what do you let your patients tell you?" However, communication is more than listening. Getting to know the patient as a person is essential. Learning about significant areas of the patient's life such as family, work, or school and chatting about common interests are the most natural. Like anybody else these individuals get self-respect from a sense that others value them for what they have done and for their personal qualities. Allowing dying persons to tell their own stories helps build a balanced relationship. Patients want to be dealt with as a real person, not as a dying patient. It is important to take conversational cues from the patient whenever possible. Communication is more than verbal. For example, a pat on the arms, a wave, or a wink communicates reassurances [41].

Physicians can communicate their pledge to provide continued care for dying patients by discussing with patients and families the availability of supportive measures such as pain control and nutrition. They should also have an understanding of the patients' perceptions of their stages of illness and be flexible in providing care outside the hospital [2].

When the diagnosis is made and the patient should be informed of it, it is best to begin by sitting down with the patient in a private place. Spouses and other family members can be included in the discussion of the diagnosis and treatment. An opening statement should include delivering them calmly and briefly, encouraging further dialogue and reassuring continued attention and care [41].

24.7 Countertransference

Countertransference reactions can occur at any time during physicians' treatment of cancer patients. For example, physicians may have fantasy for cancer treatment and omnipotent feeling for caring for patients coping with impending death. However, physicians may have guilt and depression over providing no more help to the patient, especially over not preventing recurrence of cancer [42]. At this time, the physician's depression as a reaction to disappointment may be a factor that alienates patients. In particular, therapists with fear of death may try to avoid cancer patients facing impending death. Such distancing therapist may not only have pessimistic communication but also reinforce his/her sense of isolation and disappointment [9]. Sometimes patients may identify with their therapists or react negatively to them [43].

In addition, it should be cautioned that therapists may have overconcern about patients' medical issues, visit patients more often, spend more time on talking with them, provide overinterpretation, try to give them so much emotional support, and contact them physically [43, 44]. Such physicians' overactive care and the physicians' unresolved emotion over death of their parents, relatives, or friends are also regarded as countertransference issues [43].

Therefore, it is essential to detect countertransference from therapists in order to make psychotherapy successful. Another reason for resolving such issue is that the therapist may suffer from depression while managing cancer patients [9].

24.8 Therapeutic Approaches

24.8.1 General Treatment

The therapeutic goal is not only to help the patient adjust to cancer but resolve his/her previously existing conflicts as well as his/her emotions and problems [9]. In general, the therapeutic approaches used in cancer patients are a combination of psychotherapeutic, psychopharmacologic, and behavioral techniques [2]. Individual therapy utilizes a crisis intervention approach in which the therapist (1) encourages the patient to express feelings, (2) offers support and optimism, (3) clarifies feelings, (4) interprets thoughts in psychodynamic terms, (5) encourages the patient to act on his or her circumstances, (6) explores the current situation in the context of the past, (7) focuses on specific relevant psychodynamic issues, and (8) limits the duration of therapy [45].

The educational component of this therapeutic system includes [9]: (1) clarifying the state of the medical condition including diagnosis, prognosis, and therapeutic alternatives; (2) teaching about the effects of the cancer and its treatments; (3) teaching methods for relief of anxiety such as relaxation techniques, self-hypnosis, or biofeedback [46], (4) providing an individualized method of utilizing visual imaging to combat the cancer; (5) supporting compliance with medical regimens; (6) teaching about lifestyle, diet, and exercise; (7) teaching about the common reactions of patients, relatives, and friends to cancer; and (8) providing access to self-help groups.

Clarification of the medical condition and related treatments is important. Informed patients have less fear and anxiety, lower levels of stress, and better functioning coping responses [47]. Relaxation techniques help patients feel that they can exercise control over their bodies as well as relieve pain and anxiety without extra medication [46]. In addition, lower stress level may be associated with enhanced cancer prognosis [46, 48].

These psychotherapeutic and educational approaches are all helpful in the management of cancer patients, although whether these methods favorably alter the prognosis of the cancer remains to be seen. However, these approaches have been shown to lower psychological distress and improve treatment satisfaction and compliance [49]. The techniques of choice with each patient and family depend on individual needs and the modalities available. An integrated approach including those techniques which are differentially helpful to each individual is strongly suggested [9].

24.8.2 Cognitive Behavioral Therapy

Cognitive behavioral treatment can be used effectively for patients with cancer. The overall aim of this treatment is to correct maladaptive coping, to lower levels of distress, to reclaim personal control, to teach problem-solving methods, and to improve morale. As a short-term educational intervention focusing on the "here and now," this therapy enables the clinician and the patient to collaborate in promoting the patient's self-control and responsibility for health. Another advantage of this treatment is cost-effectiveness [6].

In an approach that focuses on problem-solving, patients are taught to recognize, confront, and solve commonly encountered cancer problems [37, 38]. The intervention consists of four sessions and follows the general principles of any short-term psychotherapy. In the first session, the patient is informed that the patient and the therapist will look at common problems faced by many cancer patients and the best and most practical ways to solve them. Ideas for problem-solving are taught, and patients are encouraged to practice these skills on their own problems. Relaxation is presented as a time-out procedure for managing stress [50]. As a way to promote self-management, the patient is given a "homework" assignment for the week which involves daily relaxation training [6].

In the second session, the therapist notes the patient's progress in relaxation training. The therapist works with the patient to generate possible problem-solving strategies for his/her particular issues and to develop ways to establish priorities among the various possible approaches. The third session places a heavy focus on problem-solving. At this point, the therapist explores current personal problems with the patient and applies this approach to these problems [6].

During the fourth session, the patient and therapist together evaluate the effectiveness of the approach for dealing with problems during the preceding week. The need for further sessions is evaluated, and then the therapist may terminate the formal sessions. The philosophy behind this cognitive intervention is that problems can be reorganized into manageable proportions [6].

Behavioral techniques include passive relaxation with visual imagery, progressive muscle relaxation, electromyographic (EMG) feedback, systematic desensitization, and cognitive distraction [51–53]. In addition, exercise intervention may have beneficial effects on health-related quality of life including physical functioning, role function, social functioning, and fatigue [54].

24.8.3 Family Therapy

Family therapy is essential for cancer patients. The best way to enable their family members to participate in treatment is to point out that the patients and their family members need to communicate to each other and to provide them with assistance in coping with cancer, while they have to live with it [5]. The therapist should help spouses of cancer patients take care of the patients and come to terms with the reality of cancer while providing them with emotional support. However, the spouses also have to be able to express their own fear, sadness, and anger, because the family members of cancer patients tend to focus on the patients' needs so that they deny their own need for help and neglect their own health. Behavioral therapy for the family includes relaxation with visual imagery, systematic desensitization, and cognitive distraction [51–53]. Teaching family members how to relax and how to cope with cancer can help lower their levels of anxiety and stress related to taking care of the patients [9]. As a result, the family members of cancer patients can reduce expression of negative emotion such as hostility and criticism toward the patients and then provide them with more support. In addition, the therapist needs to evaluate if the patient and his/her spouse can maintain their sexual relationship and then to recommend it [55, 56].

24.8.4 Group Psychotherapy

Group psychotherapy for cancer patients is not only efficient in terms of time and financial cost but also highly effective in improving quality of life; reducing psychological distress, anxiety, and depression; improving coping skills; and reducing symptoms such as pain, nausea, and vomiting [57–59]. Group psychotherapy may allow cancer patients to receive support from others (patients or nonpatients) who have experienced and conquered similar problems of medical illness [2]. In addition to providing support, the role of group psychotherapy is to provide basic information, facilitate emotional expression, and teach coping skills [57, 58].

Group psychotherapy may offer benefits not available in individual settings, such as a sense of universality, sharing a common experience and identity, a feeling helping oneself by helping others, hopefulness fostered by seeing how others have coped successfully, and a sense of belonging to a larger group (self-transcendence, meaning, common purpose) [60]. Group participation helps decrease the sense of isolation and alienation, as the cancer patient and his/her family can see that they are not alone in adjusting to the illness [2].

Group psychotherapy for cancer patients falls predominantly into the following categories: (1) patient education/psychoeducation, (2) supportive-expressive intervention, and (3) cognitive behavioral intervention [59]. Supportive-expressive group psychotherapy for women with metastatic breast cancer includes detoxifying death by direct discussion of death anxiety and other fears toward impending death, which can result in positive life changes [61, 62].

Topics for discussion in group psychotherapy to be included are grief work, coping skills, mastery, cognitive reframing, and the re-ordering of priorities [60]. A randomized trial of supportive-expressive group therapy for women with metastatic breast cancer [63] revealed that it helped build strong support bonds, express emotions, deal directly with fears of dying and death, reorder life priorities, improve relationships with their family and friends, enhance communication and shared problem-solving with physicians, and learn self-hypnosis for pain control. Over a 10-year follow-up, there was a statistically significant survival in women receiving group therapy [30].

24.8.5 *Self-Help Treatment*

Most self-help support networks (e.g., Patient to Patient Program: Reach to Recovery, ostomy clubs) for cancer patients work closely with professional medical services, thereby offering social support as an adjunct to medical care. Volunteers help decrease the sense of alienation and isolation of patients because of their unique knowledge and sensitivity, which comes with their shared experience [2]. In particular, veteran patient volunteers facilitate coping in the newly diagnosed patient by providing the patients with information, emotional support, and role model for successful adaptation and recovery [9].

24.8.6 *Biopsychosocial Effects of Psychological and Behavioral Interventions*

In many studies comparing psychotherapy groups such as crisis intervention, cognitive therapy, and supportive psychotherapy with educational and psychodynamic focus and control groups, psychotherapy groups were found to be more effective than control groups. In group therapy as well as individual therapy, patients reported less distress, higher self-esteem and self-image, less anxiety, and more self-control in post-psychotherapy compared with pre-psychotherapy [20]. In addition, the levels of satisfaction with therapy and the levels of compliance with therapy were improved [49].

Mindfulness-based stress reduction (MBSR) program was reported to be effective in decreasing mood disturbance and stress symptoms in patients with a wide variety of cancer diagnoses and stages of illness [64]. In another study, after an 8-week MBSR program that incorporated relaxation, meditation, gentle yoga, and daily home practice, significant improvements were noted in overall quality of life, symptoms of stress, and sleep quality in breast and prostate cancer patients. In addition, T-cell production of IL-4 increased and IFN-gamma decreased, whereas NK-cell production of IL-10 decreased. These results were consistent with a shift in immune profile from one associated with depressive symptoms to a more normal profile [65].

However, it was suggested that the significant variation that was observed across participants, mode of delivery, discipline of "trained helper," and intervention content in the existing studies make it difficult to arrive at a firm conclusion regarding the effectiveness of psychosocial interventions for cancer patients [66].

24.8.7 Psychopharmacotherapy

Benzodiazepine antianxiety agents are used for patients with anxiety, whereas antidepressants or beta-blocker such as propranolol are used in phobic or panic patients. In hepatic cancer patients with anxiety, short-acting lorazepam is recommended. However, in terminal cancer patients with delirium, low-dose neuroleptics are preferred instead of benzodiazepine antianxiety agents which may enhance confusion. Particularly in cancer patients with serious respiratory impairment, benzodiazepine antianxiety agents should not be used because of the risk for suppression of the respiratory center. For these patients, however, antihistamines can be used [2].

Mild or moderate depression often resolves spontaneously [67], with resolution of a precipitating stressor. However, severe depression, such as major depressive disorder (MDD), may significantly benefit from pharmacotherapy, psychotherapy, or a combination of both [68]. Moreover, the combination of antidepressant therapy and cognitive therapy may enhance long-term recovery from depression compared with cognitive therapy alone [69].

Tricyclic antidepressants are recommended in cancer patients with anorexia and weight loss. In contrast, selective serotonin reuptake inhibitors (SSRIs) and venlafaxine tend to lose weight [70]. These drugs may often cause side effects such as nausea and should be used with caution in patients with gastrointestinal cancer and those undergoing chemotherapy [71].

Particularly amitriptyline with sedative action is known to be effective in cancer patients with insomnia or emotional instability. This drug also helps relieve pain. However, anticholinergic side effects of this drug can make aged patients or those recovering from surgery difficult to tolerate. For these patients, especially those with stomatitis caused by radiotherapy, it is better to use either trazodone or paroxetine which has sedative action but few anticholinergic effects [72].

Tricyclic antidepressants, trazodone, and MAO inhibitors should be cautiously used in patients with anemia caused by bleeding because they may potentiate orthostatic hypotension. In particular, a combination of MAO inhibitors and meperidine is contraindicated due to the risk of hypertension [72].

SSRIs (e.g., paroxetine) can be effectively used in cancer patients with depression, although they may cause nausea and vomiting [73]. It is desirable to use the drugs, starting with a low dose and then gradually increasing the dosage [72]. Serotonin-norepinephrine reuptake inhibitors (e.g., mirtazapine) may also be effective in improving depression [74].

Therapists should be careful that corticosteroid, prednisone, and dexamethasone frequently used in cancer patients can cause mood disorders such as depression and mania [2]. In cancer patients with pain, analgesics such as aspirin, acetaminophen, narcotic agonist or antagonist, and antidepressants can be used. However, it is recommended that analgesics be administered at fixed regular intervals rather than as prn. Moreover, placebo should be avoided [75].

24.9 Conclusions

To live with cancer is much more than adapting to the treatments and their side effects. In the assessment and treatment of cancer patients, the importance of psychosocial factors is emphasized. The necessity for psychiatric treatment and assessment of therapies is increased in order to improve side effects of treatment and enhance quality of life. Treatment team members need to be careful of the possibility that psychiatric problems may occur regardless of the progress of illness. In case such problems occur, psychiatric consultation should be considered. The therapeutic approaches used in cancer patients are a combination of psychotherapeutic, behavioral, and psychopharmacologic techniques. Psychotherapeutic approaches include cognitive therapy, family therapy, group therapy, and self-help treatment. Behavioral approaches, such as relaxation, biofeedback, systematic desensitization, hypnosis, and guided imagery, are helpful for pain and anxiety during procedures, nausea and vomiting, and cancer-related eating disorders. Psychopharmacologic approach is effective for anxiety, depression, delirium, pain, nausea, vomiting, and insomnia. An integrated approach including those therapeutic techniques tailored to each individual's need is strongly suggested.

References

1. Fallowfield LJ, Hall A, Maguire GP, et al. Psychological outcomes of different treatment policies in women with early breast cancer outside a clinical trial. Br Med J. 1990;301:575–80.
2. Lesko LM, Massie MJ, Holland JC. Oncology. In: Stoudemire A, Fogel BS, editors. Principles of medical psychiatry. Orlando: Grune & Stratton; 1987.
3. Holland JC, Rowland J, Lebovits A. Reactions to cancer treatment: assessment of emotional response to adjunct radiotherapy. Psychiatr Clin N Am. 1979;2:347–58.

4. Holland JC. Psychological issues in the care of the terminally ill. In: Flach F, editor. Directions in psychiatry. New York: Hatherleigh; 1982.
5. Wellisch D. Psychosocial problems of cancer. In: Haskell CM, editor. Cancer treatment. Philadelphia: WB Saunders; 1980.
6. Worden JW. Cognitive therapy with cancer patients. In: Freeman A, Greenwood V, editors. Cognitive therapy: applications in psychiatric and medical settings. New York: Human Science Press; 1987.
7. Peck A. Emotional reactions to having cancer. Radium Ther Nucl Med. 1972;114:591–9.
8. Plumb MM, Holland J. Comparative studies of psychological functions in patients with advanced cases of self-reported depressive symptoms. J Psychosom Med. 1979;39:264–76.
9. Kaufman E, Micha VG. A model for psychotherapy with the good-prognosis cancer patient. Psychosomatics. 1987;28:540–7.
10. Abrams RD. The patient with cancer: his changing pattern of communication. N Engl J Med. 1966;274:317–22.
11. Singer BA. Psychosocial trauma, defense strategies and treatment consideration in cancer patients and their families. Am J Fam Ther. 1983;11:15–21.
12. Koh KB, Kim KW. A comparison of psychopathology between cancer patients on radiotherapy and noncancer patients. J Korean Neuropsychiatr Assoc. 1990;29:662–8.
13. Koh KB, Kim ST. Coping strategy of cancer patients. J Korean Neuropsychiatr Assoc. 1988;27:140–50.
14. Koh KB. Stress and coping strategy in family members of cancer patients. J Korean Neuropsychiatr Assoc. 1988;27:693–702.
15. Kaplan HI, Sadock BJ. Synopsis of psychiatry. 5th ed. Baltimore: Williams & Wilkins; 1988. p. 100.
16. Moos RH, Tsu VD. The crisis of physical illness: an overview. In: Moos R, editor. Coping with physical illness. New York: Plenum; 1977.
17. Campell PC. Suicide among cancer patients. Community Health Bull. 1966;80:207–12.
18. Hackett TP, Cassem NH, Wishnie H. Detection and treatment of anxiety in the coronary care unit. Am Hosp J. 1969;78:729–36.
19. LeShan L. Cancer mortality rates: some statistical evidence of the effect of psychological factors. Arch Gen Psychiatry. 1962;63:333–5.
20. Kubler-Ross E. On death and dying. New York: Macmillan; 1969.
21. Lederberg MS, Holland JC. Psychooncology. In: Kaplan HI, Sadock BJ, editors. Comprehensive textbook of psychiatry. Baltimore: Williams & Wilkins; 1995.
22. Daune F. Psychological aspects of breast cancer. Rev Med Brux. 1995;16:245–7.
23. Goldfarb C, Driesen J, Cole D. Psychophysiologic aspects of malignancy. Am J Psychiatry. 1967;123:1545–52.
24. Greer S, Morris T. Psychological attributes of women who develop breast cancer: a controlled study. J Psychosom Res. 1975;19:147–53.
25. Abse DW, Wilkins MM, Van de Castle RL. Personality and behavioral characteristics of lung cancer patients. J Psychosom Res. 1974;18:101–13.
26. Joffe RT, Rubinow DR, Denicoff KD, et al. Depression and carcinoma of the pancreas. Gen Hosp Psychiatry. 1986;8:241–5.
27. Koh KB. A comparison of illness behavior between cancer and noncancer patients. J Korean Neuropsychiatr Assoc. 1991;30:739–51.
28. Perrin GM, Pierce IR. Psychosomatic aspects of cancer; a review. Psychosom Med. 1959;21:397–421.
29. Locke SE, Gorman JR. Behavior and immunity. In: Kaplan HI, Sadock BJ, editors. Comprehensive textbook of psychiatry. Baltimore: Williams & Wilkins; 1989.
30. Heim E, Augustiny KF, Schaffner L, et al. Coping with breast cancer over time and situation. J Psychosom Res. 1993;37:523–42.
31. Derogatis LR, Morrow GR, Fetting J. The prevalence of psychiatric disorders among cancer patients. JAMA. 1983;249:751–7.

32. Buckberg JB, Penman DT, Holland JC. Depression in hospitalized cancer patients. Psychosom Med. 1984;46:199–212.
33. Fox BH, Stanek EJ, Boldy SC, et al. Suicide rates among cancer patients in Connecticut. Chron Dis. 1982;35:85–100.
34. Bolund C. Suicide and cancer: 1. Demographic and social characteristics of cancer patients who committed suicide in Sweden 1973–1976. J Psychosoc Oncol. 1985;3:17–30.
35. Greer S, Morris T, Pettingale KW. Psychological response to breast cancer: effect on outcome. Lancet. 1979;2:785–7.
36. Chen CC, David A, Thompson K, et al. Coping strategies and psychiatric morbidity in women attending breast assessment clinics. J Psychosom Res. 1996;40:265–70.
37. Janis E, Mann L. Decision-making. New York: Free Press; 1997.
38. Spivack G, Platt J, Schure M. The problem-solving approach to adjustment. San Francisco: Jossey-Bass; 1976.
39. Billings AG, Moos RH. The role of coping responses in attenuating the stress of life events. J Behav. 1981;4:139–57.
40. Smith LW, Patterson TL, Grant I. Avoidant coping predicts psychological disturbance in the elderly. J Nerv Ment Dis. 1990;178:525–30.
41. Cassem NH. The dying patient. In: Cassem, editor. MGH handbook of general hospital psychiatry. St. Louis: Mosby Year Book; 1991.
42. Bleeker JAC. Brief psychotherapy with lung cancer patients. Psychosom Med. 1978;29:282–7.
43. Renneker RE. Countertransference reactions to cancer. Psychosom Med. 1957;19:409–18.
44. Druss RG. Psychotherapy of patients with serious intercurrent medical illness. Bull Assoc Psychoanal Med. 1984;23:163–8.
45. Marmor J. Short-term dynamic psychotherapy. Am J Psychiatry. 1979;136:149–55.
46. Fiore N. Fighting cancer: one patient's perspective. N Engl J Med. 1979;300:284–9.
47. Bloom JR, Ross RD, Burnell G. The effect of social support on patient adjustment after breast surgery. Patient Couns Health Educ. 1978;1:50–9.
48. La Barba RC. Experimental and environmental factors in cancer. Psychosom Med 1970;32:259–269.
49. Jerse MA, Whitman HH, Gustafson JP. Cancer in adults. In: Roback HB, editor. Helping patients and their families cope with medical problems. San Francisco: Jossey-Bass; 1984.
50. Benson H. The relaxation response. New York: Morrow; 1975.
51. Burish TG, Lyles JN. Effectiveness of relaxation training in reducing adverse reactions to cancer chemotherapy. J Behav Med. 1981;4:65–78.
52. Morrow GR, Morrell BS. Behavioral treatment for the anticipatory nausea and vomiting induced by cancer chemotherapy. N Engl J Med. 1982;306:1476–80.
53. Redd WH, Andresen GV, Minagawa Y. Hypnotic control of anticipatory emesis in patients receiving cancer chemotherapy. J Consult Clin Psychol. 1982;50:14–9.
54. Mishra SI, Scherer RW, Snyder C, et al. Exercise interventions on health-related quality of life for people with cancer during active treatment. Cochrane Database Syst Rev. 2012;8:CD008465. https://doi.org/10.1002/14651858.CD008465.pub2.
55. Pfeffenbaum G, Pasnau R, Jamison K. A comprehensive program of psychosocial care for mastectomy patients. Int J Psychiatry Med. 1977;8:65–71.
56. Schain WS. Sexual problems of patients with cancer. In: Devita VT, Hellman S, Rosenberg SA, editors. Cancer: principles and practices of oncology. Philadelphia: JB Lippincott; 1982.
57. Fawzy FI, Fawzy NW. Group therapy in the cancer setting. J Psychosom Res. 1998;45:191–200.
58. Fawzy FI, Fawzy NW. Psychoeducational interventions. In: Holland JC, editor. Textbook of psychooncology. London: Oxford University Press; 1998. p. 676–93.
59. Spiegel D, Stein SL, Earhart TZ, et al. Group psychotherapy and the terminally ill. In: Chochinov H, Breitbart W, editors. The handbook of psychiatry in palliative medicine. New York: Oxford Univ. Press; 2000. p. 241–51.
60. Breitbart W. Spirituality and meaning in supportive care: spirituality and meaning-centered group psychotherapy interventions in advanced cancer. Support Care Cancer. 2002;10:272–80.

61. Kissane D, Block S, Miach P, et al. Cognitive existential group therapy for patients with primary breast cancer – techniques and themes. Psychooncology. 1997;6:25–33.
62. Spiegel D, Spira J. Supportive-expressive group psychotherapy: a treatment manual of psychosocial intervention for women with recurrent breast cancer. Stanford: Psychosocial Treatment Lab, Stanford Univ. School of Medicine; 1991.
63. Spiegel D, Bloom JR, Yalom ID. Group support for patients with metastatic cancer: a randomized prospective outcome study. Arch Gen Psychiatry. 1981;38:527–33.
64. Carlson LE, Ursuliak Z, Goodey E, et al. The effects of a mindfulness meditation-based stress reduction program on mood and symptoms of stress in cancer outpatients: 6-month follow-up. Support Care Cancer. 2001;9:112–23.
65. Carlson LE, Speca M, Patel KD, et al. Mindfulness-based stress reduction in relation to quality of life, mood, symptoms of stress, and immune parameters in breast and prostate cancer outpatients. Psychosom Med. 2003;65:571–81.
66. Galway K, Black A, Cantwell M, et al. Psychosocial interventions to improve quality of life and emotional wellbeing for recently diagnosed cancer patients. Cochrane Database Syst Rev. 2012;11:CD007064. https://doi.org/10.1002/14651858.CD007064.pub2.
67. Williams JW, Barrett J, Oxman T, et al. Treatment of dysthymia and minor depression in primary care: a randomized controlled trial in older adults. JAMA. 2000;284:1519–26.
68. Fann JR, Thomas-rich AM, Katon WJ, et al. Major depression after breast cancer: a review of epidemiology and treatment. Gen Hosp Psychiatry. 2008;30:112–26.
69. Maguire P, Hopwood P, Tarrier N, et al. Treatment of depression in cancer patients. Acta Psychiatr Scand Suppl. 1985;320:81–4.
70. Cunningham LA, Borison RL, Carman JS. A comparison of venlafaxine, trazodone and placebo in major depression. J Clin Psychopharmacol. 1994;14:99–106.
71. Koh KB. Stress and psychosomatic medicine. Seoul: Ilchokak; 2011.
72. Cunningham LA. Depression in the medically ill: choosing an antidepressant. J Clin Psychiatry. 1994;55(Suppl AJ):90–7.
73. Morrow GR, Hickok JT, Roscoe JA, et al. Differential effects of paroxetine on fatigue and depression: a randomized, double-blind trail from the University of Rochester Cancer Center Community Clinical Oncology Program. J Clin Oncol. 2003;21:4635–41.
74. Thompson DS. Mirtazapine for the treatment of depression and nausea in breast and gynecological oncology. Psychosomatics. 2000;41:356–9.
75. Foley K. Pharmacologic management of pain. In: Massie MJ, Lesko LM, editors. Current concepts in psycho-oncology. New York: Gold Publishers; 1984.

Chapter 25
Approaches to Specific Cancers

25.1 Introduction

This chapter reviews specific cancers such as breast cancer, prostate cancer, and childhood cancer in which there are unique characteristics not seen in other cancers with regard to assessment and treatment, although all of them have some general characteristics in common.

25.2 Breast Cancer

25.2.1 Psychosocial Issues

Psychosocial factors are becoming increasingly important components of the assessment and management of patients with breast cancer. Clearly, the development and evaluation of psychological interventions that ameliorate side effects of treatment and enhance quality of life are needed [1].

Whatever the course of the disease, the treatment team should be alert to the ever-present possibility of psychological morbidity, which, if present, requires rigorous evaluation and judicious referral. This referral may not only help reduce morbidity but, perhaps more importantly, may also prevent disease dominance over the lives of affected women [2].

In particular, at the stage of hospitalization and operation, the major problems which patients face include the risks of surgery, the loss of a breast (including a disturbed body image and reduced self-esteem), and the prognosis, which may induce fear of a painful death, followed by anger and acceptance. During this period, women are at increased vulnerability to a number of psychological problems as the series of physiological and psychosocial stressors generated by the illness is

K. B. Koh, *Stress and Somatic Symptoms*,
https://doi.org/10.1007/978-3-030-02783-4_25

continuous. Thus, psychiatric care can be more intensely required than at any other stage. It is recommended in these circumstances to help patients gain support from those closest to them and confront their situation with a fighting spirit [3].

The times of the most frequent psychiatric referral of breast cancer patients are during initial treatment and during treatment of metastatic or recurrent disease at a radiation oncology clinic. There is a high incidence of major depressive disorder in the outpatient breast cancer population, although oncologists frequently fail to recognize it. Because psychiatric management is an important part of overall treatment, breast care services need to include clinical staff whose job it is to provide supportive care [4].

With breast cancer, a symbol of femininity may be compromised, and a woman's loss of a breast may interfere with her identity. The psychological impact of breast cancer varies from one woman to another. It depends on the patient's age, personality, life experience, social and familial relationships, and psychiatric history [5].

It has already been reported that suppression of anger is associated with a higher risk of breast malignancy [6]. Anger is found to be associated with anxiety and can be frequently directed toward physicians, hospital staff, and family members [7].

25.2.2 Psychotherapeutic Interventions

Psychological interventions have been shown to facilitate psychological adaptation to breast cancer [8]. Psychological interventions include strategies to reduce stress, improve mood, alter health behaviors, and maintain adherence to cancer treatment and care [9].

When a cancer is diagnosed, especially breast cancer in women, the overall psychological history should be taken into account [5]. The therapist should help the patient adjust to surgery and disfigurement and should encourage a return to prior activities without fear of what others are thinking [10]. As later illustrated in a case report, concerns about the loss of femininity can sometimes be overcome by the therapist's helping the patient express her emotion and encouraging the husband to assist her without being confrontational [11].

Breast conservation surgery can be considered in patients with severe disturbance of body image [12], since, compared to mastectomy, this operation is associated with a less negative body image [2]. In readjusting to normal life, diversions from the illness and self-validation (or relativizing) seem to be helpful during periods of convalescence and chemo-/radiotherapy [3].

Anger as well as anxiety and depression can be appropriately managed, sometimes with the help of a psychiatrist. Effective psychotherapeutic treatment of depression has been found to affect the course of cancer. Psychotherapy also resulted in longer survival time for patients with breast cancer. Psychotherapeutic effects include changes in health maintenance behavior, health-care utilization, endocrine environment, and immune function. Specifically, effective treatment of depression in cancer patients results in better adjustment to the illness, remitted symptoms, and reduced cost of care and may influence the disease course. Thus, the treatment of depression in these patients may be considered part of medical treatment [13].

Patients with persistent concerns about body image, sexual desire, and sexual function should be referred to professionals who are trained in sexual rehabilitation. Treatment techniques include supportive psychotherapy, behavioral techniques such as relaxation, and gradual reeducation in sexual functioning [14].

Case

A woman in her late 30s with breast cancer who had undergone radical mastectomy became depressed, along with a perceived loss of femininity and loss of self-esteem caused by the mastectomy. After being discharged from the hospital, the patient was encouraged by her sister to see a psychiatrist. She said, "I can't tolerate living with only one breast" and complained of insomnia and a lack of interest in life. She also showed strong resentment and anger toward her husband, recalling that he had shown little concern about her situation and had returned home late at night a few times several months earlier. Accompanied by the patient, her husband said apprehensively, "My wife is trying to avoid sleeping in the same bed with me." During her sessions, the patient was allowed to vent her emotions, including anger toward her husband's negligence. Antidepressant (fluoxetine) and antianxiety (ethyl loflazepate) agents were administered twice daily. Her anger level was assessed using a hostility questionnaire. She recorded high scores on the anger subscale, saying "I seemed to get sick because I had a bad temper." Then, a variety of coping strategies were reviewed, including a few considered good for her situation. Through the application of the strategies, she began to introspectively search her inner self.

She found herself egotistic and self-centered, and she regretted getting into religion only extrinsically but not intrinsically. In addition, with her husband's understanding of the situation and his active assistance, the patient began to accept her own reality, to forgive her husband for mistreating her, and to regain her emotional stability and self-confidence. The issue relevant to her loss of femininity was not directly confronted by the psychiatrist. Rather, she was encouraged to vent her anger and do her limited daily activities, while she would deal with issues surrounding her illness. Also, the therapist encouraged her husband to actively participate in the therapeutic session. Such the therapist's effort and the husband's assistance helped the patient overcome her depression caused by the loss of femininity and anger toward her spouse and return to her routine activities.

25.2.3 Biopsychosocial Effects of Psychological Interventions

Psychological interventions were reported to have a number of favorable effects on biopsychosocial parameters in patients with breast cancer. For example, psychological interventions can attenuate emotional distress such as anxiety and depression manifested during radiotherapy treatment [15]. In addition, psychological interventions can influence neuroendocrine (e.g., cortisol) and immune function indicators, especially lymphocyte proliferation and Th1 cytokine production [7]. For example, those assigned to a 10-week group-based cognitive behavioral stress management program evidenced better psychosocial adaptation (reduced anxiety symptoms) and physiological adaptation (lower cortisol and greater Th1 cytokine interleukin-2 (IL-2) and interferon-γ (IFN-γ) production) after adjuvant treatment compared to those in the control group [16]. In another study, immune responses paralleled psychological and behavioral improvements from psychological interventions. T-cell proliferation in response to PHA and Con A remained stable or increased for the intervention patients, whereas both responses declined for assessment-only patients [17]. Experiential-existential group psychotherapy reduced levels of plasma cortisol and prolactin compared to those in a waiting list control group [18].

However, it was suggested that behavioral rather than immunity change was influential in achieving weaker symptoms and higher functional status. Therefore, distress reduction is highlighted as an important mechanism by which health can be improved in breast cancer patients [19]. Moreover, psychological adaptation in women with breast cancer can reduce anxiety and depressive mood and improve quality of life, which affects immune functions, such as increased production of the Th1 cytokine IL-2, IFN-γ, and tumor necrosis factor-α (TNF-α) [6].

Psychological interventions can also improve survival. Psychological intervention patients were found to have reduced risks of breast cancer recurrence and death from breast cancer compared with the assessment-only patients [9]. However, the relationship between supportive-expressive group therapy and longer survival was not replicated in another study [20].

25.3 Prostate Cancer

25.3.1 Psychosocial Issues

Prostate cancer has been a neglected area in psycho-oncology for decades [21]. However, as the incidence and prevalence of prostate cancer continue to rise, the number of men who need help and support in coping with the disease and treatment-related symptoms is increasing [22]. Prostate cancer is unique in some aspects: it affects only males, especially older males [23]. Contrary to other types of cancer, prostate cancer is growing slowly so that it will sometimes make the patients do nothing but monitor closely. As a result of treatment, prostate cancer patients often will experience specific problems such as micturition disturbance, incontinence, erectile disorders, and bowel problems, apart from problems that accompany cancer in general such as fatigue, anxiety, and pain [24]. Quality of life in prostate cancer patients needs to be emphasized because treatments not only provide a good survival rate but also cause adverse side effects [25]. Prostate cancer patients also have needs for support in the psychological, informational, and daily living domains [26]. At diagnosis of prostate cancer, low-to-moderate psychological distress was the most common, with distress decreasing after treatment [27].

25.3.2 Psychosocial Interventions

Overall, psychosocial interventions such as cognitive behavioral therapy, psychoeducational approach, supportive therapy, and counseling may have short-term beneficial effects on certain domains of well-being, as measured by the physical component of quality of life (QOL) when compared with usual care. In addition, they help enhance knowledge of the prostate. However, these interventions failed to demonstrate a significant effect on other domains such as symptom-related QOL, self-efficacy, uncertainty, distress, and depression [22]. Another prospective study found that men who were undecided about what treatment to receive experienced greater decision-related distress, although psychological and decision-related distress decreased over time, regardless of treatment modality. Therefore, interventions for prostate cancer patients should target decision-related distress and in-depth psychological support for those who experience ongoing difficulties [27].

25.4 Childhood Cancer

25.4.1 Psychosocial Issues

Patients with childhood cancer such as leukemia, lymphadenoma, and tumor of the central nervous system have psychosocial problems related to long-term treatment (e.g., chemo- and radiotherapy) as well as psychological responses to cancer [28]. These patients are known to have a higher prevalence of mental disorders than non-cancer patients [29]. They show separation anxiety, regressive behavior, and symbiotic relationship with their mothers [30]. Anxiety of children with cancer is usually associated with chronic uncertainty about survival [31].

Complications of cancer treatment include physical distress such as pain, nausea, vomiting, and anxiety relevant to medical procedures (e.g., bone marrow aspiration, lumbar puncture, intravenous injection) and chemotherapy [32]. Such procedures not only produce insomnia, nightmare, anorexia, interpersonal avoidance, and depression [33] but also prevent them from complying with medical procedures and treatment [32].

Side effects of treatment can cause many physical changes such as weight gain or loss, alopecia, oral ulcer, amputation, infertility, brain injury, and skeleton abnormality [34]. Therefore, such physical changes are likely to be followed by changes in body image, loss of self-esteem [35], and regressive behavior [36]. Finally the children may face many difficulties in psychosocial adaptation, avoiding play with peers and showing fear about attending school [36].

Children with cancer can experience hospitalization as separation, thereby clinging to their parents and showing signs of distress, disappointment, interpersonal avoidance, and depression [37]. Moreover, the use of an isolation room for preventing infections can cause psychological problems such as anxiety, depression, sleep disturbance, and behavioral problems [38].

Psychosocial issues and treatment of cancer patients are related to separation, loss, control, and competence. Facing a life-threatening illness such as cancer means separation from or loss of a loved one. In addition, it includes the loss of health, of the body, and of one's ordinary life. Children also experience changes in self-perception and in their relationships with others, so that the illness affects their development to a great extent; such changes may deprive them of their learned abilities of self-control and competence [34, 39].

25.4.2 Children's Coping with and Adaptation to Cancer

Childhood cancer patients' efforts to cope with cancer-related stress can cause a variety of psychosocial problems. They often have emotional and behavioral problems such as anxiety, fear, depression, extreme dependence on parents, sleep disturbance, regression, anger, and interpersonal avoidance [40]. In addition, developmental problems occur because their basic developmental process can be affected by cancer-related stress [34].

Childhood cancer patients do not express their positive as well as negative emotions freely and show more passive attitude in their social contact and more prevalent learning disorder than the healthy controls [41]. They often hate to go to school due to changes in their external features, the potential loss of contact with their peers, difficulty in complying with their school curriculum, and severe separation anxiety [34].

Good copers usually use open communication, honesty, maintenance of hope, and denial effectively [42]. In particular, denial is regarded as playing an important role in confronting reality and maintaining a positive perspective of the future [43].

The effects of coping strategies used can vary depending on the patterns of stress, situations, and individual characteristics. Major determinants of adaptation to childhood cancer include characteristics of the illness, the child's developmental levels, and social (environmental) factors [44].

Most survivors appear to lead normal adult lives, obtain high school degrees, and have good jobs, and some even have families and children. However, a small number of survivors show psychological and social problems, such as anxiety, fear over the future or over relapse, or sterility. The most vulnerable among the survivors are known to be females, people in poor financial conditions, the unemployed, and those with low education levels [45].

25.4.3 Psychotherapeutic Interventions

For childhood cancer patients, ambulatory treatment at the outpatient clinic is recommended rather than hospitalization, because the former can reduce emotional side effects, facilitate return to their home, friends, school, and community [34] and help them return to normal life.

Open communication between parents, physicians, and teachers is crucial for children with cancer who have difficulty in adapting to their school life [34]. It helps the children maintain close relationships with their parents and express a sense of basic satisfaction toward themselves. Therefore, their teachers should be given information on the illness and treatment in order to offer emotional support to the children. At the same time, psychosocial treatment for childhood cancer patients focuses on helping their family and treatment team provide emotional support to them and promoting development at maximum level by encouraging normal activities.

The family's emotional support consists of being able to communicate emotions, such as fear and hope, openly and freely and to share concerns about the illness [34]. Children who openly discuss their illness do not show defensive attitudes but maintain close relationships with their parents and express a sense of basic satisfaction toward themselves. Therefore, open communication enables the patients to cope with the illness effectively and to gain access to the resources of support within the family. Methods of communication that are fit for their age and stimulate open communication include play programs, art therapy, group therapy, and counseling [34, 46]. In particular, team approach is recommended for treatment of childhood cancer patients in which pediatricians, child psychiatrists, nurses, social workers, teachers, and chaplains are involved [28].

25.5 Social Support for Breast, Prostate, and Childhood Cancer Patients

Social support for cancer patients has a great influence on the course of the illness. For example, marital status or perceived social support in patients with breast cancer is closely associated with their survival. In one 7-year follow-up study, mortality rate in married patients was found to be lower than in unmarried patients [47].

The death rate was even lower among those who shared their feelings with more than one confidant. Thus, the availability of social support through marriage and friends proved to be a robust predictor of survival [48]. Social support from a spouse, another intimate, or a physician, as well as actively seeking social support, has been shown to be related to higher natural killer (NK)-cell activity in patients with stage I and II breast cancer [49].

Breast cancer patients need psychological care for their feelings of sadness, anxiety, and depression. In particular, younger women need more psychosocial care than older women. In addition to psychological needs, women with breast cancer have needs for support and for information [50, 51]. The needs for support comprise support from the family, treatment team, support groups, and professionals (e.g., counseling) as well as informal support. In addition, they may have unmet needs; they want to know whether they can talk freely to a caregiver about the cancer, the degree to which the cancer interferes with social activities, and how much financial burdens they experience [52].

On the other hand, men with prostate cancer have needs related to psychological, health-care system, sexual, and physical issues [53]. Therefore, therapeutic team members should give attention to the physical, psychological, social, and sexual needs of cancer patients [54]. Patients with childhood cancer and their family, especially parents, need psychosocial support because they experience significant psychological distress throughout the course of the illness [55]. It was proposed that psychosocial palliative care standards for them be developed and established [56].

25.6 Psychopharmacotherapy of Depression in Breast, Prostate, and Childhood Cancer Patients

Selective serotonin reuptake inhibitors (SSRIs) (e.g., paroxetine) and serotonin-norepinephrine reuptake inhibitors (e.g., mirtazapine) may be effective in improving depression [57, 58] and decreasing menopausal symptoms in breast cancer survivors [59–65]. The mechanisms for these effects are likely mediated by the serotonergic effects of these agents. In addition, the norepinephrine reuptake inhibitor reboxetine is known to be effective in breast cancer patients with major depressive disorder [66]. A study of bupropion in early-stage breast cancer patients on hormonal therapy following chemotherapy showed improvement in both sexual functioning and Beck Depression Inventory (BDI) depression scores [67]. In patients with stomatitis and urinary retention following radiotherapy or chemotherapy, antidepressants such as SSRIs and tricyclic antidepressants (e.g., nortriptyline or desipramine) with low anticholinergic effects are recommended [14].

Estrogen may also serve as an adjunct to the treatment of depression in postmenopausal women [68]. A few studies [69, 70] found that depressed postmenopausal women taking SSRIs had better improvement in depressive symptoms and quality of life if they received estrogen replacement therapy. Therefore, clinicians should be careful of the possibility that antidepressant efficacy will be lower in women taking an estrogen antagonist, such as tamoxifen [68].

In cancer patients with anorexia, tricyclic antidepressants are recommended. For nausea and vomiting following chemotherapy and radiotherapy, a combination of antiemetics, antianxiety agents such as alprazolam and lorazepam, and muscle relaxation can be used [14].

A variety of antidepressants can be used in depressed patients with prostate cancer. In particular, venlafaxine [71] and paroxetine [72] proved to be effective in reducing hot flushes, the most common complaints reported by men undergoing androgen suppression treatment for prostate cancer.

SSRIs are known to have modest effects on childhood depression. However, SSRIs may be associated with behavioral activation, self-harm, or suicidal ideation or attempts. Therefore, antidepressants including SSRIs should be used with caution in depressed children and adolescents, and the use of SSRIs for them requires careful diagnostic assessment, evaluation of comorbid conditions, and monitoring, especially within the 1st week of treatment [73, 74].

25.7 Conclusions

Breast cancer, prostate cancer, and childhood cancer have unique characteristics not seen in other cancers with regard to assessment and treatment. Breast cancer patients with persistent concerns about body image, sexual desire, and sexual function should be referred to professionals. Quality of life in prostate cancer patients needs to be emphasized because treatments not only provide a good survival rate, but also cause adverse side effects. Prostate cancer patients also need support in psychological, informational, and daily living domains. Open communication between parents, physicians, and teachers is crucial for children with cancer who have difficulty in adapting to their school life. Psychosocial treatment for childhood cancer patients focuses on helping their family and treatment team provide emotional support to them and promoting development at maximum level by encouraging normal activities. Team approach is recommended for treatment of these children in which pediatricians, child psychiatrists, nurses, social workers, teachers, and pastors are involved. A variety of antidepressants can be used in depressed patients with breast cancer, prostate cancer, and childhood cancer. However, clinicians should be careful of the possibility that antidepressant efficacy will be lower in women taking an estrogen antagonist, such as tamoxifen.

References

1. Walker LG, Eremin O. Psychological assessment and intervention: future prospects for women with breast cancer. Semin Surg Oncol. 1996;12:76–83.
2. Kissane DW, Clarke DM, Ikin J, et al. Psychological morbidity and quality of life in Australian women with early-stage breast cancer: a cross-sectional survey. Med J Aust. 1998;169:192–6.
3. Heim E, Augustiny KF, Schaffner L, et al. Coping with breast cancer over time and situation. J Psychosom Res. 1993;37:523–42.
4. Pendlebury SC, Snars J. Role of a psychiatry liaison clinic in the management of breast cancer. Australas Radiol. 1996;40:283–6.
5. Daune F. Psychological aspects of breast cancer. Rev Med Brux. 1995;16:245–7.
6. Blomberg BB, Alvarez JP, Diaz A, et al. Psychosocial adaptation and cellular immunity in breast cancer patients in the weeks after surgery: an exploratory study. J Psychosom Res. 2009;67:369–76.
7. Peck A. Emotional reactions to having cancer. Radium Ther Nucl Med. 1972;114:591–9.
8. McGregor BA, Antoni MH. Psychological intervention and health outcomes among women treated for breast cancer: a review of stress pathways and biological mediators. Brain Behav Immun. 2009;23:159–66.
9. Andersen BL, Yang HC, Farrar WB, et al. Psychologic intervention improves survival for breast cancer patients: a randomized clinical trial. Cancer. 2008;113:3450–8.
10. Worden JW. Cognitive therapy with cancer patients. In: Freeman A, Greenwood V, editors. Cognitive therapy: applications in psychiatric and medical settings. New York: Human Science Press; 1987.
11. Koh KB. Psychosocial aspects of breast cancer: focus on interventions. In: Koh KB, editor. Somatization and psychosomatic symptoms. New York: Springer; 2013.
12. Mamelock AE. Psychiatry and surgery. In: Kaplan HI, Sadock BJ, editors. Comprehensive textbook of psychiatry. Baltimore: Williams & Wilkins; 1995.
13. Spiegel D. Cancer and depression. Br J Psychiatry. 1996;30(Suppl):109–16.
14. Lesko LM, Massie MJ, Holland JC. Oncology. In: Stoudemire A, Fogel BS, editors. Principles of medical psychiatry. Orlando: Grune & Stratton; 1987.
15. Nunes DF, Rodriguez AL, da Silva Hoffmann F, et al. Relaxation and guided imagery program in patients with breast cancer undergoing radiotherapy is not associated with neuroimmunomodulatory effects. J Psychosom Res. 2007;63:647–55.
16. Antoni MH, Lechner S, Diaz A, et al. Cognitive behavioral stress management effects on psychosocial and physiological adaptation in women undergoing treatment for breast cancer. Brain Behav Immun. 2009;23:580–91.
17. Andersen BL, Farrar WB, Golden-Krreutz DM, et al. Psychological, behavioral, and immune changes after a psychological intervention: a clinical trial. J Clin Onclo. 2004;22:3570–80.
18. van der Pompe G, Duivenvoorden HJ, Antoni MH, et al. Effectiveness of a short-term group psychotherapy program on endocrine and immune function in breast cancer patients: an exploratory study. J Psychosom Res. 1997;42:453–66.
19. Andersen BL, Golden-Kreutz D, Emery CF, et al. Distress reduction from a psychological intervention contributes to improved health for cancer patients. Brain Behav Immun. 2007;21:953–61.
20. Spiegel D, Butler LD, Giese-Davis J, et al. Effects of supportive-expressive group therapy on survival of patients with metastatic breast cancer: a randomized prospective trial. Cancer. 2007;110:1130–8.
21. Visser A, van Andel G. Psychosocial and educational aspects in prostate cancer patients. Patient Educ Couns. 2003;49:203–6.
22. Parahoo K, McDonough S, McCaughan E, et al. Psychosocial interventions for men with prostate cancer. Cochrane Database Syst Rev. 2013;12:CD008529. https://doi.org/10.1002/14651858.CC008529.pub3.

23. Facts and Figures of the Integraal Kankercentrum Nederland n.d.. http://www.cijfersover-kanker.nl/selecties. Accessed 1 Nov 2011.
24. Voerman B, Fischer M, Visser A, et al. Prostate cancer: a review of the literature on psychosocial problems and psychosocial interventions. Gedrag en Gezondh: Tijdschr Psychol Gezondh. 2004;32:251–70.
25. van Andel G, Bottemley A, Fossa SD, et al. An international field study of the EORTC QLQ-PR25: a questionnaire for assessing the health-related quality of life of patients with prostate cancer. Eur J Cancer. 2008;44:2418–24.
26. Sanson-Fisher R, Girgis A, Boyes A, et al. The unmet supportive care needs of patients with cancer. Cancer. 2000;88:226–37.
27. Steginga SK, Occhipinti S, Gardiner RA, et al. Prospective study of men's psychological and decision-related adjustment after treatment for localized prostate cancer. Urology. 2004;63:751–6.
28. Lederberg MS, Holland JC. Psycho-oncology. In: Kaplan HI, Sadock BJ, editors. Comprehensive textbook of psychiatry. 5th ed. Baltimore: Williams & Wilkins; 1989.
29. Howarth RV. The psychiatry of terminal illness in children. Proc R Soc Med. 1972;65:1039–40.
30. Lansky SB, Gendel M. Symbiotic regressive behavior patterns in childhood malignancy. Clin Pediatr. 1978;17:133–8.
31. Spinetta JJ, Deasy-Spinetta P. Living with childhood cancer. St. Louis: CV Mosby; 1981.
32. Kellerman J, Varni JW. Psychosocial aspects of pediatric hematology-oncology. In: Willoughby M, Siegel SE, editors. Hematology and oncology. London: Butterworth Scientific; 1982.
33. Kashani J, Hakami N. Depression in children and adolescents with malignancy. Can J Psychiatr. 1982;27:474–7.
34. van Dongen-Melman JEWM, Sanders-Woudstra JAR. Psychosocial aspects of childhood cancer: a review of the literature. J Child Psychol Psychiatry. 1986;29:145–80.
35. Bach SR. Spontaneous picture of leukemic children as an expression of the total personality, mind and body. Acta Paedopsychiatr. 1975;41:86–104.
36. Kagen-Goodheart L. Reentry: living with childhood cancer. Am J Orthop. 1977;47:651–8.
37. Bozeman MF, Orbach CE, Sutherland AM. Psychological impact of cancer and its treatment:III. The adaptation of mothers to the threatened loss of their children through leukemia. Cancer. 1955;8:1–19.
38. Kellerman J, Rigler D, Siegel SE. The psychological effects of isolation in protected environments. Am J Psychiatry. 1977;134:563–5.
39. Brunnquell C, Hall MD. Issues in the psychological care of pediatric oncology patients. Am J Orthop. 1982;52:32–44.
40. Frienman SB, Chodoff P, Mason JW, et al. Behavioral observations on parents anticipating the death of a child. Pediatrics. 1963;32:610–25.
41. Deasy-Spinetta P. The school and the child with cancer. In: Spinetta JJ, Deasy-Spinetta P, editors. Living with childhood cancer. St. Louis: CV Mosby; 1981.
42. Slavin LA, O'Malley JE, Koocher GP, et al. Communication of the cancer diagnosis to pediatric patients: impact on long-term adjustment. Am J Psychiatry. 1982;139:179–83.
43. Beisser AR. Denial and affirmation in illness and health. Am J Psychiatry. 1979;136:1026–30.
44. Katz ER. Illness impact and social reintegration. In: Kellerman J, editor. Psychological aspects of childhood cancer. Springfield: Charles Thomas; 1980.
45. Massimo L, Zarri D, Caprino D. Psychosocial aspects of survivors of childhood cancer or leukemia. Minerva Pediatr. 2005;57:389–97.
46. Adams MA. A hospital play program: helping children with serious illness. Am J Orthop. 1976;46:416–24.
47. Maunsell E, Jacques B, Deschenes L. Social support, a survival among women with breast cancer. Presented at the annual Psycho-oncology meeting, Memorial-Sloan Ketteri Cancer Center. 1993.
48. Spiegel D, Kato PM. Psychosocial influences on cancer incidence and progression. Harvard Rev Psychiatry. 1996;4:10–26.

49. Levy SM, Herberman RB, Whiteside T, et al. Perceived social support and tumor- estrogen/progesterone receptor status as predictors of natural killer cell activity in breast cancer patients. Psychosom Med. 1990;52:73–85.
50. Visser A, Breed W, Geluk W, et al. The value of open walking-in houses for cancer patients and their proxies: history, use, needs and evaluation. Nederl Tijdschr Oncol. 2009;6:248–55.
51. Thewes B, Butow P, Girgis A, et al. The psychosocial needs of breast cancer survivors; a qualitative study of the shared and unique needs of younger versus older survivors. Psycho-Oncology. 2004;13:177–89.
52. Soothill K, Morris SM, Harman J, et al. The significant unmet needs of cancer patients: probing psychosocial concerns. Support Care Cancer. 2001;9:597–605.
53. Daeter L Visser A, Van der Hooft-Lemans T. Determinants of seeking psychosocial care in Dutch men with prostate cancer. Master thesis. Report De Vruchtenburg, Rotterdam; 2012.
54. Visser A. Cancer in a psychosomatic perspective. In: Koh KB, editor. Somatization and psychosomatic symptoms. New York: Springer; 2013.
55. Steele AC, Mullins LL, Mullins AJ, et al. Psychosocial interventions and therapeutic support as a standard of care in pediatric oncology. Pediatr Blood Cancer. 2015;62(Suppl 5):S585–618.
56. Weaver MS, Heinze KE, Bell CJ, et al. Establishing psychosocial palliative care standards for children and adolescents with cancer and their families: an integrative review. Palliat Med. 2016;30:212–23.
57. Morrow GR, Hickok JT, Roscoe JA, et al. Differential effects of paroxetine on fatigue and depression: a randomized, double-blind trail from the University of Rochester Cancer Center Community Clinical Oncology Program. J Clin Oncol. 2003;21:4635–41.
58. Thompson DS. Mirtazapine for the treatment of depression and nausea in breast and gynecological oncology. Psychosomatics. 2000;41:356–9.
59. Loprinzi CL, Kugler JW, Sloan JA, et al. Venlafaxine in management of hot flashes in survivors of breast cancer: a randomized controlled trial. Lancet. 2000;356:2059–63.
60. Loprinzi CL, Sloan JA, Perez EA, et al. Phase III evaluation of fluoxetine for treatment of hot flashes. J Clin Oncol. 2002;20:1578–83.
61. Stearns V, Issacs C, Rowland J, et al. A pilot trial assessing the efficacy of paroxetine hydrochloride (Paxil) in controlling hot flashes in breast cancer survivors. Ann Oncol. 2000;11:17–22.
62. Soares CN, Poitras JR, Prouty J, et al. Efficacy of citalopram as a monotherapy or as an adjunctive treatment to estrogen therapy for perimenopausal and postmenopausal women with depression and vasomotor symptoms. J Clin Psychiatry. 2003;64:473–9.
63. Kimmick GG, Lovato J, McQuellon R, et al. Randomized, double-blind, placebo-controlled, crossover study of sertraline (Zoloft) for the treatment of hot flashes in women with early stage breast cancer taking tamoxifen. Breast J. 2006;12:114–22.
64. Stearns V, Beebe KL, Iyengar M, et al. Paroxetine controlled release in the treatment of menopausal hot flashes: a randomized controlled trial. JAMA. 2003;289:2827–34.
65. Gordon PR, Kerwin JP, Boesen KG, et al. Sertraline to treat hot flashes: a randomized controlled, double-blind, crossover trial in a general population. Menopause. 2006;13:568–75.
66. Grassi L, Biancosino B, Marmai L, et al. Effect of reboxetine on major depressive disorder in breast cancer patients: an open-label study. J Clin Psychiatry. 2004;65:515–20.
67. Mathias C, Cardeal Mendes CM, Ponde de Sena E, et al. An open-label, fixed-dose study of bupropion effect on sexual function scores in women treated for breast cancer. Ann Oncol. 2006;17:1792–6.
68. Fann JR, Thomas-rich AM, Katon WJ, et al. Major depression after breast cancer: a review of epidemiology and treatment. Gen Hosp Psychiatry. 2008;30:112–26.
69. Schneider LS, Small GW, Clary CM. Estrogen replacement therapy and antidepressant response to sertraline in older depressed women. Am J Geriatr Psychiatry. 2001;9:393–9.
70. Schneider LS, Small GW, Hamilton SH, et al. Estrogen replacement and response to fluoxetine in a multicenter geriatric depression trial. Fluoxetine Collaborative Study Group. Am J Geriatr Psychiatry. 1997;5:97–106.

71. Irani J, Salomon L, Oba R, et al. Efficacy of venlafaxine, medroxyprogesterone acetate, and cyproterone acetate for the treatment of vasomotor hot flushes in men taking gonadotropin-releasing hormone analogues for prostate cancer: a double-blind, randomized trial. Lancet Oncol. 2010;11:147–54.
72. Naoe M, Ogawa Y, Shichijo T, et al. Pilot evaluation of serotonin reuptake inhibitor antidepressants in hot flash patients under androgen-deprivation therapy for prostate cancer. Prostate Cancer Prostatic Dis. 2006;9:275–8.
73. Scahill L, Hamrin V, Pachler ME. The use of selective serotonin reuptake inhibitors in children and adolescents with major depression. J Child Adolesc Psychiatr Nurs. 2005;18:86–9.
74. Moreno C, Roche AM, Greenhill LL. Pharmacotherapy of child and adolescent depression. Child Adolesc Psychiatr Clin N Am. 2006;15:977–98.

Part IV
Religion, Spirituality, and Psychosomatic Medicine

Chapter 26
The Role of Religion and Spirituality in Health and Illness

26.1 Historical Development

There has historically been tension between psychiatry and religion in relation to alternative explanations for mental disorders. Psychiatry tended to portray religion negatively; religion/spirituality was used to illustrate psychopathology [1]. Conversely, religious thinkers tended to express skepticism toward psychiatry, especially psychoanalysis, calling it the morbid product of Freud's coarse materialism [2].

During the past few decades this historical antagonism has been waning. Diagnostic and Statistical Manual (DSM)-IV added a diagnostic category for religious and spiritual problems, recognizing that religious/spiritual beliefs are not inherently pathological [3]. Later the World Psychiatric Association also established a section on psychiatry and religion [4]. Mental health workers increasingly value close cooperation with community clergy and patients' belief systems [5]. These developments suggest that the historic division between psychiatry and religion may be narrowing and that the appreciation for the clinical importance of religion/spirituality in psychiatry is growing [6].

During physical illnesses, 40% or more of older hospitalized patients experience clinical depression [7, 8]. Poorer health status and perceptions, less social support, and lower spiritual well-being were related to significant depressive symptoms [9]. Among older medically ill hospitalized patients with depression, the severity of depression was associated with a lower religious attendance, prayer, scripture reading, and lower intrinsic religiosity [10].

Psychiatrists are more open to engaging patients on religious and/or spiritual matters than are other physicians. Psychiatrists generally have a positive attitude toward the influence of religion/spirituality on health, although they recognize that religion/spirituality may have negative effects [11]. However, most psychiatrists receive little professional training about religious matters [12].

K. B. Koh, *Stress and Somatic Symptoms*,
https://doi.org/10.1007/978-3-030-02783-4_26

This chapter reviews the role of spirituality as coping with stress, the relation between religious involvement and mental/physical well-being, effects of religious coping, the relation between spirituality and social support, and the role of religion and spirituality in depression of the medically ill.

26.2 Definition of Religion and Spirituality

Religion can be described as a set of beliefs about the transcendent shared by a community, often associated with common sacred writings and practices [13, 14]. Spirituality can be characterized as an individual's relationship to and experience of the transcendent, whether through religion or other paths [13]. Spirituality is often equated with religious faith. However, a broader and more inclusive definition is the way in which people understand their lives in view of their ultimate meaning and value [15].

Some scholars have employed the terms 'religion' and 'religiosity' to describe institutional or formal traditions and expressions [16]. Conversely, the term 'spirituality' has been used more recently to describe an individual's sense of purpose and meaning and personal connectedness to the divine or to the truth. In this view, the conception of spirituality relies more on the individual context than the institutional context [9].

26.3 Spirituality as Coping with Stress

Although researchers interested in coping overlooked the role of religion for years, there is mounting evidence that religious cognitions and behaviors can offer effective resources for dealing with stressful events and conditions [17]. In particular, much attention has focused on the role of spirituality as a buffer from the impact of negative life events, and as a coping mechanism to deal with life strains and hassles [18–22].

Nonetheless, mental illness can be negatively understood in terms of a spiritual framework as themes of guilt and persecution dominate. However, spirituality can be evoked in a manner that enhances one's hope and confidence so that life will improve [19, 23]. Furthermore, maintaining a spiritual belief system seems to be associated with a greater sense of well-being and with the use of more effective coping strategies in times of stress [19, 20, 24, 25]. In general, coping strategies that build self-efficacy, or that involves a higher power as a partner, are more effective than simple deferring strategies (i.e., it's all in God's hands) [26].

26.4 Effects of Religious Coping

Researchers have documented positive associations between religious involvement (e.g., religious attendance and private piety) and self-esteem or personal efficacy [27, 28]. People who profess stronger spiritual beliefs seem to resolve their grief more rapidly and completely after the death of a close person than do people with no spiritual beliefs [29]. Religious cognitions and behaviors, especially those focusing on prayer, meditation, and other devotional pursuits, seem to be valuable in dealing with bereavement as well as serious health problems [17, 30, 31]. Studies of families coping with the death of a child [32, 33] and research into the adaptation of older people to widowhood [34] suggest that religious belief affects the outcome of bereavement. In addition, studies on the health effects of religion/spirituality have linked it to reduced depression and anxiety, increased longevity, and other physical and psychological health benefits [35–37].

Some coping styles (e.g., coping in collaboration with a divine other) were found to yield positive results by bolstering feelings of control, enhancing confidence in the ability to manage difficulties, and producing desirable health outcomes [21, 38]. According to some studies, religion can help individuals adjust the self-concept so that physical frailties and other problems are less threatening to personal identity [30]. In addition, religious cognitions and practices may aid in coping with stressors. For example, prayer and other intrapsychic religious coping efforts may alter primary appraisals, leading religious persons to reassess the meaning of potentially problematic conditions as opportunities for spiritual growth or learning or as part of a broader divine plan rather than as challenges to fundamental aspects of personal identity [39].

However, certain aspects of religiosity (e.g., beliefs in original sin and divine omnipotence) may undermine self-esteem and feelings of personal mastery [40, 41]. Religious coping styles such as passively leaving the responsibility for resolving crises entirely up to divine intervention are likely to yield pathological health-related consequences [17]. In particular, maladaptive coping responses (e.g., those that are poorly matched with the features and requirements of specific stressful situations) can be destructive. Other unproductive or counterproductive religious coping responses, such as those that focus on righteous anger and prayers for divine vengeance and feelings of divine abandonment, were also documented [42] .

26.5 Religious Involvement and Mental and Physical Well-Being

Religious involvement may lead to positive emotions such as forgiveness [43], contentment, and love, as well as to negative emotions such as guilt and fear. These religiously engendered emotions may provide possible linkage with health status. The practice of religion, particularly prayer and worship may lead to the experience or expression of certain emotions that, through psychoneuroimmunological or neuroendocrine pathways, could affect physiological parameters [35].

Religious involvement may promote better health by enhancing feelings of self-esteem, or a sense of intrinsic moral self-worth, feelings of efficacy, or perception that one can master or have control over one's personal affairs, promoting constructive coping responses, or enhancing social support [35].

Religious involvement, especially participation in religious communities, may promote mental and physical well-being by regulating health-related behaviors in ways that decrease the risks of diseases. This includes (1) discouraging behaviors that increase the risk of health problems and (2) encouraging positive and low-stress lifestyle choices. Actually numerous studies document an inverse relationship between religious involvement and alcohol, tobacco, and substance use and abuse [44, 45]. In addition, the effects of religious involvement on health behaviors and lifestyles may be explained as follows [46, 47]. First, individuals may internalize strong religio-ethical norms so that the prospect of violating these internalized religious norms may evoke feelings of guilt and shame or even fear of divine punishment. Second, members of religious communities may conform to religious norms because they fear the threat of embarrassment and possible social sanctions. Third, religious persons may alter their lifestyles to make them consistent with those of reference group members (e.g., influential church members) they consider worthy of emulation [44].

How might religious involvement enhance these important dimensions of self-perception? Through devotional activities (e.g., prayer, scriptural studies) and other spiritual practices and pursuits, individuals may construct personal relationships with a divine other in the same way that they develop relationships with concrete social others [48, 49]. By identifying with figures portrayed in religious texts and media, individuals may come to define their own life circumstances in terms of a biblical figure's situation and then begin to interpret their situations from the point of view of the God-role (e.g., what a divine other might expect in the way of human conduct). Thus, individuals may gain a sense of self-worth and control by developing a close personal relationship with a potent divine other who loves and cares for each person unconditionally and can be engaged interactively in a quest for solace and guidance. They may also enjoy a sense of vicarious control over their affairs through their alliance with an omniscient and omnipotent deity (e.g., with God, all things are possible) [50].

26.6 Spirituality and Social Support

Religious communities help mold values and shape behavior in not only the domain of marital and family life but also other domains (e.g., work and financial dealings, interpersonal relations) in ways that may reduce the risk of stressful events and conditions [35]. Spirituality (e.g., sharing of religious thoughts and insights, praying for others) [51, 52] is a source of social support that goes far beyond the bounds of actual contact with a congregation or a formal religious institutions [26]. Shared values within religious communities may provide the basis for a common discourse and set of shared meanings concerning human suffering, adjustment, and support [47, 52].

As mentioned earlier, social pressures within religious congregations may reduce the risk of exposure to unhealthy lifestyles. However, it is possible that these social norms and pressures can also increase the negative consequences of certain stressors (e.g., by framing them as sin and thus ascribing responsibility for events or conditions to the flawed character of the individuals involved rather than to the interplay of contextual or other factors) [47]. Such framing may foster feelings of guilt and shame, erode feelings of competence, self-worth, and hopefulness and distract persons from more productive coping responses (e.g., through excessive worry) and encourage the withdrawal of community support. As a result, health might be negatively affected [53, 54].

26.7 Role of Religion and Spirituality in Depression of the Medically Ill

Religious beliefs and behavior are reported to serve as coping strategies to help manage emotional distress [55–58]. Religious involvement helps older persons with chronic medical problems cope better with these conditions and then may protect older patients from depression [12]. Depressed older medical inpatients with heart failure or chronic pulmonary diseases who are active in their religious communities, especially those who pray and read religious scriptures regularly and have strong personal religious commitment and intrinsic motivation, remit more quickly from depression after hospital discharge [59]. Helping address the spiritual needs of patients in the medical or community setting may be one way to decrease depressive symptoms in patients with HIV/AIDS [11]. However, depression itself may impact religious involvement, making it more difficult for older adults with medical illnesses to engage in religious activities [12].

Religion is likely to have both positive and negative effects on coping through a number of pathways in older medical patients. Religion may give these patients a sense of purpose and meaning in life despite health problems [60], provide hope and optimism about the future [61], increase a sense of control (through prayer), provide role models and inspiration (through scripture reading), and improve decision-making (by adhering to doctrines that discourage excessive alcohol use) [62]. In addition, religion may enhance social support outside their immediate family. These effects enable older patients to cope better with their illnesses [63]. In particular, among outpatients with heart failure, greater spiritual well-being, particularly meaning/peace, was strongly associated with less depression. This result suggests that enhancement of patients' sense of spiritual well-being might reduce or prevent depression and thus improve quality of life in this population [64].

However, religion at times may increase guilt and neurosis [65]. As religion often stigmatizes depression, highly religious people may be less comfortable admitting they are depressed. There may also be subtle messages promoted by religious groups that depression is due to a lack of faith or lack of appreciation for what God has to offer. In those cases, religion may be a source of negative emotions, particularly guilt [59].

Depressed patients who are not religious may be at greater risk for persistent depression. Nonetheless, it is inappropriate to encourage such patients to become more religiously involved, because there is no research showing that becoming religious for mental health reasons alone has any mental health benefits. However, whether religiously inclined or not, clinicians need to see religious community as potential source of support and healing, particularly for severely ill patients who have few other options [59].

26.8 Conclusions

There is mounting evidence that religious cognitions and behaviors can offer effective resources for dealing with stress. Religious involvement may promote better health by enhancing feelings of self-esteem, or a sense of intrinsic moral self-worth, feelings of efficacy, or perception that one can master or have control over one's personal affairs, promoting constructive coping responses, or enhancing social support. In particular, participation in religious communities may promote mental and physical well-being by regulating health-related behaviors in ways that decrease the risks of diseases. Spirituality such as sharing of religious thoughts and insights and praying for others is a source of social support. Studies on the health effects of religion/spirituality have linked it to reduced depression and anxiety, increased longevity, and other physical and psychological health benefits. Religion/spirituality may give depressed patients with physical diseases a sense of purpose and meaning in life as well as social support despite health problems. These effects may protect the patients from depression by enabling them to cope better with their illnesses. However, certain aspects of religiosity may undermine self-esteem and feelings of personal mastery. Religious coping styles such as passively leaving the responsibility for resolving crises entirely up to divine intervention are likely to yield pathological health-related consequences.

References

1. Lukoff D, Lu F, Turner R. Toward a more culturally sensitive DSM-IV: psychoreligious and psychospiritual problems. J Nerv Ment Dis. 1992;180:673–82.
2. Colombo D. Psychoanalysis and the Catholic Church in Italy: the role of Father Agostino Gemelli, 1925–1953. J Hist Behav Sci. 2003;39:333–48.

3. Turner RP, Lukoff D, Barnhouse RT, Lu FG. Religious or spiritual problem: a culturally sensitive diagnostic category in the DSM-IV. J Nerv Ment Dis. 1995;183:435–44.
4. O'Connell RA. The church and psychiatry. National Cathol Wkly. 2001;185:15–7.
5. Greenberg D, Witztum E. Problems in the treatment of religious patients. Am J Psychother. 1991;45:554–65.
6. Curlin FA, Lawrence RE, Odell S, et al. Religion, spirituality, and medicine: psychiatrists' and other physicians' differing observations, interpretations, and clinical approaches. Am J Psychiatry. 2007;164:1825–31.
7. Kitchell MA, Barnes RF, Veith RC, et al. Screening for depression in hospitalized geriatric medical patients. J Am Geriatr Soc. 1982;30:174–7.
8. Koenig HG, Meador KG, Cohen HJ, et al. Depression in elderly hospitalized patients with medical illness. Arch Intern Med. 1988a;148:1929–36.
9. Yi MS, Mrus JM, Wade TJ, et al. Religion, spirituality, and depressive symptoms in patients with HIV/AIDS. J Gen Intern Med. 2006a;21:S21–7.
10. Koenig HG. Religion and depression in older medical inpatients. Am J Geriatr Psychiatry. 2007a;15:282–91.
11. Baetz M, Bowen R, Marcoux G. Spirituality and psychiatry in Canada: psychiatric practice compared with patient expectations. Can J Psychiatr. 2004;49:265–71.
12. Sansone RA, Khatain K, Rodenhauser P. The role of religion in psychiatric education: a national survey. Acad Psychiatry. 1990;14:34–8.
13. Sulmasy DP. The rebirth of the clinic: an introduction to spirituality in health care. Washington, DC: Georgetown University Press; 2007.
14. Koenig HG. Medicine, religion, and health: where science and spirituality meet. West Conshohocken: Templeton Foundation Press; 2008.
15. Muldoon M, King N. Spirituality, health care, and bioethics. J Relig Health. 1995;34:329–49.
16. Hill PC, Pargament KI. Advances in the conceptualization and measurement of religion and spirituality. Implications for physical and mental health research. Am Psychol. 2003;58:64–74.
17. Pargament KI. The psychology of religion and coping. New York: Guilford; 1997a.
18. Crawford M, Handal P, Weiner R. The relationship between religion and mental health/distress. Rev Relig Res. 1989;31:16–22.
19. Ellison C. Religious involvement and subjective well-being. J Health Soc Behav. 1991;32:80–99.
20. Hathaway W, Pargament K. Intrinsic religiousness, religious coping, and psychosocial competence: a covariance structural analysis. J Sci Study Relig. 1990;29:423–41.
21. Pargament K, Kennell J, Hathaway W, et al. Religion and the problem-solving process: three styles of coping. J Sci Study Relig. 1988;27:90–104.
22. Ross C. Religion and psychological distress. J Sci Study Relig. 1990;29:235–45.
23. Maton R. Spiritual discernment in psychiatric patients. J Relig Health. 1987;26:125–30.
24. Donahue M. Intrinsic and extrinsic religiousness: review and meta-analysis. J Pers Soc Psychol. 1985;48:400–19.
25. Petersen L, Roy A. Religiosity, anxiety, and meaning and purpose: religion's consequences for psychological well-being. Rev Relig Res. 1985;27:49–62.
26. Sullivan WP. It helps me to be a whole person: the role of spirituality among the mentally challenged. Psychosoc Rehabil J. 1993;16:125–34.
27. Bergin AE. Religiosity and mental health: a critical reevaluation and meta-analysis. Prof Psychol Res Pract. 1983;14:170–84.
28. Gartner JD, Larson DB, Allen GD. Religious commitment and mental health: a review of the empirical literature. J Psychol Theol. 1991;19:6–25.
29. Walsh K, King M, Jones L, et al. Spiritual beliefs may affect outcome of bereavement: prospective study. BMJ. 2002;324:1551–6.
30. Idler EL. Religion, health, and non-physical senses of self. Soc Forces. 1995a;74:683–704.
31. Mattlin JA, Wethington E, Kessler RC. Situational determinants of coping and coping effectiveness. J Health Soc Behav. 1990;31:103–22.

32. Chopra D. Perfect health: the complete mind/body guide. New York: Harmony Books; 1991.
33. Dossey L. Healing words: the power of prayer and the practice of medicine. San Francisco: Harper; 1993.
34. Benson H. Timeless healing: the power and biology of belief. New York: Scribners; 1996.
35. Ellison CG, Levin JS. The religion-health connection: evidence, theory, and future directions. Health Educ Behav. 1998;25:700–20.
36. Mueller PS, Plevak DJ, Rummans TA. Religious involvement, spirituality, and medicine: implications for clinical practice. Mayo Clin Proc. 2001;76:1225–35.
37. Matthews DA, McCullough ME, Larson DB, et al. Religious commitment and health status: a review of the research and implications for family medicine. Arch Fam Med. 1998;7:118–24.
38. Pargament K, Ensing DS, Falgout K, et al. God help me: (1) religious coping efforts as predictors of the outcomes to significant negative life events. Am J Community Psychol. 1990;18:793–824.
39. Foley DP. Eleven interpretations of personal suffering. J Relig Health. 1988;27:321–8.
40. Ellis AL. Reason and emotion in psychotherapy. Secaucus: Lyle Stuart; 1992.
41. Branden N. The six pillars of self-esteem. New York: Bantam; 1994.
42. Pargament K, Ishler K, Dubow EF, et al. Methods of religious coping with the Gulf war: cross-sectional and longitudinal analyses. J Sci Study Relig. 1994;33:347–61.
43. Kaplan BH, Monroe-Blum H, Blazer DG. Religion, health, and forgiveness: traditions and challenges. In: Levin JS, editor. Religion in aging and health: theoretical foundations and methodological frontiers. Thousand Oaks: Sage; 1994. p. 52–77.
44. Cochran JK, Beeghley L, Bock EW. Religiosity and alcohol behavior: an exploration of reference group theory. Sociol Forum. 1988;3:256–76.
45. Koenig HG, George LK, Meador KG, et al. Religious practices and alcoholism in a Sothern adult population. Hosp Community Psychiatry. 1994;45:225–31.
46. Ellis L. Religiosity and criminality: evidence and explanations complex relationships. Sociol Perspect. 1985;28:501–20.
47. Grasmik HG, Bursik RJ, Cochran JK. Render unto Caesar what is Caesar's: religiosity and taxpayers' inclinations to cheat. Sociol Q. 1991;32:251–66.
48. Pollner M. Divine relations, social relations, and well-being. J Health Soc Behav. 1989;30:92–104.
49. Ellison CG. Religion, the life stress paradigm, and the study of depression. In: Levin JS, editor. Religion in aging and health: theoretical foundations and methodological frontiers. Thousand Oaks: Sage; 1994. p. 78–121.
50. Poloma MM, Gallup G. Varieties of prayer: a survey report. Philadelphia: Trinity Press International; 1991.
51. Taylor RJ, Chatters LM. Church members as a source of informal social support. Rev Relig Res. 1988;30:193–202.
52. Maton KI. Community settings as buffers of life stress? Highly supportive churches, mutual help groups, and senior centers. Am J Community Psychol. 1989;17:203–32.
53. Sorenson AM, Grindstaff CF, Turner RJ. Religious involvement among unmarried adolescent mothers: a source of emotional support? Sociol Relig. 1995;56:71–81.
54. Strawbridge WJ, Shema SJ, Cohen RD, et al. Religiosity buffers effects some stressors on depression but exacerbates others. J Gerotol Soc Sci. 1998;53B:S118–S26.
55. Koenig HG, Smiley M, Gonzales JP. Religion, health and aging: a review and theoretical integration. Westport: Greenwood Press; 1988. p. 13–21.
56. Swanson WC, Harter CL. How do elderly blacks cope in New Orleans? Int J Aging Hum Dev. 1971;2:210–6.
57. Rosen CC. Ethnic differences among impoverished rural elderly in use of religion as a coping mechanism. J Rural Community Psychol. 1982;3:27–34.
58. Conway K. Coping with the stress of medical problems among black and white elderly. Int J Aging Hum Dev. 1985–1986;21:39–48.

59. Koenig HG. Religion and remission of depression in medical inpatients with heart failure/pulmonary disease. J Nerv Ment Dis. 2007b;195:389–95.
60. George LK, Larson DB, Koenig HG, et al. Spirituality and health: what we know, what we need to know. J Soc Clin Psychol. 2000;19:102–16.
61. Breitbart W. Spirituality and meaning in supportive care: spirituality and meaning-centered group psychotherapy interventions in advanced cancer. Support Care Cancer. 2002;10:272–80.
62. Koenig HG. Faith and mental health. Philadelphia: Templeton Foundation Press; 2005.
63. Koenig HG. Religious beliefs and practices of hospitalized medically ill older adults. In J Geriatr Psychiatry. 1998;13:213–24.
64. Bekelman DB, et al. Spiritual well-being and depression in patients with heart failure. J Gen Intern Med. 2007;22:470–7.
65. Freud S. Future of an illusion (1927). In: Stachey J, editor. Standard edition of the complete psychological works of Sigmund Freud. London: Hogarth Press; 1962. p. 43.

Chapter 27
Practical Application of Spirituality in Terminally Ill Patients

27.1 Introduction

Impending death can cause anxiety in not only cancer patients but also their family and caretakers. Fear related to death include (1) the sense of helplessness and loss of control, (2) the sense of guilt and being punished, (3) physical or symbolic injury (castration), and (4) self-abandonment [1, 2].

The stage of the life cycle in which terminal illness occurs has a strong impact on how death will be perceived, since both attitudes and views toward death change with age [3]. Adolescents and young adults recognize the finality of death. During these periods, death is viewed as an adversary that must be fought, and anger, hostility, and bitterness may be strong in terminal stages. The older adults feel that death must be faced, but not yet. The elderly adults usually have a realistic view of life expectancy and may be more concerned about the stages of terminal illness and the manner of dying than about death itself [4].

In addition to these developmental life stages, physical factors in the course of illness such as pain and relapse, cultural attitudes about death, and coping mechanisms influence patients' perception of terminal illness. In particular, patients' and family's acceptance of terminal illness depends on cultural and religious factors [4].

People may have greater spiritual needs during illnesses. Addressing the spiritual needs of patients may enhance recovery from illnesses. Most studies have shown that religious involvement and spirituality are associated with better health outcomes, including greater longevity, coping skills, and health-related quality of life (even during terminal illnesses) and less anxiety, depression, and suicide [5].

This chapter reviews the role of religion and spirituality in terminally ill patients, spiritual assessment, and interventions for spiritual suffering of patients with terminal illnesses, especially meaning-centered psychotherapy for advanced cancer patients.

K. B. Koh, *Stress and Somatic Symptoms*,
https://doi.org/10.1007/978-3-030-02783-4_27

27.2 Role of Religion and Spirituality in Terminally Ill Patients

With physical decline and death in view, many patients with advanced illnesses seek hope [6–8], meaning [9, 10], and comfort [10–12] in their connection to the transcendent. The majority of patients with advanced illnesses view religion and/or spirituality as personally important [13–16] and experience spiritual needs [17–19].

Advancing age and life-threatening illnesses such as cancer can be stimuli for expansion of one's previous concepts of self-boundaries, leading to changes in personal life purpose and meaning. Therefore, the diagnosis of a terminal illness may be seen as either a crisis or an opportunity for growth and meaning, as one learns to cope with it [20].

Some studies have found that religion or spirituality generally plays a positive part in patients' coping with illnesses such as cancer or HIV [16, 21, 22]. In particular, spiritual well-being and meaning have been demonstrated to play central roles as buffering agents, protecting against depression, hopelessness, and desire for hastened death among terminally ill cancer patients [16, 23]. In contrast, depression and hopelessness are associated with poorer survival in cancer patients [24]. Kissane et al. [25] have described a syndrome of demoralization in the terminally ill, which is distinct from depression and characterized by a triad of hopelessness, loss of meaning, and desire for death. These data suggest the critical need for the development of interventions that address depression, hopelessness, and loss of meaning and impact desire for death and demoralization in terminally ill cancer patients [26].

27.3 Assessment of Spiritual Beliefs and Activities

Dombreck and Karl [27] provide a basic three-factor model of assessment that focuses on (1) an individual's placement in a religious community; (2) the personal meanings one attaches to symbols, rituals, beliefs, and divine figures; and (3) one's relationship to religious resources. In particular, attention should be devoted to changes in spiritual activity and beliefs over time [28]. It is argued that an assessment of spiritual beliefs and activities should be a regular feature of helping endeavors [29].

27.3.1 Taking a Spiritual History

The spiritual history helps the physician recognize the spiritual needs of patients. Furthermore, the patients may need sources of spiritual care (e.g., chaplains) available to address their spiritual needs [5]. However, referral to pastoral counselors, clergy, and others trained to address spiritual needs of patients may be complicated if productive interchanges have not been established between the clergy, faith communities, patients, families, and professional helpers [29].

Recognizing the spiritual needs of patients can be done by taking a spiritual history. Similar to the social history, the spiritual history informs the physician of the importance of spiritual matters in the life of the patient and how the patient's spirituality can be used as a source of strength and coping. For terminally ill patients, the spiritual history is regarded as a crucial component of palliative medicine [30–32].

Several formats for taking a spiritual history have been suggested [33–35]. The FICA spiritual history, one easy-to-use and practical questionnaire [36], is as follows: (Faith) Do you consider yourself spiritual? Do you have a religious faith?; (Importance) How important are your religious beliefs and spirituality, and how might they influence decisions related to your health?; (Community) Are you part of a religious or spiritual or other community? If so, how does this community support you?; (Address) How might I address your spiritual needs? In addition, the following questions might be considered: "What helps you get through tough times?"; "To whom do you turn when you need support?"; "What meaning does this illness have for you?"; and "What are your hopes (expectations, fears) for the future?" [37, 38].

Spiritual history can help clinicians learn about how religion affects patients' coping with illness, social support, and medical decisions. Clinicians need to become more comfortable discussing religion and spirituality and make use of the support they provide to many older patients [39].

27.3.2 Sources of Spiritual Care

Spiritual history itself can be a form of spiritual care. Allowing patients to voice their spiritual doubts, needs, and concerns may be reassuring and comforting to them [40]. Informing patients of and making available sources of spiritual care may also be reassuring, minimize the isolation caused by illness, and facilitate recovery. Chaplains are an important source of spiritual care. Other important sources of spiritual care include family and friends, readily available religious texts, artifacts, hospital chapels, and special rooms devoted to prayer and meditation [5].

27.4 Care of the Terminally Ill

In the care of the terminally ill, a combination of the science and the art such as medicine and psychiatry is essential. The art often depends on the caregiver's own personality, the past history of the patient and family, and their psychosocial values and issues [41]. Conflicts that arise regarding decisions about care may lead to requests for psychiatric consultation and intervention [4].

Psychiatric consultation can be beneficial in the care of patients with terminal stage of cancer and their families. Such consultants should address a variety of issues in the care of the patients: the patient's and family's understanding of terminal illness, their coping mechanisms, cultural or religious mind set, preexisting psychiatric disorders, family functioning (cohesion), family resources (e.g., social support, physical and psychologic stamina, and financial support), and family's open communication [4].

Treatment for the terminally ill is aimed at providing maximal comfort during their remaining life span. When the label "dying" is assigned to a patient, attitudes and behaviors of staff, family, and friends often assume a different character that tends to isolate or alienate patients from those they need most at that crucial time. Therapists need to make them aware that the person who is dying has not changed; only his/her life expectancy has changed, and his/her emotional needs may intensify [4].

27.4.1 Principles of Interventions for Spiritual Suffering at the End of Life

Care of the terminally ill has traditionally been delegated to various religious groups. St. Christopher's Hospice was founded by Cicely Saunders in London, which was the beginning of the hospice movement [4]. During the terminal stage, support from those close to the patients and religion both appear to play critical roles in helping patients cope with the process of dying [42].

Psychotherapeutic interventions for spiritual suffering of patients with terminal illnesses are aimed at improving spiritual well-being and a sense of meaning while diminishing hopelessness, demoralization, and distress at the end-of-life care. Such interventions can be implemented as individual or group psychotherapy interventions. However, group psychotherapy interventions may be more effective than individual psychotherapies for cancer patients [43].

As Rousseau [26] outlined, a step-by-step approach for the treatment of spiritual suffering is as follows: (1) controlling physical symptoms; (2) providing a supportive presence; (3) encouraging life review to assist in recognizing purpose, value, and meaning; (4) exploring guilt, remorse, forgiveness, and reconciliation; (5) facilitating religious expression; (6) reframing goals; and (7) encouraging meditative practices and focusing on healing rather than cure. This kind of psychotherapy intervention has utilized the concept of self-transcendence and meaning as developed by Victor Frankl [44–47]. Self-transcendence (i.e., expansion of personal boundaries) is one aspect of logotherapy which works as a means of understanding man's will to meaning and utilizing meaning (i.e., having a sense of meaning and purpose in life) [20].

Addressing spiritual needs and existential questions among the dying is generally neglected in palliative care practice but could be a crucial aspect of psychological functioning [48]. In particular, spiritual care from the medical system seems to help patients transition to hospice and improve their well-being near death. Furthermore, among highly religious coping patients, spiritual support seems to reduce the risk of receiving aggressive interventions at the end of life [49].

Mental health care for the terminally ill would probably benefit from a more thorough incorporation of pastoral care principles and practices [9]. Chaplains play an essential role as professional providers of spiritual care. In addition, other medical providers can have a crucial role in spiritual assessment and making pastoral care referral [49]. Experimental work [50] and clinical experience indicate that an extrinsic value system, without internalization, seems to offer no assistance in coping with a fatal illness. However, a religious commitment that is intrinsic appears to offer considerable stability and strength to those who possess it. Consultation with the chaplain needs to be discussed with a patient with a firm religious conviction. The patient's own minister can not only provide many valuable facts and insights about the patient and family but also help reduce their distress by softening the dying process [51]. Therefore, an interdisciplinary approach is important in palliative care [9].

Promoting religion in an effort to deal with patients' spiritual concerns or suffering at the end of life is not universally applicable to all patients. However, interventions based on the "meaning" component of spirituality are likely to be more universally applicable to patients and accepted by health-care providers as well as patients [20].

27.4.2 Meaning-Centered Psychotherapy for Advanced Cancer Patients

As described below, Breitbart [20] applied meaning-centered group psychotherapy to advanced cancer patients by using Frankl's concept of logotherapy (meaning and spirituality). The premise of logotherapy is that failure to find meaning in life results in psychological distress. This therapy is designed to help patients with advanced cancer sustain or enhance a sense of meaning, peace, and purpose in their lives even as they approach the end of life. Individual logotherapy can be adapted to patients with terminal illnesses who have six 45-min sessions over a 2-week period.

This therapeutic intervention utilizes a mixture of didactics, discussion, and experiential exercises focused around particular themes related to meaning and advanced cancer. The session themes include (1) concepts of meaning and sources of meaning; (2) cancer and meaning; (3) meaning and historical context of life; (4) storytelling and life project; (5) limitations and finiteness of life; (6) responsibility, creativity, and deeds; (7) experience, nature, art, humor; and (8) termination, goodbyes, and hopes for the future. Patients are assigned readings and homework that are specific to each session's theme and are utilized in each session. Addressing a limited prognosis, support, and expression of emotion is inevitable in the context of each group session.

The logotherapist helps the patients discover for themselves who they are, how they wish to interpret their present situation, and what they want to become. Importance is placed on the individual's acceptance of the freedom to change his/her attitude toward the difficulties experienced, to develop a new perspective on their identity, and to reinterpret the significance of his/her life's contributions in a positive way. The steps undertaken include (1) enhancing rapport with the therapist, (2) eliciting sources (e.g., activities, relationships) that provided meaning in each patient's life, (3) focusing on the impact of illness, (4) dealing with the fear of dying using the technique of dereflection (i.e., directing a person's attention away from his/her problem and towards something important to the person), and finally (5) enhancing a sense of closure with significant others in life as death approaches.

27.5 Limitations of Research and Perspective on Future Studies

Inconsistent results of many studies may be due to methodological weaknesses. A particular issue is how religious coping was conceptualized and measured. Any effect of church attendance may be confounded by social support. Further, many studies used general coping instruments that do not identify the content of prayer or the cognitions used. Other limitations and methodological shortcomings are that many were cross-sectional and used mixed cancer groups at different stages of the illnesses [52].

Future studies need to take a multidimensional approach and examine both positive and potentially negative religious coping strategies with specific cancers. In order to fully understand the role of religious coping with cancer, future studies need to examine religious coping, using specific cancer groups that are similar in terms of length of illnesses (e.g., newly diagnosed patients with one type of cancer only). Studies should be longitudinal in design, informing researchers of the short- and long-term effects of both positive and negative coping strategies. Studies should also consider a systematic control for other possible variables such as perceived social support and illness variables such as cancer stage and treatment. In addition, religious coping with cancer across different cultures needs to be explored [64]. The need for education of physicians for spiritual care and the importance of integrating pastoral care into multidisciplinary medical teams will be more emphasized in the future [49].

27.6 Conclusions

Spiritual well-being and meaning have been demonstrated to play central roles as buffering agents, protecting against depression, hopelessness, and desire for hastened death among terminally ill cancer patients. Spiritual history helps physicians recognize the spiritual needs of patients. Meaning-centered group psychotherapy may help patients with advanced cancer sustain or enhance a sense of meaning, peace, and purpose in their lives. Medical providers can have a crucial role in spiritual assessment and pastoral care referral. In this respect, an interdisciplinary approach is important in palliative care. The need for education of physicians for spiritual care and the importance of integrating pastoral care into multidisciplinary medical teams will be more emphasized in the future.

References

1. Freud S. The ego and the id. In: Strachey J, editor. Standard edition, vol. 19. London: Hogarth Press; 1961.
2. Deutsch F. Euthanasia: a clinical study. Psychoanal Q. 1933;5:347–68.
3. Holland JC, Rowland J, Lebovits A. Reactions to cancer treatment: assessment of emotional response to adjunct radiotherapy. Psychiatr Clin N Am. 1979;2:347–58.
4. Lesko LM, Massie MJ, Holland JC. Oncology. In: Stoudemire A, Fogel BS, editors. Principles of medical psychiatry. Orlando: Grune & Stratton; 1987.
5. Mueller PS, Plevak DJ, Rummans TA. Religious involvement, spirituality, and medicine: implications for clinical practice. Mayo Clin Proc. 2001;76:1225–35.
6. Reynolds MA. Hope in adults, ages 20–59, with advanced stage cancer. Palliat Support Care. 2008;6:259–64.
7. Saleh US, Brockopp DY. Hope among patients with cancer hospitalized for bone marrow transplantation: a phenomenologic study. Cancer Nurs. 2001;24:308–14.
8. Fanos JH, Gelinas DF, Foster RS, et al. Hope in palliative care: from narcissism to self-transcendence in amyotrophic lateral sclerosis. J Palliat Med. 2008;11:470–5.
9. McClain CS, Rosenfeld B, Breitbart W. Effect of spiritual well-being on end-of-life despair in terminally-ill cancer patients. Lancet. 2003;361:1603–7.
10. Gall TL, Cornblat MW. Breast cancer survivors give voice: a qualitative analysis of spiritual factors in long-term adjustment. Psychooncology. 2002;11:524–35.
11. Johnson SC, Spika B. Coping with breast cancer: the role of clergy and faith. J Relig Health. 1991;30:21–33.
12. Sodestrom K, Martinson IM. Patients' spiritual coping strategies: a study of nurse and patient perspective. Oncol Nurs Forum. 1987;14:41–6.
13. Koenig HG. Religious beliefs and practices of hospitalized medically ill older adults. Int J Geriatr Psychiatry. 1998;13:213–24.
14. Roberts JA, Brown D, Elkins T, et al. Factors influencing views of patients with gynecologic cancer about end-of-life decisions. Am J Obstet Gynecol. 1997;176:166–72.
15. Balbori TA, Vanderwerker LC, Block SD, et al. Religiousness and spiritual support among advanced cancer patients and associations with end-of-life treatment preferences and quality of life. J Clin Oncol. 2007;25:555–60.
16. Nelson CJ, Rosenfeld B, Breitbart W, et al. Spirituality, religion, and depression in the terminally ill. Psychosomatics. 2002;43:213–20.
17. Astrow AB, Wexler A, Texeira K, et al. Is failure to meet spiritual needs associated with cancer patients' perceptions of quality of care and their satisfaction? J Clin Oncol. 2007;25:5753–7.
18. Moadel A, Morgan C, Fatone A, et al. Seeking meaning and hope: self-reported spiritual and existential needs among an ethnically-diverse cancer patient population. Psychooncology. 1999;8:378–85.
19. Hermann CP. The degree to which spiritual needs of patients near the end of life are met. Oncol Nurs Forum. 2007;34:70–8.

20. Breitbart W. Spirituality and meaning in supportive care: spirituality and meaning-centered group psychotherapy interventions in advanced cancer. Support Care Cancer. 2002;10:272–80.
21. Baider L, Russak SM, Perry S, et al. The role of religious and spiritual beliefs in coping with malignant melanoma: an Israeli sample. Psychooncology. 1999;8:417–28.
22. Breitbart W, Rosenfeld B. Physician-assisted suicide: the influence of psychosocial issues. Cancer Control. 1999;6:146–61.
23. Breitbart W, Rosenfeld B, Pessin H, et al. Depression, hopelessness, and desire for hastened death in terminally ill cancer patients. JAMA. 2000;284:2907–11.
24. Watson M, Haviland JJ, Greer S, et al. Influence of psychological response on survival in breast cancer population-based cohort study. Lancet. 1999;354:1331–6.
25. Kissane D, Block S, Miach P, et al. Cognitive existential group therapy for patients with primary breast cancer – techniques and themes. Psychooncology. 1997;6:25–33.
26. Rousseau P. Spirituality and the dying patient. J Clin Oncol. 2000;18:2000–2.
27. Dombreck M, Karl J. Spiritual issues in mental health care. J Relig Health. 1987;26:183–93.
28. Titone A. Spirituality and psychotherapy in social work practice. Spiritual Soc Work Commun. 1991;2:7–9.
29. Sullivan WP. It helps me to be a whole person: the role of spirituality among the mentally challenged. Psychosoc Rehabil J. 1993;16:125–34.
30. Schuetz B. Spirituality and palliative care. Aust Fam Physician. 1995;24:775–7.
31. Bollwinkel EM. Role of spirituality in hospice care. Ann Acad Med Singap. 1994;23:261–3.
32. Rummans TA, Bostwick JM, Clark MM. Mayo Clinic Cancer Center quality of life working group, maintaining quality of life at the end of life. Mayo Clin Proc. 2000;75:1305–10.
33. Koenig HG. Religion, spirituality, and medicine: application to clinical practice. JAMA. 2000;284:1708.
34. Maugans TA. The SPIRITual history. Arch Fam Med. 1996;5:11–6.
35. Anandarajah G, Hight E. Spirituality and medical practice: using the HPE questions as practical tool for spiritual assessment. Am Fam Physician. 2001;63:81–9.
36. Puchalski C, Romer AL. Taking a spiritual history allows clinicians to understand patients more fully. J Palliat Med. 2000;3:129–37.
37. Post SG, Puchalski C, Larson DB. Physicians and patient spirituality: professional boundaries, competency, and ethics. Ann Intern Med. 2000;132:578–83.
38. Gioiella ME, Berkman B, Robinson M. Spirituality and quality of life in gynecologic oncology patients. Cancer Pract. 1998;6:333–8.
39. Koenig HG. Religion and depression in older medical inpatients. Am J Geriatr Psychiatry. 2007;15:282–91.
40. Taylor EJ, Outlaw FH, Bernardo TR, et al. Spiritual conflicts associated with praying about cancer. Psychooncology. 1999;8:386–94.
41. Holland JC. Psychological issues in the care of the terminally ill. In: Flach F, editor. Directions in psychiatry. New York: Hatherleigh; 1982.
42. Heim E, Augustiny KF, Schaffner L, et al. Coping with breast cancer over time and situation. J Psychosom Res. 1993;37:523–42.
43. Greenstein M, Breitbart W. Cancer and the experience of meaning: a group psychotherapy program for people with cancer. Am J Psychother. 2000;54:486–500.
44. Frankl VF. The doctor and the soul. New York: Random House; 1955/1986.
45. Frankl VF. Men's search for meaning. 4th ed. Boston: Beacon Press; 1959/1992.
46. Frankl VF. The will to meaning. Foundations and applications of logotherapy. Expanded edition. New York: Penguin; 1969/1988.
47. Frankl VF. Men's search for ultimate meaning. New York: Plenum Press; 1975/1997.
48. Kearney M, Mount B. Spiritual care of the dying patient. In: Chochinov H, Breibart W, editors. Handbook of psychiatry in palliative medicine. New York: Oxford University Press; 2000. p. 357–73.

49. Balboni TA, Paulk ME, Balboni MJ, et al. Provision of spiritual care to patients with advanced cancer: association with medical care and quality of life near death. J Clin Oncol. 2010;28:445–52.
50. Magni KG. The fear of death. In: Godin A, editor. Death and presence. Brussels: Lumen Vitae; 1972. p. 125–38.
51. Cassem NH. The dying patient. In: Cassem, editor. MGH handbook of general hospital psychiatry. St. Louis: Mosby Year Book; 1991.
52. Thune-Boyle IC, Stygall JA, Keshtgar MR, et al. Do religious/spiritual coping strategies affect illness adjustment in patients with cancer?: a systematic review of the literature. Soc Sci Med. 2006;63:151–64.

Correction to: Cognitive Behavioral Approach to Stress

Correction to:
Chapter 7 in: K. B. Koh, *Stress and Somatic Symptoms*, https://doi.org/10.1007/978-3-030-02783-4_7

The published version of this book had missed to include the reference number [11] as follows: 7.6.2 Examples of Interventions [11] in page 78. This has now been updated.

The updated online version of this chapter can be found at https://doi.org/10.1007/978-3-030-02783-4_7

K. B. Koh, *Stress and Somatic Symptoms*,
https://doi.org/10.1007/978-3-030-02783-4_28

Index

K. B. Koh, *Stress and Somatic Symptoms*,
https://doi.org/10.1007/978-3-030-02783-4

D

MIX
Papier aus verantwortungsvollen Quellen
Paper from responsible sources
FSC® C105338

If you have any concerns about our products,
you can contact us on
ProductSafety@springernature.com

In case Publisher is established outside the EU,
the EU authorized representative is:
Springer Nature Customer Service Center GmbH
Europaplatz 3, 69115 Heidelberg, Germany

Printed by Libri Plureos GmbH
in Hamburg, Germany